School Health Services and Programs

Julia Graham Lear

Stephen L. Isaacs

James R. Knickman

Foreword by Risa Lavizzo-Mourey

⟿ School Health Services and Programs

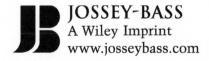

JOSSEY-BASS
A Wiley Imprint
www.josseybass.com

Published by Jossey-Bass
A Wiley Imprint
989 Market Street, San Francisco, CA 94103-1741   www.josseybass.com

Jossey-Bass books and products are available through most bookstores. To contact Jossey-Bass directly call our Customer Care Department within the U.S. at 800-956-7739, outside the U.S. at 317-572-3986, or fax 317-572-4002.

Jossey-Bass also publishes its books in a variety of electronic formats. Some content that appears in print may not be available in electronic books.

Library of Congress Cataloging-in-Publication Data

School health services and programs /Julia Graham Lear, Stephen L. Isaacs, James R. Knickman [editors] ; foreword by Risa Lavizzo-Mourey.— 1st ed.
    p. cm.
   Includes bibliographical references and index.
   ISBN-13: 978-0-7879-8374-1
   ISBN-10: 0-7879-8374-8
    1. School health services—United States.   I. Lear, Julia Graham.   II. Isaacs, Stephen L.   III. Knickman, James.
   LB3409.U5S373 2006
   371.710973—dc22   2006041710

Printed in the United States of America
FIRST EDITION
PB Printing   10 9 8 7 6 5 4 3 2 1

— Contents

—ₘ— Sources

Chapter Two: Kort M. The delivery of primary health care in American public schools, 1890-1980. *J Sch Health.* 1984;54(11):453–457.

Chapter Three: Sedlak MW, Schlossman S. The public school and social services: reassessing the progressive legacy. *Educ Theory.* 1985;35(4):371–383.

Chapter Four: Yankauer A. An evaluation of the effectiveness of the Astoria Plan for medical service in two New York City elementary schools. *Am J Public Health.* 1947;37:853–859.

Chapter Five: Costante CC. School health nursing: framework for the future, part I. *J Sch Nurs.* 2001;17(1):3–11.

Chapter Six: Costante CC. School health nursing: framework for the future, part II. *J Sch Nurs.* 2001;17(2):64–72.

Chapter Seven: Hootman J. The importance of research to school nurses and school nursing practice. *J Sch Nurs.* 2002;18(2):18–24.

Chapter Eight: Institute of Medicine. Executive summary of the Report of the Committee on Comprehensive School Health Programs in Grades K–12. In: Allensworth DD, Lawson E, Nicholson L, Wyche JH, eds. *Schools and Health: Our Nation's Investment.* Washington, DC: National Academy Press; 1997.

Chapter Nine: Kolbe LJ, Kann L, Brener ND. School health policies and programs study 2000: overview and summary of findings. *J Sch Health.* 2001;71(7):253–259.

Chapter Ten: Dryfoos JG. Schools as places for health, mental health, and social services. *Teachers Coll Rec.* 1993;94(3):540–567.

Chapter Eleven: Adelman HS, Taylor L. Addressing barriers to learning: beyond school-linked services and full-service schools. *Am J Orthopsychiatry.* 1997;67(3):408–421.

Chapter Twelve: Morone JA, Kilbreth EH, Langwell KM. Back to school: a health care strategy for youth. *Health Aff.* 2001;20(1):122–136.

Chapter Thirteen: Schlitt JJ, Santelli JS, Juszczak L, Brindis CD, Nystrom R, Klein JD, Kaplan DW, Seibou MD. *Creating Access to Care for Children and Youth: School-Based Health Center Census 1998–1999.* Washington, DC: National Assembly on School-Based Health Care; 2000.

Chapter Fourteen: National Assembly on School-Based Health Care. *School-based health centers: a blueprint for healthy learners. Data from the 2001–2002 School-Based Health Center Census.* Washington, DC: National Assembly on School-Based Health Care; 2003.

Chapter Fifteen: Kaplan DW, Calonge BN, Guernsey BP, Hanrahan MB. Managed care and school-based health centers: use of health services. *Arch Pediatr Adolesc Med.* 1998;152:25–33.

Chapter Sixteen: Webber MP, Carpiniello KE, Oruwariye T, Lo Y, Burton WB, Appel DK. Burden of asthma in inner-city elementary schoolchildren: do school-based health centers make a difference? *Arch Pediatr Adolesc Med.* 2003;157:125–129.

Chapter Seventeen: Brodeur P. School-based health clinics. In: Isaacs SL, Knickman JR, eds. *To Improve Health and Health Care: The Robert Wood Johnson Foundation Anthology.* San Francisco: Jossey-Bass; 2000:chap 1.

Chapter Eighteen: Rones M, Hoagwood K. School-based mental health services: a research review. *Clin Child Fam Psychol Rev.* 2000;3(4):223–241.

Chapter Nineteen: Weist MD. Expanded school mental health services: a national movement in progress. *Adv Clin Child Psychol.* 1997;19: 319–351.

Chapter Twenty: Hoyt HH, Broom BL. School-based teen pregnancy prevention programs: a review of the literature. *J Sch Nurs.* 2002;18(1): 11–17.

Chapter Twenty-One: Tiezzi L, Lipshutz J, Wrobleski N, Vaughan RD, McCarthy JF. Pregnancy prevention among urban adolescents younger than 15: results of the "In Your Face" program. *Fam Plann Perspect.* 1997;29:173–176.

Chapter Twenty-Two: Armbruster P, Andrews E, Couenhoven J, Blau G. *Clinical Psychology Review,* Collision or collaboration? School-based health services meet managed care. 1999;9(2):221–237.

Chapter Twenty-Three: Adams EK, Johnson V. An elementary school–based health clinic: can it reduce Medicaid costs? *Pediatrics.* 2000;105(4):780–788. Copyright © 2000.

~~~ The Editors

Julia Graham Lear, PhD, directs the Center for Health and Health Care in Schools at the School of Public Health and Health Services within the George Washington University Medical Center. She is also a research professor in its Department of Prevention and Community Health, where she teaches school health and safety. During the past two decades, she has contributed to the development of new models of health care at school, including the school-based health center and school-based mental health programs. Together with colleagues at the center, she has developed a Web-based resource that highlights effective school health programs (http://www.healthinschools.org). The site records more than 60,000 visits monthly. Lear graduated from Brown University and received her master's degrees and doctorate from Tufts University.

Stephen L. Isaacs, JD, is a partner in Isaacs/Jellinek, a San Francisco–based consulting firm, and a president of Health Policy Associates, Inc. A former professor of public health at Columbia University and founding director of its Development Law and Policy Program, he has written extensively for professional and popular audiences. His book, *The Consumer's Legal Guide to Today's Health Care,* was reviewed as "the single best guide to the health care system in print today." His articles have been widely syndicated and have appeared in law reviews and health policy journals. He also provides technical assistance internationally on health law, civil society, and social policy. A graduate of Brown University and Columbia Law School, Isaacs served as vice president of International Planned Parenthood's Western Hemisphere Region, practiced health law, and spent 4 years in Thailand as a program officer for the U.S. Agency for International Development.

James R. Knickman, PhD, is vice president for research and evaluation at the Robert Wood Johnson Foundation. He oversees a range of grants and national programs supporting research and policy analysis to better understand forces that can improve health status and delivery of health care. In addition, he is in charge of developing formal evaluations of national programs supported by the foundation. During the 1999–2000 academic year, he held a Regents' Lectureship at the University of California, Berkeley. Previously, Knickman was on the faculty of the Robert Wagner Graduate School of Public Service at New York University. At NYU, he was founding director of a university-wide research center focused on urban health care. His publications include research on a range of health care topics, with particular emphasis on issues related to financing and delivering long-term care. He has served on numerous health-related advisory committees at the state and local levels and spent a year working at New York City's Office of Managment and Budget. Currently, he chairs the board of trustees of Robert Wood Johnson University Hospital in New Brunswick, New Jersey. He completed his undergraduate work at Fordham University and received his doctorate in public policy analysis from the University of Pennsylvania.

~~ First Authors

E. Kathleen Adams, PhD, is Associate Professor of Health Policy and Management at Emory University School of Medicine in Atlanta, Georgia.

Howard S. Adelman, PhD, is Professor of Psychology and Co-Director of the School Mental Health Project and its federally supported National Center for Mental Health in Schools at the University of California, Los Angeles.

Paula Armbruster, PhD, is Associate Clinical Professor and Director of Outpatient Services at the Child Study Center, Yale School of Medicine, New Haven, Connecticut.

Paul Brodeur was a staff writer at the New Yorker for nearly forty years. He is now an independent journalist living in Cape Cod.

Carol C. Costante, RN, MA, NCSN, FNASN, is a past president of the National Association of School Nurses. She is supervisor of school nursing with the Baltimore County Public Schools, Baltimore, Maryland.

Joy G. Dryfoos is an independent researcher and writer whose work has been supported by the Carnegie Corporation. She lives in Boston.

Janis Hootman, RN, PhD, NCSN, is past president of the National Association of School Nurses and a school nurse in Gladstone, Oregon.

Helina H. Hoyt, RN, MSN, is a school nurse at Holtville Unified School District in Holtville, California.

David W. Kaplan, MD, MPH, is Professor of Pediatrics and Head of Adolescent Medicine at the University of Colorado School of Medicine and The Children's Hospital, Denver, Colorado.

Lloyd J. Kolbe, PhD, is Professor of Applied Health Science at Indiana University, Bloomington.

Michael Kort, PhD, is Professor of Social Science at Boston University's College of General Studies.

James A. Morone, PhD, is Professor of Political Science at Brown University, Providence, Rhode Island.

Michelle Rones was, at the time the article was written, a graduate student in the Department of Clinical Psychology at the George Washington University, Washington D.C. She is currently at Children's Hospital in Boston.

Michael W. Sedlak, PhD, is Professor of the History of Education and Associate Dean for Academic Affairs in the College of Education, Michigan State University, East Lansing, Michigan.

Lorraine Tiezzi is Director of the Center for Community Health and Education and Associate Clinical Professor of Population and Family Health at Columbia University in New York.

Mayris P. Webber, DrPH, is an Associate Professor in the Department of Epidemiology and Public Health, AIDS Research Program, at Montefiore Medical Center in New York.

Mark D. Weist, PhD, is Professor and Director of the Center for School Mental Health Assistance at the University of Maryland School of Medicine, Baltimore.

Alfred Yankauer, MD, was Professor in the Department of Pediatrics and Family and Community Medicine at the University of Massachusetts Medical School, Worcester, Massachusetts.

⎯⎯ Foreword

School-based health care represents one of the Robert Wood Johnson Foundation's most sustained, if lesser-known, commitments. The Foundation's interest in advancing school-based health care dates back to 1972, when the newly established national philanthropy made grants to several school-based health programs. In 1977, the foundation funded the School Health Services Program, a seven-year, $6 million initiative that brought nurse-practitioners into thirty-three elementary schools in four states. We increased our investments in the 1980s and 1990s with our support of two large national demonstration programs: the $17 million School-Based Adolescent Health Care Program and the $25 million Making the Grade program. The foundation's commitment, which furthers our goal of improving access to quality health care, continues through the present day with our support of the George Washington University's Center for Health and Health Care in Schools. Indeed, the Robert Wood Johnson Foundation has been intimately connected with the growth and development of the field of school-based health services.

Given this close connection, school-based health care is a logical topic for this, the second volume of the Robert Wood Johnson Foundation Health Policy Series. The idea behind the series is to give readers an understanding of some of the fields in which the Robert Wood Johnson Foundation has made sustained and substantial investments. To do this, we have developed a unique vehicle: a book that includes an original comprehensive review article by a leading expert; reprints of outstanding articles and reports; a relevant chapter from *To Improve Health and Health Care: The Robert Wood Johnson Foundation Anthology;* and summaries from the foundation's grants results reports.

At the Robert Wood Johnson Foundation, we pride ourselves on being an organization that learns from its programs and its grantees and that shares with the field and the public what we have learned about improving health and health care. With that in mind, in 2004, we produced *Generalist Medicine and the United States Health System,* the first in the Robert Wood Johnson Foundation Health Policy Series. We hope that *School Health Services and Programs* will be a worthy successor to that book and will be a valuable resource for those working in school-based health care as well as for those interested in the field. This effort to advance learning about school-based health reflects our commitment to our colleagues in the field and, even more important, to improving the health and health care of all Americans—especially the most vulnerable among us, our children and their families.

Princeton, New Jersey   Risa Lavizzo-Mourey
October 2005

⟿ Editors' Introduction

There were two main challenges in editing *School Health Services and Programs*. The first was deciding which, of the many outstanding articles and reports, were so important or influential that they deserved to be among the twenty-two pieces that space permits us to reprint. Although the final decisions were ultimately those of the editors, we sought the guidance of many of the foremost figures in the field of school-based health care in trying to meet this challenge. In winnowing the list of reprints down from roughly seventy-five to twenty-two, we looked for pieces that were widely considered to have been important to the field or were written by influential authors, and we tried to include both articles that provided wide-ranging analyses of specific topics and case studies of particular programs. Clearly, some important pieces were not reprinted. People will have differing perspectives on which articles and reports should have been included and which should have been omitted. In the end, guided by the expert advice we received, we fashioned the reprint list using our best judgment.

The second challenge was organizing the material in a clear and logical manner that will be useful to both professionals in the field and the wider public. The theory behind school-based health care is pretty simple: take services to where the kids are. Putting theory into practice is somewhat tricky, however. It raises issues, including the role of schools, parents' control of their children's education, what services to offer and how and where to provide them, the scope of nursing and medical practice, and paying for school-based care. For the sake of clarity, we have organized the book into seven sections.

Section One contains a comprehensive examination of the entire field of school-based health care. This original contribution was written by Julia Graham Lear, the director of the Center for Health and Health Care in Schools at the George Washington University School of Public Health and Health Services, one of the editors of this book. The Robert Wood Johnson Foundation has funded the center since its establishment in 2001. The chapter offers readers a comprehensive guide that covers all relevant aspects of school-based health care, including its early beginnings and justification, its growth and development, the issues it raises, and the challenges it faces.

Although school-based health care received considerable attention in the third quarter of the twentieth century, the concept actually dates back to the late nineteenth century, when a Massachusetts physician suggested that schools should have regular physicians, just as almshouses and prisons did. Section Two contains reprints of three articles that trace the historical roots of school-based health care and its growth and development.

Chapter Two, by Michael Kort, provides a broad historical analysis of the delivery of primary care in the public school system, beginning in the 1890s and continuing through the 1970s.

In the next chapter, Michael Sedlak and Steven Schlossman offer a different perspective on the historical development of school-based health care, focusing on its early-twentieth-century roots in the Progressive movement, with its vision of the school as a place to provide a wide variety of social services.

The third chapter in this section, by Alfred Yankauer, offers a case study of one of the most influential early school-based health care programs, begun in Astoria, Queens, New York City, in 1940. The article assesses the program's effectiveness after its first six years of operation.

Nursing has long been the backbone of school-based health. There are now an estimated 57,000 nurses working in public schools. Today's school-based health services evolved from the concept of the school nurse. Thus, to understand health services in schools, it is first necessary to explore the history and potential of school nursing. This is the subject of Section Three. In it, we reprint a two-part series by Carol Costante, published in 2001, that looks at the trends and issues affecting the future of school nursing and offers a framework for the twenty-first century. These two review pieces are followed by a reprint of an article by Janis Hootman that focuses on research related to school nurses and the practice of school nursing.

Building on the historical context set forth in Section Two and the role of nursing examined in Section Three, Section Four explores some basic questions about school-based health care. What is the rationale for providing care in schools? What kinds of health care services should be provided in the nation's public schools? What kinds of services are being provided? What is the current status of school-based health care, and what is known about its effectiveness? What is the potential of schools as places to provide other kinds of social services? We have chosen to reprint four pieces that address these basic questions.

In the early 1990s, the National Academy of Sciences' Institute of Medicine (IOM) appointed a committee, chaired by Diane Allensworth and James Wyche, to assess the status of school-based health care programs, determine the factors that led to success or failure, and identify ways of expanding successful approaches. The report of the IOM Committee on Comprehensive School Health Programs in Grades K–12, whose charge was modified in the course of its investigation, provides a solid summary of the rationale for and the promise of school-based health care programs. The executive summary is reprinted here.

Debate continues regarding what elements a school-based health program should contain. The traditional model of comprehensive care contained three components: health education, health services, and a healthful environment. The Centers for Disease Control and Prevention (CDC) expanded the model to one with eight components: health education, physical education, health services, nutrition services, health promotion for staff, counseling and psychological services, a healthy school environment, and parent and community involvement.

In 1994, the CDC conducted the School Health Policies and Programs Study (SHPPS) to monitor the impact of school-based health programs. It conducted a second SHPPS in 2000. The report of the 2000 SHPPS, whose overview and summary by Lloyd Kolbe, Laura Kann, and Nancy Brener is reprinted, provides detailed information about state, district, and school policies and practices.

Some children's health activists argue that schools should go beyond providing just health services and offer a full range of social services to children and their families. Joy Dryfoos, one of the pioneers of school-based health programs, has been an articulate advocate for the concept of "full-service schools." We reprint her article "Schools as Places for Health, Mental Health, and Social Services."

The final chapter in Section Four, by Howard Adelman and Linda Taylor, calls for an approach that goes beyond full-service schools. These authors propose school community partnerships that will bring about what they term a "total transformation" in the way schools are able to service children and their families.

One approach to providing comprehensive school-based health care is through a center or clinic located within the school. Nurse practitioners, physician assistants, and physicians generally provide a range of preventive, curative, and first-aid services at the clinic, often backed up by mental health care professionals. In the more than 90,000 public schools in the United States, there are about fifteen hundred school-based health centers, a large percentage of which are located in schools in poorer neighborhoods. In Section Five, we reprint five reports and articles, and one book chapter. Taken together, they provide a comprehensive picture of school-based health centers, how they operate, how effective they have been, and the challenges they face.

Chapter Twelve, "Back to School: A Health Care Strategy for Youth," by James Morone, Elizabeth Kilbreth, and Kathryn Langwell, traces the history of school-based health centers from their renaissance in the late 1960s and early 1970s through the present. The authors discuss the political challenges faced by school-based health clinics—moral opposition triggered by concern about reproductive health services offered in schools, funding in a managed care era, and partisan politics—and how these challenges have been addressed.

Chapter Thirteen is the National Assembly on School-Based Health Care's 1998–1999 census, formally titled "Creating Access to Care for Children and Youth: School-Based Health Center Census, 1998–1999" Written by John Schlitt, John Santelli, Linda Juszczak, Claire Brindis, Robert Nystrom, Jonathan Klein, David Kaplan, and Michelle DuBray Seibou, the census provides a detailed narrative analysis of the characteristics, staffing, scope of services, and policies of school-based health centers.

The National Assembly on School-Based Health Care conducted a follow-up census in 2001–2002 and issued a statistical report, called "School-Based Health Centers: A Blueprint for Healthy Learners." This short report, reprinted in Chapter Fourteen, provides more recent data on the status of school-based health centers.

These chapters, which provide a broad perspective, are followed by two chapters offering a closer look at school-based health centers. The first, Chapter Fifteen, compares the use of health care services in Denver by adolescents with access to school-based services and those enrolled in managed care plans without such access. The authors—David Kaplan, Ned Calonge, Bruce Guernsey, and Maureen Hanrahan—found, among other things, that students with access to school-based centers were ten times more likely to seek substance abuse or mental health treatment counseling.

Chapter Sixteen examines whether the availability of a school-based health clinic improved the health and school performance of children with asthma. The authors—Mayris Webber, Kelly Carpiniello, Tosan Oruwariye, Yungtai Lo, William Burton, and David Appel—compared results from four Bronx, New York, elementary schools with clinics with results from two comparison schools without clinics. They found that asthmatic children attending schools with a clinic had strikingly lower rates of both absenteeism and hospitalization for asthma-related conditions than their counterparts in the comparison schools.

The next chapter, by Paul Brodeur, published in the 2000 volume of *To Improve Health and Health Care: The Robert Wood Johnson Foundation Anthology,* looks at the role of the Robert Wood Johnson Foundation in shaping school-based health care. It is followed by summaries of reports on relevant foundation grants.

Section Six examines the specifics of school-based mental health services and teenage pregnancy prevention programs. School health programs address a wide range of health issues—everything from nutrition to physical education and from environmental health to substance abuse. Two components of school-based health programs have attracted special attention in the academic and popular literature: mental health and reproductive health services—mental health because so much of the care provided in school-based programs is directed toward children with emotional or mental health problems (in fact, insofar as children receive any mental health services at all, schools are the primary place where they receive them) and reproductive health because it has long been the most controversial part of school-based health programs. Although mental health and reproductive health services may not be more significant than other services offered by school-based programs, the fact that they have received so much attention demands that we, too, give them a special look. We therefore include two articles on mental health and two on reproductive health.

In Chapter Eighteen, Michelle Rones and Kimberly Hoagwood report on the results of a computerized search of evaluations of school-based mental health care programs published between 1985 and 1999. The authors identify a group of school-based mental health programs that have been effective in addressing a variety of emotional and behavioral problems in children.

In the next chapter of this section, Mark Weist examines what he calls "expanded" school-based mental health programs—those offering a full range of mental health services. Arguing that such programs represent a burgeoning national movement, Weist's wide-ranging piece covers the need for and advantages of school-based mental health programs, the applicable laws, the models of full-range school-based mental health services, and the critical issues facing programs and school-based clinicians.

Many pilot school-based health programs begun in the 1960s, 1970s, and 1980s were justified on the grounds that they would reduce teenage pregnancy and cut the rates of sexually transmitted diseases, including HIV/AIDS, among young people. Chapter Twenty, by Helina Hoyt and Betty Broom, summarizes the state of knowledge about school-based teen pregnancy programs as of 2002 and identifies nine characteristics of effective programs.

Chapter Twenty-One—by Lorraine Tiezzi, Judy Lipshutz, Neysa Wrobleski, Roger Vaughan, and James McCarthy—examines a school-based program attempting to reduce unintended pregnancies among junior high school students in a largely Latino northern Manhattan neighborhood. The authors describe the operation of the program in some detail and present findings of an evaluation showing that the pregnancy rate among students in the four schools participating in the program declined by 34 percent between 1992 and 1996.

How to pay for school-based health services has been and remains a challenge. Insofar as the health care needs of poor children (the ones mainly served by school-based programs) are covered at all, it is through government programs such as Medicaid and the State Children's Health Insurance Program. Managed care, which tends to have a businesslike perspective and to avoid covering mental health and preventive care, has complicated the financial challenges faced by school districts. In Section Seven, we present two chapters that provide a clear picture of the financing issues and how they are being addressed.

The first, Chapter Twenty-Two, by Paula Armbruster, Ellen Andrews, Jess Couenhoven, and Gary Blau, raises the question of whether schools will be able to collaborate with managed care organizations or whether the different mind-sets of the two will inevitably lead to clashes. The authors offer the experience in Connecticut as a case study that others might build on.

The final chapter, by Kathleen Adams and Veda Johnson, addresses the question of whether school-based health services can reduce Medicaid costs. Based on data from Atlanta, Georgia, school districts, the study found that children with access to services at school had significantly lower medical costs than those without access to school-based health services.

One of the ways in which the Robert Wood Johnson Foundation carries out its mission of improving the health and health care of all Americans is to develop and strengthen fields. One such field, that of generalist medicine, was the subject of the first volume in The Robert Wood Johnson Foundation Health Policy Series. School-based health is the subject of this volume. Another field in which the foundation has made substantial investments over a long period of time is tobacco policy research. That will be the subject of the next volume of the Health Policy Series.

Washington, D.C.   Julia Graham Lear
San Francisco, California   Stephen L. Isaacs
Princeton, New Jersey   James R. Knickman
October 2005

⟶ Acknowledgments

We are grateful to the many experts in the field of school-based health whose wisdom has guided us in the development of this book. We acknowledge in particular Joy Dryfoos, Linda Juszczak, Lloyd Kolbe, John Schlitt, Mark Weist, and Trina Anglin, all of whom were generous in sharing their insights into the field and their suggestions about the most appropriate articles to reprint.

At the Robert Wood Johnson Foundation, we offer special thanks to David Morse, who has been a full partner in this endeavor. We are very appreciative of the encouragement and support of Risa Lavizzo-Mourey, and we wish to thank Tim Crowley, Marilyn Ernst, Deborah Malloy, Paul Moran, Barbara Sherwood, Judith Stavisky, and Hope Woodhead for their assistance.

This book would not have been possible without the outstanding research talents of Susan Godstone. Her contribution has been enormous, and we owe her a debt of gratitude for it. Our thanks, too, go to C. Pat Crow, for his usual outstanding job of editing. Finally, we would like to express our appreciation to Andy Pasternack and his staff at Jossey-Bass, and to Jon Peck at Dovetail Publishing Services.

J.G.L.
S.L.I.
J.R.K.

A Review of the Field

CHAPTER 1

Children's Health and Children's Schools

A Collaborative Approach to Strengthening Children's Well-Being

Julia Graham Lear, 2005

There are nearly 61 million American children between ages 5 and 19, and about 50 million of them attend an elementary or secondary school in the United States.[1,2] Schools are the one place where most school-age children congregate six or seven hours a day, nine months a year. Providing effective, high-quality health services in schools is the most direct, efficient means of ensuring that children receive the care they need when obstacles to community-based services bar the way to such care.

Strengthening school-based health services and linking them to community-based health care is a strategy that benefits not only children's health but also their academic well-being. Treating problems before they become serious and managing chronic conditions that can keep children out of school have cost-effective benefits. But for more than a century, school- and community-based services have not been connected in meaningful ways. Why? And what can be done about this missed opportunity?

Over the past 30 years, school-based health services have been conspicuously absent from policy discussions and research studies on improving child health. They were absent from the agenda-setting

Daytona Conference on Adolescent Health in 1987[3]; they have been absent from commonly cited articles examining children's access to health care[4–6]; and until recently they have been absent from discussions of adolescent health needs and the importance of changing the content of adolescent health care.[7] Not only has the school health field been isolated from community care, but it also has been considered irrelevant in serious discussions about how to improve health outcomes for children.

Recent developments, however, suggest that the gap between school health care and community care may be narrowing. Increased public recognition of the health problems of many young people and concerns about the relationship between unattended health problems and poor student achievement have prompted greater interest in health programs in schools. New models of health care organization, including school-based health centers and full-service schools, have offered strategies for addressing problems.[8,9] And school-based health services, especially school-based mental health care, are being examined for their potential to improve health status *and* academic achievement.[10–12] With managed care prompting some providers to work more closely with schools, and with private health care organizations taking responsibility for organizing some city school-based health services, new actors are joining the discussion about how children's health care should be delivered. The potential for change in school-based health services is greater than it has been since the first days of school health.[13]

Five elements are essential to understanding the potential for change in school-based health care: (1) the unmet health problems of school-age children, (2) the structure and the priorities of American schools and their implications for school health services, (3) the history of school health programs and their status today, (4) the emerging forces in health and education that may portend substantial changes in health care delivery in schools, and (5) approaches to reorganizing school-based health so that these services contribute to improved child well-being in the twenty-first century.

THE HEALTH STATUS OF SCHOOL-AGE CHILDREN

While most children in the United States are in excellent health and do receive needed services, a significant number experience acute and chronic health problems[14] and also lack adequate medical care. Chronic conditions, especially asthma and other respiratory problems, affect

Table 1.1   Common Health Problems of School-Age Children Ages 5 to 17, 2004.

Problem or Condition	Number	Percentage of Children Ages 5–17
Asthma		
Ever told had asthma	8,890,000	12.2
Asthma attack in past 12 months	3,975,000	5.4
Hay fever, respiratory allergies, other allergies	24,286,000	N.A.*
Learning disability and attention deficit disorder		
Ever told had learning disability	4,881,000	8.0
Ever told had attention deficit disorder	4,527,000	7.4
Medication		
Problem for which prescription medication was taken regularly for at least 3 months in past year	9,627,000	13.2

*A child may be counted more than once in this category.

large numbers of children, as do learning disabilities and attention deficit disorders (see Table 1.1).[14] Dental health problems are common. In 2000, it was estimated that 4 million children aged 2 to 17 had unmet dental needs because their families could not afford care. Mental health problems, including anxiety, depression, and other disorders, are also reported as common. According to the Surgeon General's Report on Mental Health, one in five children aged 9 to 17 experienced symptoms of a mental health problem. One in ten experienced significant impairment, but it was estimated that three-quarters of those needing care did not receive it.[12,14,15]

As with adults, medications play a substantial role in treatment. Slightly more than 13% of children and adolescents were reported as taking prescription medications for at least 3 months in the previous year.

An additional number of children and young people are harmed or die prematurely as a result of behavior-related problems, including substance abuse, fighting, and risky sexual behavior (see Table 1.2).[16]

The implications of these data for school-based services are threefold. First, a substantial number of school-age children experience health problems that might be ameliorated if they were addressed in the school setting. And these health problems have direct academic consequences. The National Health Interview Survey conducted by the Centers for Disease Control and Prevention (CDC) for 2004 reports that 10.7% of schoolchildren missed 6 to 10 days of school, 5% missed

Table 1.2   Youth Risk Behavior Survey, 2003.

Risk Behavior	1997	2003
Frequent cigarette use (smoked one or more cigarettes every day for the 30 days preceding the survey)	16.7%	15.8%
Episodic heavy drinking (drank five or more drinks on at least one occasion during 30 days preceding survey)	34.4	28.3
Current cocaine use (one or more times during 30 days preceding survey)	3.3	4.1
Did not use condom during sexual intercourse (one or more times during 30 days preceding survey)	N.A.	37.0
Threatened or injured with a weapon on school property (one or more times in the 12 months preceding survey)	4.0	9.2
Felt too unsafe to go to school	7.4	5.4

11 days or more, and 1% do not attend school at all.[14] Second, children with health problems, especially untreated problems, are more likely to be poorer, members of minority groups, and uninsured. Thus it is possible to direct services to schools in those communities that are most in need. Third, all schools must consider the substantial number of prescription medications required by their student populations and evaluate the adequacy of their systems to support children who require medication during the school day.

THE SCHOOL CONTEXT FOR SCHOOL-BASED HEALTH SERVICES

The Importance of Health in the School Setting

Approximately 50 million children aged 5 to 19 attend the nearly 120,000 elementary and secondary schools in the United States. These young people require clean air, a physically safe environment, and education about how to promote their own safety and health. They also require prompt, effective emergency care; need safe administration of medications during school; need protection from communicable diseases; and for younger children especially, require treatment and timely responses to the injuries common to playgrounds and school corridors.

School health programs vary greatly from school district to school district and from state to state, but nearly all communities agree with four basic propositions:

1. There is an obligation to guarantee the safety of the public, including children, when gathered in public buildings. Either the school system or the health department must ensure the safety of the school building and its grounds.

2. There is an obligation to provide emergency services and essential medical services to people in the school building.

3. Because children are in school to learn, there is broad support for the notion that schools should educate children about keeping their bodies safe and healthy. Many states and school districts believe that a good school health program includes a strong health education curriculum.

where is this?!

4. All communities have a legal obligation under Section 504 of the 1973 Rehabilitation Act, the Individuals with Disabilities Education Act, and the Americans with Disabilities Act to provide for such care as is necessary to enable a child with a physical or mental disability to benefit from a free, appropriate public education.

An increasing number of communities also believe that it makes sense to invest in school health programs that go beyond the basic components. These communities find several arguments to be persuasive in supporting a broader range of school-based health programs:

1. That health programs facilitate learning and may increase test scores

2. That there are gaps in the health care system, especially for low-income children and adolescents, and that there are cost savings to be achieved by providing early intervention and treatment for unserved or underserved children

different for low-income, unfortunately. They need it more than others in a lot of cases.

school taking on the role of parents

3. That children's parents are frequently not available to schools and that caring for sick children for at least part of the day will fall to school staff members

The arguments in support of more effective school-based health programs—and more of them—continue to grow. And an increasing number of communities and several states have taken specific steps to expand the scope of school-based health services. What has frequently been a surprise to those who have been enthusiastic about the potential for such services is how complex the school environment is and how many factors must be considered in pursuing links between community-based health care systems and school-based activities.

The Organization of Schools

The school environment is quite different from that found in health care. Authority tends to flow from the bottom up—from school district to state education agency, and from locally elected public officials to state and federal policymakers. Notwithstanding the move toward state standards and national guidelines, education remains a locally driven enterprise with a tradition of local decision-making and engaged power brokers that must be taken into account when attempting to change existing programs.

In contrast to health care, where strong federal agencies such as the Center for Medicare and Medicaid Services set standards of care and define eligible providers, no single federal agency establishes standards for curricula, pupil support services, facilities, or staff. Program priorities are mostly determined by 15,000 local school boards and superintendencies.

Fifty state legislatures, state education agencies, and state boards of education provide a second layer of direction for school systems. At the federal level, many federally funded discretionary programs come under federal oversight. However, the most extensive federal mandates are generated by federal legislation protecting the rights of physically disabled and learning-disabled children to "free, appropriate education." Federal enforcement of the legislation has generated an extensive set of special education requirements that shape both classroom arrangements and school-based health services.

Passage of the No Child Left Behind Act of 2001, the most recent revision of the federal Elementary and Secondary Education Act, has sharpened requirements that state and local governments must meet to secure federal funding and has increased the perception of federal oversight elementary and secondary schools. While federal funding constitutes less than 10% of K–12 spending, it supports services for low-income students, purchases of instructional materials, and development of state-level education programs.[17]

During the 1999–2000 school year, there were nearly 90,000 elementary and secondary public schools in the United States, enrolling about 46.9 million students (see Table 1.3).[18] Five million students attended 27,000 private schools, of which a third were Catholic schools.[19(tab7)]

Student enrollment among these schools varies considerably. The smallest public elementary schools are found in South Dakota, where total enrollment averages 160 students; the largest are found in Florida, where they average 694. High schools, typically larger than

Table 1.3 Schools by Level and Type of Institution.

	Total	Public	Private
Elementary	79,362	62,739	16,623
Secondary	24,169	21,682	2,487
Combined	11,412	3,120	8,292
Total	114,943	87,541	27,402

elementary schools, average an enrollment of 369 in Wyoming but 1,468 in Hawaii.[19(tab5)] Urban high schools in large school districts frequently exceed 1,500 students.[20]

As indicated in Table 1.4, nearly half (7,193) of the school districts have fewer than 1,000 students each, but the 25 largest districts enroll 12% of all public school students in the United States.[18] Indeed, 5.7% of all school districts (817 school districts) enroll half of all public school students in the nation.

Policies, Funding, and School Health

At the state level, governors, legislators, and members of state boards of education all contribute to shaping school policies and school programs, including those that relate to health. A few states help fund health services directly, but most contribute indirectly through general financial support to school districts. Many states also establish mandates for specific services or require student documentation that they

Table 1.4 Public School Districts in the United States by Student Enrollment, 1999–2000.

District Size	Districts	Percentage of Districts	Percentage of Student Enrollment
Total, United States	**14,571**	**100.0%**	**100.0%**
100,000 or more	25	0.2	12.4
25,000–99,999	213	1.5	19.7
10,000–24,999	579	4.0	18.7
5,000–9,999	1,036	7.1	15.4
1,000–4,999	5,524	37.9	27.8
1–999	7,193	49.3	6.0

have received services such as immunizations. However, as Table 1.5 indicates, school district requirements tend to be more extensive than those of state governments.[21(pp295–297)]

One of the most useful insights concerning children's health programs is provided by Table 1.6, which describes the current availabil-

Table 1.5 Most Frequently Required Health Mandates: States and District Requirements by Type of Service.

	Percentage of States	Percentage of Districts
Health Services		
Administration of medications	64.0%	93.7%
First aid	48.0	92.1
CPR	42.0	81.5
Identification of or referral for physical, sexual, or emotional abuse	64.7	75.7
Crisis intervention for personal problems	20.4	64.8
Alcohol or other drug use prevention	22.0	64.2
Immunizations		
Kindergarten or First Grade Entry		
Diphtheria	100.0	99.1
A measles-containing vaccine	100.0	99.1
A polio vaccine	100.0	98.9
Tetanus	98.0	97.7
Hepatitis B	72.6	75.6
Middle or Junior High School Entry		
A second measles-containing vaccine	68.6	81.0
Tetanus	43.8	60.6
Senior High School Entry		
A second measles-containing vaccine	44.9	66.8
Tetanus	36.8	61.4
Screenings		
Hearing	70.6	88.4
Vision	70.6	90.4
Scoliosis	45.1	68.8
Height, weight, or body mass	26.0	38.4

Brener ND, Burstein GR, DuShaw ML, Vernon ME, Wheeler L, Robinson J.. Health services, results from the School Health Policies and Programs Study 2000. *J Sch Health*. 2001;71(7):294–303. Reprinted with permission. American School Health Association, Kent, Ohio.

ity of some basic health equipment in schools as reported by the CDC's periodic School Health Policies and Programs Study.[21(p300)] That one-third of all schools report not having a separate locked medication storage cabinet and that fewer than 60% have a refrigerator reserved for health purposes suggest the constraints that some schools face in implementing school-based health services.

Current arrangements for school financing support the dominant role of state and local governments in decision making. Despite obligations of the No Child Left Behind Act, the limited funding provided by the federal government suggests that except for the unique requirements related to services for students with disabilities, the federal government is unlikely to be proscriptive about policies and programs related to school health. In fiscal year 2003–2004, of $501.3 billion spent on public elementary and secondary schools, state funding supported 46% of the cost and local support amounted to 37%. Only 8.2% of the public schooling budget came from federal agencies. The remaining 9% came from private sources and was directed primarily to private schools.[22] Federal support for education remains well below that for health. In 2002, federal health expenditures amounted to 33% of the total.[23]

Table 1.6   Percentage of Schools with Facilities or Equipment for Health Services.

Type of Facility or Equipment	Percentage of Schools
Portable first aid kit	92.7%
Sick room, nurse's office, or other area reserved for health services	81.1
Medical supply cabinet with lock	73.9
Vision test, eye chart, cards, or anything else to measure vision	70.6
Scale	69.8
Separate medicine cabinet with lock	65.4
Refrigerator reserved for health services	57.3
Audiometer	48.5
Peak flow meter	27.2
Examining table	24.0
Answering machine or voice mail reserved for health services staff	20.5
Glucose meter not just for a specific individual's use	17.8
Nebulizer not just for a specific individual's use	13.0

Brener ND, Burstein GR, DuShaw ML, Vernon ME, Wheeler L, Robinson J.. Health services, results from the School Health Policies and Programs Study 2000. *J Sch Health*. 2001;71(7):294–303. Reprinted with permission. American School Health Association, Kent, Ohio.

School System Capacity to Address Health Issues

While the complexity of school systems and their limited financial resources may create barriers to strengthening school-based health services, greater impediments are likely to be the absence of a structure within education to address health issues and the low priority that superintendents and school boards assign to health services. In the main, neither superintendents nor school boards view health issues as worth a fight. School board members assigned to oversee school health programs are frequently the most recently elected or appointed officials. Among school system administrators, the assistant superintendents for pupil support—those who generally have responsibility for school-based services—are frequently not part of the school district's leadership team.

[handwritten margin note: Suggesting health isn't important]

The issues that currently consume school system leadership focus on students' educational achievement and mechanisms for holding principals and teachers accountable for student outcomes. Since the primary accountability mechanism in schools is testing, many schools focus on the things that affect student performance on tests. And in many districts, school health does not make that list.

A BRIEF HISTORY OF
SCHOOL-BASED HEALTH SERVICES

Historically, school health services evolved separately from community-based health care. For much of the twentieth century, the medical community in the United States opposed the expansion of health services in schools. At the same time, other potential health partners, such as social reformers and welfare professionals concerned about poor children's well-being or hospitals that served large numbers of poor children, did not press the issue of linking school-based and community-based services. Recently, however, the separation between school-based and community-based systems has begun to narrow, and the potential for a new era in school-based health services has emerged.

[handwritten margin note: historically school health separate from community health]

[handwritten margin note: narrowing the gap]

School Health: The First Seventy-Five Years

School health developed in tandem with the expansion of public school systems at the end of the nineteenth century. As is the case today, school-based health services achieved their greatest depth and significance in urban centers where large numbers of schoolchildren, frequently recent arrivals from other countries, came to school with unmet needs and untreated problems.

The first programs were launched in the large cities—Boston, New York, Chicago, and Philadelphia—when health department nurses and physicians began to vaccinate schoolchildren and to screen them for infectious diseases. In 1910, the Russell Sage Foundation reported that 337 city school systems had initiated some form of medical screening. In addition to city efforts, state governments began to establish health requirements for schools. In 1899, Connecticut began requiring teachers to test students' eyesight every 3 years. By the end of World War I in 1918, almost every state had enacted legislation related to school health.[24],[25]

Initially, school health services, especially in the large cities, were weighted heavily toward physician screenings and nursing services. Nurses not only helped families get medical care for children who had been excluded from school but also provided continuing help for health problems. Larger cities, especially those with substantial immigrant populations, made medical, dental, and social services available in the schools. Vacation schools, school lunches, and visiting school nursing all became part of the services that might be found in a school during the first two decades of the twentieth century.[8]

As the twentieth century progressed, however, school health services began to contract. The opposition of private medical practice to the provision of services in schools was overwhelming. To a great degree, school health was thought of as a component of public health, and the provision of health care to needy communities by public health authorities was losing ground to a sustained attack from the American Medical Association.[26]

When the New York City Health Department hired a chief medical inspector and 150 part-time inspectors to make daily examinations of children suspected of being sick, the department promised that the inspectors would provide no medical service but would refer the children to physicians, hospitals, or dispensaries. In 1915, when the health department closed five special nose and throat clinics for schoolchildren, the New York Academy of Medicine congratulated the department's Bureau of Child Hygiene, saying, "The functions of the Department of Health should be restricted to the prevention of disease, and no therapeutic activities should be undertaken."[26]

By the 1920s, the separation of medical treatment from preventive care was complete. Except in the narrowest circumstances, public

[handwritten margin note: referrals vs providing/attention medical]

health would not provide medical services. For the most part, public health limited its focus to health education, personal hygiene, and environmental health. School health followed suit.

Until the 1970s, school health focused primarily on health education, with health services limited to emergency care, first aid, documentation of student compliance with district or state health requirements, and periodic student screenings. Only as the century entered its final quarter did potentially significant new themes begin to emerge in the types of services.[8]

The Next Twenty-Five Years: New Directions

During the latter part of the twentieth century, three factors emerged with the potential for altering the shape and the direction of school-based health services: (1) an expansion of school-based efforts to accommodate the health care needs of children with disabilities, (2) an increased awareness of the health problems of low-income children and a willingness to use schools to address these problems, and (3) a reconsideration of the separation of school-based health services from community-based care, with activities emerging that linked in-school and community-based systems.

PROVIDING HEALTH CARE TO CHILDREN WITH DISABILITIES. Passage of federal legislation to protect and support Americans with disabilities opened the door once more to expanded school-based health services. Section 504 of the 1973 Rehabilitation Act, the Education for the Handicapped Act of 1975, and the Americans with Disabilities Act of 1990 (ADA) created federally protected rights for disabled children. These rights included access to a variety of supportive services in schools, including certain health services. As a result, over the final quarter of the twentieth century, a major expansion occurred in school-based health services provided, the number of health professionals who worked for or contracted with schools, and the political acceptability of schools as sites for health care.

Section 504 of the 1973 Rehabilitation Act declared that discrimination because of disability was prohibited in federally funded programs, including the public schools. When the Americans with Disabilities Act was passed in 1990, the right to protection from discrimination was extended beyond federally funded programs to programs in the private sector and government agencies that do not receive federal funding. Consequently, private schools as well as public schools must comply with federal requirements. Local governments, whether they accept federal dollars or not, must also comply. Under Section 504, school districts must make an effort to identify students with disabilities and provide services to enable the students to participate in or benefit from "any program or activity receiving Federal financial assistance."[27] Students eligible for services under Section 504 may also be eligible for services under the Individuals with Disabilities Education Act, the current version of the Education for All Handicapped Children Act. Beginning with the Education for the Handicapped Act of 1975, the federal government mandated that states ensure that children with certain disabilities receive the services necessary to secure free, appropriate education in the least restrictive environment possible. Children who are eligible for services under Section 504 because they are disabled may not be eligible for services under IDEA if their disabilities are determined not to interfere with learning. Under both laws, however, school systems are required to provide a range of related health services that commonly include speech therapy, physical and occupational therapy, and counseling. Other services that might be offered include psychological services, social work services, school health services, and early identification and assessment of disabilities.[28]

PROVIDING HEALTH CARE TO HIGH-NEED CHILDREN AND ADOLESCENTS. Until passage of Section 504 and Education for the Handicapped legislation, the twentieth century had witnessed a retreat from the provision of health services to children in school. In schools with nurses, the nurses provided first aid but referred children requiring more extensive acute or chronic care to a physician. Supporters of this "link and refer" strategy argued that schools were not open 52 weeks a year and in any event did not have the dollars to provide medical care as well as educational services.[29,30] Opponents countered that "link and refer" strategies often did not result in needed services and that money was wasted in finding and refinding the same problems, untreated, each year. They noted that in poor neighborhoods, where children are more likely to have untreated or inadequately treated asthma, dental problems, diabetes, or other serious health problems, school nurses could not find sufficient numbers of physicians, dentists, and other providers to guarantee care. With many children needing referrals, nurses were also less likely to have time to follow up on recommended services.[8]

By the late 1970s, some school districts began to take a broader view toward health services. In addition to expanded services for disabled

Figure 1.1   School-Based Health Center Initiatives, 2001–2002, by State.

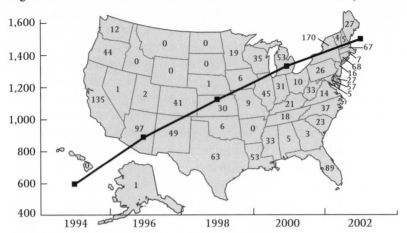

From *2002 State Survey of School-Based Health Center Initiatives.* Center for Health and Health Care in Schools. Washington DC.

children, the emergence of the nurse practitioner as a new and accepted type of provider made possible the hiring of a lower-cost primary care provider. Nurse practitioners, who were increasingly authorized by state licensing authorities to diagnose common illnesses and prescribe medications, enabled school-based practices to treat students without requiring a physician referral.

Another innovative model for health care in school—the school-based health center—was built on the availability of nurse practitioners and thus expanded the services provided in schools.[8] The long-term isolation of school-based health services began to diminish. The health centers, sponsored by mainstream health care organizations—hospitals, public health departments, and community health centers—first appeared in the 1970s and grew slowly over the next 10 years with funds from local and national philanthropies. In the 1980s, the centers expanded more rapidly as local and state governments began to offer support. In the 1990s, their growth became exponential (see Figure 1.1).[31]

As these changes occurred in the school health field, societal changes—the War on Poverty, the civil rights movement, increases in single-parent families, concerns about young people's drug use—all contributed to an awareness of the many children who had not benefited from the general economic prosperity. Serious untended health problems, coupled with concern about the large number of children and adolescents who had no health insurance, created a more sympathetic political climate for providing health care in schools.

Government policy changes also facilitated expanded school-based services in some communities. Congressional passage of Medicaid legislation in 1966 had provided federal support for health insurance for low-income children, among others. In 1988, the federal Medicaid director informed the states that they could establish relationships with school systems that would allow those systems to be reimbursed for services provided to Medicaid beneficiaries.[32] The services would include those specified in the Medicaid legislation, whether provided to IDEA-enrolled students or to students in the general school population.

In 1997, school participation in health care received another boost through the passage of the State Children's Health Insurance Program (SCHIP). Although this program did not directly encourage school-delivered services, SCHIP administrators worked hard during the program's first 5 years to engage the schools as partners in enrolling children in the program. And the notion that schools had a role to play in securing safety-net services received a modest measure of reinforcement and support.

LINKING SCHOOL-BASED SERVICES WITH COMMUNITY-BASED SYSTEMS OF CARE. Some of the most interesting and perhaps most powerful changes affecting school-based services have occurred in the past 10 years. Perhaps most profoundly, the widespread introduction of managed care has shifted the standards by which health care services are measured. The health care system, driven by managed care, has adopted the notion that its services should meet performance standards. Moreover, building on efforts by the National Academy of Sciences to improve patient safety and quality of care, there is a growing belief among policymakers and health care analysts that services should be assessed in terms of the extent to which the providers either follow evidence-based, recommended procedures or achieve preestablished quality outcomes. Also understood is the expectation that patients and communities have a right to be informed about health care providers' performance in terms of these quality measures.[13] The increasing emphasis on quality measures in health care, the related importance of patient safety, and the vital role of evidence-based practice will inevitably influence the way that community stakeholders think about school health services. School-based health programs will be asked to define their services, costs, and value in terms that take these concepts into account.

In addition to altering the health policy context for school-based health services, managed care is creating incentives for organizational links between community-based and school-based care. In states where managed care is the dominant mode of practice, and especially in states where Medicaid managed care arrangements are characterized by tight control of access to services, managed care companies have incentives (and occasional state mandates) to consider how school-based health services might enhance their ability to either constrain costs or achieve objectives specified in their state contracts.

At the same time, the drive toward school reform—especially efforts focused on accountability and student performance—have brought low-performing schools to public attention and raised questions about what can be done to help students from poor neighborhoods succeed academically. The recognition that health problems can impair student achievement has prompted some communities to offer greater support for health programs in schools.[13,33]

SCHOOL-BASED HEALTH CARE AT THE BEGINNING OF THE TWENTY-FIRST CENTURY

Across the nation, a significant number of health professionals, clinical challenges, and dollars are involved in providing health care in school. The services and their funding can be only imperfectly described, since no single entity at the state or national level collects standardized data on health care in schools. Only school-based health centers, recent arrivals on the school health scene, are well documented. However, reports from professional organizations and estimates published in professional journals, as well as reports from individual states and school districts, provide a sense, if not a clear picture, of the health services found in many schools.

Clinical Care: Providers

SCHOOL NURSES. In 2000, a federally funded sample survey of nurses in the United States estimated that 56,239 nurses were working in the public schools. Another 5,132 worked in private schools, and an additional 5,519 worked in "other school health services." An unknown percentage of those nurses worked full time, while others were part time.[34] Given nursing shortages across the United States and climbing nursing salaries in competitive health care organizations, the likelihood of a serious school nurse shortage is real and suggests the need to develop new approaches to stretching the available nursing resources.

Depending on the state or the school district, school nurses' educational credentials and responsibilities vary widely. Some school nurses are licensed practical nurses who have completed a 6-month training course. They may also be registered nurses with a 4-year bachelor of science degree, or as in the case of Vermont school nurses, they may be nurse specialists with master of science degrees. Typically, school nurse responsibilities include some or all of the following services: documenting immunization status, conducting screening examinations, administering medications, enrolling students in health insurance programs, finding a medical home for students, providing case management to children involved with several public agencies, caring for disabled students as well as children with chronic health conditions, and providing first aid and emergency care to all students.

An emerging debate regarding the future of school nursing is the degree to which this position should focus on the care of individual children or whether the role of the school nurse is to ensure the health of the school's overall physical and social environment. Under the latter approach, the school nurse would concentrate primarily on such activities as tracking and containing outbreaks of flu, ensuring a fully immunized student body, and identifying threats to students and faculty from air, food, and water quality problems, as well as monitoring the emotional and behavioral environment of the school.

Although school nursing is frequently viewed as synonymous with school health services, an increasing number of other in-school health professionals and aides play key roles in addressing individual student health care needs and the public health challenges confronted at schools.

UNLICENSED PERSONNEL. Whether because of budget shortfalls or nursing shortages, schools have frequently turned to unlicensed personnel to serve as assistants or alternatives to school nurses. Estimates of their numbers are not available. They may be referred to as health aides or health assistants, and they may also have additional duties in the school—secretary, clerk, volunteer. If a nurse is assigned to a school, the assistant works under the nurse's direction and license. The skills of unlicensed assistants are inconsistent across school sites, as are the training, supervision, and support made available to these staff members.[35] A 2001 study by the General Accounting Office (now the General Accountability Office) that examined the administration of attention disorder drugs at school found that nurses were the most frequent providers of medications (59%) but that non–health care personnel were the second most common providers (28%).[36]

Another theme in school health regards the appropriate delegation of responsibility from nurses to unlicensed personnel. Some nurses express concern that school policies toward the use of unlicensed personnel can put a nurse's license in jeopardy. Others question the adequacy of training provided to these assistants, especially when they are frequently the ones charged with medication management for all schoolchildren during school hours.[37]

SCHOOL-BASED HEALTH CENTERS. Although most school health services are managed by public school systems or, to a lesser extent, by local health departments, school-based health centers are predominantly organized by private, nonprofit institutions that are already providing health services to young people in the community. These include hospitals, which sponsor 32% of the school-based health centers; community health centers (17%); nonprofit agencies (12%); and universities and medical schools (5%). School systems, in charge of 15% of the centers, frequently subcontract with a variety of nonprofit health agencies to provide direct care. Local health departments are responsible for 17% of the centers; a small number of other agencies (2%) organize the remaining centers.[38]

From the standpoint of providing care, the primary distinctions between school-based health centers and traditional school health services are that the health centers are staffed with professionals who are licensed to diagnose and treat medical problems and that the services themselves are arranged by community-based organizations. With combinations of nurse practitioners, physician assistants, clinical social workers, psychologists, physicians, and health aides, the centers can identify and treat most problems without the need to make referrals and arrange transportation. Most centers prescribe medications if needed; a smaller number even dispense medications.

While nearly all the centers offer basic medical services, 61% of them also employ mental health professionals—primarily psychologists and clinically trained social workers—to address mental health concerns among students. Using individual sessions as well as group work and family counseling, the centers report providing crisis interventions, case management, assessments, and peer support, as well as grief counseling and the assessment of learning problems.[38]

The school-based health centers bridge the divide between community-based care and school health. Since they are sponsored by community-based organizations, they have access to well-established referral networks and are able to get specialty care for their patients from colleagues in the sponsoring organization. The challenge for the centers has been the absence of adequate funding within health care budgets at the state and federal levels. This lack places clear limits on the expansion of the health centers.

Data from a 2001 finance survey conducted by the National Assembly on School-Based Health Care (as yet unpublished) describe then-current funding arrangements for the centers: 9% of revenue came from the federal government; 28% from state governments; 19% from private sources such as foundations; 13% from patient care revenue, primarily Medicaid and private insurance; and 18% from in-kind contributions from the school districts and other organizations.

In 2002, it was estimated that 1,500 school-based health centers provided care in public schools—in a nation of nearly 90,000 public schools. And while rough estimates project that 10,000 schools are high-need candidates for the centers and that 7,500 of those have would have the space for and the interest in pursuing a school-based health center, there is still a considerable distance to go.[39] Although entrepreneurial state and local health officials have been particularly creative in helping communities patch together enough money to keep the centers multiplying, limited federal dollars and small-scale state and county grant programs may deter all but the hardiest champions of school-based health centers.

SCHOOL-BASED MENTAL HEALTH AND SOCIAL SERVICES. A widely quoted comment from a team of mental health researchers in the mid-1990s was that schools function as the "de facto mental health system" for children and adolescents.[40(p155)] Surveys conducted in the 1990s documented that about 20% of the children and adolescents had diagnosable mental disorders, and yet only a small portion of those children received the help they needed.[10] According to a RAND Corporation analysis, on average, only one-fourth of children and adolescents who needed mental health care got that help.[15] To the extent that children with mental health problems received treatment, the majority of that care was provided at school.[15,40]

Relying on the School Health Policy and Programs Survey of 2000, the CDC reports that three-fourths of schools have a part-time or full-time guidance counselor, two-thirds of schools have a part-time or full-time psychologist, and slightly more than 40% have a part-time or full-time social worker.[41] Other estimates, developed early in the

1990s, are that mental health professionals in schools include 81,000 guidance counselors, between 20,000 and 22,000 psychologists, and 12,000 social workers.[8]

School-based mental health services represent some of the most established school health services as well as some of the newest school-based health interventions. Unlike school nurses, however, who provide care to the general student population, mental health professionals in schools may be available only to certain groups of students. Substantial mental health staff time is dedicated to assessing and caring for students who may be eligible for federally required Section 504 or IDEA services. School social workers may also be assigned to work specifically with schools that have large numbers of low-income students, and counselors, found in nearly all schools, may be primarily responsible for academic guidance and have limited time to devote to developmental support. Thus, the total mental health resources available to all students are very much in doubt.

That said, there is increasing interest in the role that mental health professionals can play in creating safe, nurturing school environments and providing direct services to students with emotional or behavioral health problems. Violent tragedies in schools during the latter part of the 1990s called attention to acute mental health problems among some students. Neighborhood violence during that same time affected many more students and their families, prompting concern about young people who had witnessed violence. In response, some school districts, as well as some state governments, have established grant-funded initiatives to test new models for providing mental health services. At the federal level, the Department of Education launched the Safe Schools, Healthy Students program in conjunction with the Department of Health and Human Services and the Office of Juvenile Justice to test expanded models for school-based mental health services.

Three particular challenges confront these new programs. First, given the pressure that schools face in providing assessments for students with disabilities, it can be difficult to keep mental health services from being absorbed into the school's special education efforts. Second, the new school-based mental health services are typically stand-alone efforts that must overcome the still-present fear of stigma for receiving mental health care. Special attention is required to ensure that students have confidential access to these services. Third, while it is important to protect mental health professionals from being

absorbed into serving only the Section 504– and IDEA-related populations, it is also important that mental health professionals—some
of whom will come from community-based mental health organizations—learn about the school system and individual schools. In addition to working with students in one-on-one encounters, mental
health professionals need to work with teachers and other staff members through classroom-based and schoolwide initiatives to create
healthy learning environments.[42]

CURRENT ISSUES IN
SCHOOL-BASED CLINICAL CARE

The delivery of health services in schools has raised a number of issues
with clinical, policy, and legal ramifications. Some of these issues are
similar to those occurring in community-based settings; others are
different because of the limited resources or the political sensitivities
found at the school site.

Do Not Resuscitate Orders

Do Not Resuscitate (DNR) orders have emerged as a newly troubling
issue for school-based services. The presence of a number of medically
fragile and sometimes terminally ill students in schools has increased
the likelihood that schools may be asked to honor orders directing that
cardiopulmonary resuscitation should not be used in the event of cardiac or respiratory arrest.[43] Despite a reported sense among school
nurses that requests for schools to honor DNR orders have become
more frequent, most states and school districts do not appear to have
policies regarding DNR orders. According to a 1998 survey, 11 of 42
responding states indicated that they had policies for addressing DNR
orders in schools. Three of those states supported accepting DNR
orders, 6 were opposed, and 2 gave ambiguous responses. Twelve states
reported that some local school districts had policies in the absence
of state guidance.[43]

Medication Management

In 2000, some 13.4% of children aged 5 to 17 had a health problem
that required them to take a prescription medication for at least 3
months.[14(tab4)] A substantial portion of those children bring their

medications to schools. Nurses report that their duties in administering medication have increased dramatically, in part because of the growing role of pharmaceuticals in medical practice generally and in part because of the growing number of students who have conditions such as asthma and attention deficit or hyperactivity disorder. Since many schools do not have trained health professionals on site on a full-time basis, administering medication in a safe and reliable way is a critical and unresolved challenge.[44] The contrast in standards between administering medication in a health facility and giving medication at school can be profound.

Minor Consent

Many states authorize minors to give their consent for "confidential services," variously defined by states as including some or all of the following: contraceptive services, testing and treatment for sexually transmitted infections, drug and alcohol abuse, and outpatient mental health services. For the past two decades, efforts have been made within federal and state legislatures to reimpose parental notification or consent for some of these services.[45] At the federal level, the former congressional representative and attorney general John Ashcroft sponsored legislation that would have made parental consent requirements for abortion and contraception for minors part of federal law.[46] Although the legislation was not reintroduced in the next Congress, it does reflect the perspective of key policymakers. Congressional conservatives have also frequently labored to require either parental notification or consent before a minor may receive contraceptive services from a federally funded Title X or family planning clinic. To date, these bills have succeeded in the House of Representatives and failed in the Senate. Efforts to roll back minor consent statutes have been more successful at the state level.

In general, states recognize the right of parents to make health care decisions for their minor children. In the 1970s and 1980s, however, states expanded the rights of minors to consent to their own care in areas related to sex, alcohol or drug treatment, and mental health services. In recent years, social conservatives have argued that parental rights have been abridged by minor consent legislation. Their legislative advocates have successfully narrowed the scope of these laws at the state level so that new constraints may limit minor consent provisions. With laws varying across the nation, school-based providers must pay careful attention to what their state law allows. Since states may adopt laws that specifically limit what services may be provided in schools, all school-based providers need to review state statutes carefully.[45]

Confidentiality and Student Health Data

Two pieces of federal legislation—the 1974 Family Educational Rights and Privacy Act (FERPA) and the 1996 Health Insurance Portability and Accountability Act (HIPAA)—complicate the handling of student health information. Under FERPA, family members and school staff members who have a "legitimate educational interest," as defined in school district policy, may have access to student health records.[47] Under HIPAA, a law intended to assure that individuals have access to their health records and that information in those records is not available to unauthorized persons, the Department of Health and Human Services issued rules that specify criminal and civil penalties for "those who knowingly obtain or disclose individually identifiable information." However there has been little litigation involving HIPAA. The lack of clarity presents difficult challenges for the schools.

For school-based health centers, the legislation is less a legal problem than a political one. Since the centers are organized by health care organizations outside the school system, FERPA does not apply to the centers' medical records, but HIPAA does. Health center staff members have an unambiguous obligation not to share individually identifiable information. A political issue for the centers, however, is that people employed by the schools, accustomed to the older FERPA statute, may resent an unwillingness on the part of health center staff people to share information about students. As providers covered by HIPAA, the centers must handle medical records carefully and avoid unintentional disclosures. Both school-based health centers and schools that bill Medicaid and other third-party payers must learn the importance of well-organized records that reflect properly followed privacy policies and procedures.[48]

Personnel involved in traditional school nursing services or school-sponsored mental health services may face a difficult challenge. At present, the FERPA mandate to share information in the student record and the HIPAA obligation *not* to share student health information conflict. Until there are defining court cases, further congressional action, or U.S. Department of Health and Human Services rulings, school districts will need to issue their own guidelines for school health personnel.

Quality of Care

Since the publication of the Washington-based Institute of Medicine reports *To Err Is Human* and *Crossing the Quality Chasm,* there has been a growing focus on medical errors and the extent to which health care quality is compromised by a failure to adopt procedures that guarantee the safety of patient care.[49,50] This focus on reducing errors and increasing safety has reinforced the importance of measuring and documenting quality outcomes. When quality measures are linked with a commitment to public accountability, they can bring about broad improvements in health services.

To the extent that health care quality has been discussed in relation to school-based services, quality has been defined in terms of the ratio of school nurses to numbers of students. The staff-to-student ratio recommended by the National Association of School Nurses has been 1 nurse for every 750 students. However, with measurements of health quality process and outcome increasingly common in community-based health care, school-based health programs may also be asked to report on performance rather than personnel or other data. The Seton Health System, a group of not-for-profit hospitals that has managed the Austin, Texas, school health program for the past 8 years, has developed a combination of process and outcome measures that it uses to track system performance. Results are reported internally and to the public annually.[51]

School-based health centers have become linked to the quality movement through the development and the dissemination of a continuous quality improvement tool for the centers.[52] This tool, developed over a 3-year period with participation by the school-based health center field, is focusing the centers' attention on the content of their services and on the outcomes achieved.

Traditional school-based health or nursing services as well as health centers may also be affected by quality measures used by managed care plans. Health plans that contract with state Medicaid programs are often required to report on their performance in terms of specific quality measures. Those plans that contract with school districts or school-based health centers may require their school partners to provide data on services that will enable plans to meet Medicaid quality standards.[53,54] Thus as health plans explore partnerships with school-based health services, quality measurement and accountability will inevitably enter into the discussions.[55]

COSTS AND FINANCING

Because school health services are mostly determined and paid for locally and because there is little consistency among district health programs, there are no consistent state or national data on school health spending. However, several local and state examples, together with a national estimate of spending on specific health service providers, suggest that significant dollar amounts are involved.

In 1998, the Seattle school system, serving 50,000 students, spent $7.5 million on nursing services, counseling, psychological testing, and substance abuse programs. An additional $2 million supported comprehensive school-based health centers in eight Seattle high schools.[56] That same year, Florida's Palm Beach County school system, serving 137,000 students, estimated that it required $10 million to meet the physical, mental health, and preventive health needs of its students. A year later, in 1999, the Chicago Public Schools, a school district with 430,000 students, reported that it employed 2,500 health professionals to care for 53,000 students with disabilities and spent $209 million on general health services as well as the related health services for special needs students.[57] Under a Pennsylvania program, state general funds support a percentage of documented local expenditures on school nursing. To receive state dollars, localities submit an accounting of their expenditures on school nurses. In the school year 1996–1997, the 501 school districts of Pennsylvania reported spending $105 million on school nursing services, with the state reimbursing communities for $40 million of those expenditures.

The Center for Health and Health Care in Schools at the George Washington University developed a rough estimate of recent annual national expenditures on school-based health service providers using the assumptions in Table 1.7. National school system expenditures for the health services they provide to children with special health care needs are not available. However, in April 2000, the General Accounting Office reported that school-based claims on behalf of Medicaid-enrolled children in 47 states plus the District of Columbia totaled $2.3 billion for fiscal year 1999.[60] The GAO noted that not all these dollars are returned to the providers of health services.

The growing amounts included in school budgets for school-based services and special education–related services, plus the health dollars associated with school-based health centers, have captured the attention of public officials, educators, and health care executives, all of

Table 1.7   Estimated Total Costs for School-Based
              Health Services in the United States.

Staff	Number	Annual Salary	Cost
School nurses[34]	56,239	$38,204	$2,148,554,756
Psychologists	22,000	$50,000[58]	$1,250,000,000
Guidance counselors*	22,000	$44,100[58]	$970,200,000
Social workers	15,000	$41,700	$625,000,000
School-based health centers (1,500 centers at $175,000 each)			$262,500,000
Total			$5,256,254,756

*Estimated full-time equivalent for nonacademic counseling services provided by school guidance counselors.

whom have reason to be either concerned or interested in the allocation of those dollars and the effectiveness of school health.

Despite the considerable resources involved, critics suggest that school health services are ill-planned, lack clear and achievable goals, and have failed to keep up with the changing needs of the school population. Although new approaches to health care in school, such as school nurse practitioners and school-based health centers, have offered alternative ways of organizing physical health care and the expansion of mental health services has suggested new priorities, these new approaches have left unanswered questions about what health activities should be undertaken in schools, who should do them, and who or what organization should control the resulting program and be accountable for its performance. The emergence of managed care and its focus on nonduplicative care and accountability in spending and performance sharpen questions about the role of school-based health care. And in every instance, the unanswered question is raised: How should we pay for these services?

THE FUTURE OF SCHOOL HEALTH

School-based health services are in a different place from where they were as recently as 10 years ago. The development of school-based health centers has interested observers and engaged a new group of child health professionals and state government officials in planning how school-based health services might more effectively collaborate with the community-based delivery system for child health care.[61] Children's mental health advocates, long frustrated by the failure of mental health systems to provide early intervention services for children, see new hope in recent federal efforts to address a range of mental health concerns through school-based interventions.[10] Fifteen years of CDC funding for state departments of education to promote attention to school health programs within the education policy establishment has created a critical knowledge base.[62] And the continued growth in school health spending—for services to both disabled and learning-disabled students and the general student population—has drawn attention from school board members, potential service providers, and third-party payers for health services, who are interested in learning how additional dollars might contribute to better health and educational outcomes for children.

The Challenge of Organizational Change

Because school health programs have been isolated from community-based health services, maintaining a high-performance system has proved difficult. School-based health professionals have only limited access to continuing education, and health services managers have infrequent contact with colleagues in other school districts and rare communication with managers in community-based health services. Yet they both care for the same children. Funding difficulties and leadership lapses result in meager equipment, insufficient staff, and inadequate planning for a better system.

In 1994, during the debate on the Clinton health care reform proposals, a small group of health professionals assembled in Washington to discuss the future of school health within the context of health care reform. That group called for a coming together of community stakeholders at the state and local levels "to assess the needs of school-age children, analyze available resources, and agree on what should be done at the school site, who should do it, and who should pay for it."[63] How that might occur was only vaguely sensed, but the participants had a clear vision that school health could no longer remain apart from community health and that community health, to meet its obligations to school-age children, could no longer afford to ignore school health.[33]

One state that is attempting to strengthen school-based health services and to link those services more closely to community-based professionals is Massachusetts. Initially, the state focused on strengthening school health programs by raising standards for school nursing credentials and providing training. More recently, through its Office of School Health, the state has focused on establishing and monitoring performance standards.[64] Throughout these efforts, the state has held regional conferences for school nurses and community physicians to teach new skills and create links between the school nurses and the private pediatric community.

A more radical approach to rethinking school health services is in progress in Austin, Texas. In 1996, the superintendent of the Austin Independent School District responded to a budget crisis by terminating the 30 school nurses who served the 76,000-student school system. Only the federally mandated health services under IDEA and Section 504 of the Rehabilitation Act of 1973 would be continued. A community uproar ensued. In the end, the Seton Healthcare Network assumed responsibility for school health. The integration of school health services within the Seton system produced major changes within Austin's school health program.

The two most significant changes relate to staffing and tracking of outcomes. The first major change, which was hotly debated, was the addition of unlicensed personnel to the school health team. Operating under the principle that all health workers should function to the maximum extent of their license, nurses were relieved of administrative duties and made responsible for supervising the newly hired school health assistants. The nurses were assigned to three schools each and equipped with beepers so that they could be reached quickly by the school health assistants. The second change involved the adoption of quality measures that are tracked as the system works to increase performance. Data are reported and analyzed by school.

One of the complaints from the school system administration and the school board was that they did not know what health expenditures were buying in terms of services and results. The adoption of performance goals for common services such as administering medication and documenting immunizations has enabled the program to make the value of its services widely understood.[65]

The Challenge of Financing

Even if school systems and community-based health care institutions can join together in planning how a more integrated system of child health might come to exist, a major challenge remains. How will the reorganized or expanded services be funded? This question is particularly pressing as state governments try to cope with constrained budgets and concern over increased Medicaid expenditures.

School-based health services have been funded by a variety of sources: local tax dollars, state general funds, federal-state Maternal and Child Health block grant dollars, tobacco tax funds, federal discretionary grants, and federal and state Medicaid reimbursements. Each school district patches together its own approach to funding. And each school district periodically confronts a shortfall in anticipated revenues. One of the first targets for reduced spending inevitably appears to be the school health budget.

Increasingly, Medicaid programs have been seen as potential revenue sources to support health services provided to Medicaid-enrolled students. During the late 1980s and early 1990s, before the widespread introduction of Medicaid managed care, the Health Care Finance Administration (now the Center for Medicaid and Medicare Services) determined that Medicaid could reimburse schools for some services provided to its beneficiaries.[66,67] Not all states or school districts pursued this option because of uncertainty regarding the reimbursement rules and a risk that if the services were improperly billed, the federal government could reclaim funds down the road. However, certain states and districts began either to refinance their existing health services with help from Medicaid funding or to expand school health services with Medicaid revenues.[68]

The move of many state Medicaid programs into managed care meant that some Medicaid revenues became more difficult to obtain. Because special education "related services" are mostly carved out of the Medicaid managed care programs, school districts can continue to bill Medicaid directly for the provision of these services. But other services may no longer be directly reimbursed by the states. State governments, school districts, school heath programs, and managed care plans are just beginning to work out whether and on what terms schools will be part of managed care provider networks.

The Challenge of a Political Strategy

While much has changed in the world of school-based health services, one thing has not: the challenge of integrating school- and community-based health programs. The hot-button issues of adolescent sex and parental rights deter elected officials and school system managers from investing the energy required to redesign the way we organize health services at school. Neither the school system nor the community-based health system has found reason to elevate the issue of school-based health services to the top of its agenda. That said, a fundamental proposition remains true: linking the school-based and community-based systems of health services for children is one of the great untapped resources for strengthening the status of children's health and well-being. It is time to consider some unexplored strategies.

To date, critiques of school health services and proposals for reorganizing them have been grounded in the perspective of the health professional. Plans for reorganizing services have focused on provider arrangements, funding sources, organizational structures, and the importance of documenting greater effectiveness as a way to secure increased recognition, appreciation, and funding. But advocates of school health reform might consider another perspective, and that is that in a democratic system of government, the roles of elected officials and the voters who choose them are critical. It is possible that the health professionals who have taken the lead in thinking about the potential for school health have not thought sufficiently about the potential of politics for building support for a more effective system of school-based care.

The Austin, Texas, story provides encouragement in this regard. Performance *and* accountability persuaded the elected school board to more than double spending on the school health program within 5 years. Quarterly reports are used to keep officials informed of what is happening and to encourage a continuing dialogue. Similarly, the growth of school-based health centers suggests additional support for this perspective. James Morone, a political scientist, commenting on the reasons school-based health centers had grown rapidly over a 10-year period, concluded that it was a classic case of distributional politics. The advocates for the centers, he noted, had been very effective in enlisting constituents to make their case to members of the state legislature. Members of the legislatures saw their support for funding the centers as simply doing their job of bringing the bacon home to their districts.

Political strategizing is a different way of doing business for most of those engaged in thinking about reorganizing school-based services. But the conceptual work has been done. The objective of integrating school-based and community-based health care seems like a good fit with current priorities in the health care environment. The old opposition from private medical practices that focused on keeping all treatment services out of school has diminished. And as school-based health centers have found, advocates who can help move the school health agenda for school-based health services forward exist, but they may not be found in the usual places.[69]

The idea of blending school- and community-based health services for children is compelling. Research studies document the benefits of school-based care in areas as diverse as asthma management, insurance enrollment, access to mental health services, and the provision of primary care. Prevention programs that deter unhealthy behaviors and contribute to positive school environments have also been shown to work. Despite promising outcomes, support for school health activities that can fill gaps in community services or reinforce services that already exist has been slow to develop. A lesson from this circumstance might be that insufficient attention to advocacy and the power of a supportive citizenry can cripple a vital service. The lesson from the school-based health center experience is that doing the work required to build a base of community support can translate into more and better care for kids. In that lesson lies the hope for school health.

Notes

1. US Census Bureau. Resident population by sex and age group: 1990 and 2000. In: *Statistical Abstract of the United States.* Table 11. Washington, DC: US Government Printing Office; 2001.
2. US Department of Education. Projections of education statistics to 2013. Table 1. Available at: http://nces.ed.gov/pubs2001/proj01/tables/table01.asp. Accessed January 3, 2006.
3. Society for Adolescent Medicine. National conference on the health futures of adolescents; 1986; Minneapolis, Minn.
4. Newacheck PW, Starfield B. Morbidity and use of ambulatory care services among poor and nonpoor children. *Am J Public Health.* 1988;78:927–933.
5. St Peter RF, Newacheck PW, Halfon N. Access to care for poor children: separate and unequal? *JAMA.* 1999;267:2760–2764.
6. Perloff JD. Health care resources for children and pregnant women. *Future Child.* 1992;2:78–94.
7. Ellickson PL, Lara ME. *Forgotten Ages, Forgotten Problems: Adolescents' Health.* Santa Monica, Calif: RAND Corp; 1993.

8. Lear JG. School-based services and adolescent health: past, present and future. *Adolesc Med.* 1996;7:163–180.

9. Dryfoos JG. *Full-Service Schools: A Revolution in Health and Social Services for Children, Youth, and Families.* San Francisco, Calif: Jossey-Bass; 1994.

10. Rones M, Hoagwood K. School-based mental health services: a research review. *Clin Child Fam Psychol Rev.* 2000;3:223–241.

11. US Department of Health and Human Services. *Mental Health: A Report of the Surgeon General.* Rockville, Md: US Department of Health and Human Services; 1999.

12. US Department of Health and Human Services. *Oral Health in America: A Report of the Surgeon General.* Rockville, Md: US Department of Health and Human Services; 2000.

13. Rosenberg & Associates. *Examining the Reorganization of School Health Services: Lessons from Eight Communities.* Oakland, Calif; 1999. Available at: http://www.healthinschools.org/sh/rsh.asp. Accessed July 25, 2004.

14. National Center for Health Statistics. *Summary Health Statistics of US Children: National Health Interview Survey, 2004.* Provisional Report. Ser 10, no 227. Atlanta, Ga: Centers for Disease Control and Prevention; 2003.

15. RAND Health Communications. *Mental Health Care for Youth: Who Gets It? How Much Does It Cost? Who Pays? Where Does the Money Go?* Santa Monica, Calif: RAND Corp; 2001. Available at: http://www.rand.org/publications/RB/RB4541/. Accessed January 4, 2002.

16. Centers for Disease Control and Prevention. Youth risk behavior surveillance—United States, 2003. *MMWR Surveill Sum.* 2004;53(SS-2):1–96. Available at: http://www.cdc.gov/mmwr/PDF/SS/SS5302.pdf. Accessed September 14, 2005.

17. US Department of Education. No Child Left Behind Act of 2001: Overview. Available at: http://www.ed.gov/nclb/overview/intro/progsum/index.html. Accessed July 25, 2004.

18. National Center for Education Statistics. *Digest of Education Statistics, 2000.* Washington, DC: US Department of Education; 2000.

19. National Center for Education Statistics. *Overview of Public Elementary and Secondary Schools and Districts: School Year 1999–2000.* Washington, DC: US Department of Education; 2001. Available at: http://nces.ed.gov/pubs2001/overview/table07.asp. Accessed January 3, 2002.

20. National Center for Education Statistics. *Statistics of State School Systems; Statistics of Public Elementary and Secondary School Systems; Statistics of Nonpublic Elementary and Secondary Schools; Private Schools in American Education; Common Core Data.* Washington, DC: US Department of Education; 2000. Available at: http://nces.ed.gov/pubs2001/digest/dt087.html. Accessed January 3, 2002.

21. Brener ND, Burstein GR, DuShaw ML, Vernon ME, Wheeler L, Robinson J. Health services: results from the School Health Policies and Programs Study 2000. *J Sch Health.* 2001;71:294–304.

22. US Department of Education. 10 facts about K-12 education funding. Available at: http://www.ed.gov/nclb/landing.jhtml?src=pb. Accessed July 26, 2004.

23. Levit K, Smith C, Cowan C, Sensenig A, Catlin A, Health Accounts Team. Health spending rebound continues in 2002. *Health Aff.* 2004;23:147–159.

24. Hoag EB, Termin LB. *Health Work in the Schools.* Boston, Mass: Houghton Mifflin, 1914.

25. Kort, M. The delivery of primary health care in American public schools, 1890–1980. *J Sch Health.* 1984;54:453–457.

26. Starr P. *The Social Transformation of American Medicine.* New York, NY: Basic Books; 1982.

27. Rehabilitation Act of 1973, 29 USC § 794; Regulations at 34 CFR § 104.

28. US Department of Health and Human Services. *Medicaid Coverage of Health-Related Services for Children Receiving Special Education: An Examination of Federal Policies.* Washington, DC: US GPO; 1991.

29. Yankauer A Jr, Ballou L. The remediability of certain categories of defects. *Am J Public Health.* 1957;47:1421–1429.

30. Yankauer A Jr, Franz R, Drislane A, Katz S. A study of case-finding methods in elementary schools. *Am J Public Health.* 1962;52:656–662.

31. Center for Health and Health Care in Schools. 2002 state survey of school-based health center initiatives. Washington, DC: Center for Health and Health Care in Schools; 2003. Available at: http://www.healthinschools.org/sbhcs/survey02.htm. Accessed September 14, 2005.

32. Centers for Medicaid and Medicare Services. School-based health services programs. In: *Medicaid School-Based Administrative Claiming Guide.* Washington, DC: US Department of Health and Human Services; 2003:app.

33. Lear JG. Schools and adolescent health: strengthening services and improving outcomes. *J Adolesc Health.* 2002;31(suppl 6):310–320.

34. Spratley E, Johnson A, Sochalski J, Fritz M, Spencer W. The registered nurse population: findings from the National Sample Survey of Registered Nurses. Washington, DC: US Department of Health and Human Services; 2000. Available at: ftp://ftp.hrsa.gov/bhpr/rnsurvey2000/rnsurvey00.pdf. Accessed September 14, 2005.

35. Fryer GE, Igoe JB. Functions of school nurses and health assistants in US school health programs. *J Sch Health.* 1996;66(2):55–58.

36. US General Accounting Office. Attention disorder drugs: few incidents of diversion or abuse by schools. 2001. GAO Report 01–1011. Available at:

http://frwebgate.access.gpo.gov/cgi-bin/useftp.cgi?IPaddress=162.140.64.21 &filename=d011011.pdf&directory=/diskb/wais/data/gao. Accessed September 14, 2005.

37. Pohlman KJ. Legal framework and financial accountability for school nursing practice. In: Schwab NC, Gelfman MHB, eds. *Legal Issues in School Health Services: A Resource for School Administrators, School Attorneys, and School Nurses.* North Branch, Minn: Sunrise River Press; 2001:95–121.

38. National Assembly on School-Based Health Care. School-based health center census: national census school year 2001–02. Washington, DC: National Assembly on School-Based Health Care; 2003. Available at: http://www.nasbhc.org/EQ/2001tables.htm. Accessed September 14, 2005.

39. Lear JG. Health care goes to school: an untidy strategy to improve the well-being of school-age children. In: Garfinkel I, Hochschild JL, McLanahan SS, eds. *Social Policies for Children.* Washington, DC: Brookings Institution, 1996:173–201.

40. Burns BJ, Costello EJ, Angold A, et al. Children's mental health service use across service sectors. *Health Aff.* 1995;14:149–159.

41. Kolbe LJ, Kann L, Brener ND. Overview and summary of findings: School Health Policies and Programs Study 2000. *J Sch Health.* 2001;71:253–259.

42. Leaf JP, Alegria M, Cohen P, et al. Mental health service use in the community and schools: results from the four-community MECA study. *J Am Acad Child Adolesc Psychiatry.* 1996;37:889–897.

43. Costante CC. DNR in the school setting. In: Schwab NC, Gelfman MHB, eds. *Legal Issues in School Health Services: A Resource for School Administrators, School Attorneys, and School Nurses.* North Branch, Minn: Sunrise River Press; 2001:419–437.

44. Reutzel TJ, Patel R, Myers MA. Medication management in primary and secondary schools. *J Am Pharm Assoc (Wash).* 2001; 41:67–77.

45. Boonstra H, Nash E. Minors and the right to consent to health care. *Guttmacher Report on Public Policy,* August 2000. New York, NY: Alan Guttmacher Institute. Available at: http://www.agi-usa.org/pubs/ ib_minors_00.html. Accessed September 14, 2005.

46. Putting Parents First Act (S2380), introduced in the US Senate July 30, 1998.

47. Bergren MD. Electronic records and technology. In: Schwab NC, Gelfman MHB, eds. *Legal Issues in School Health Services: A Resource for School Administrators, School Attorneys, and School Nurses.* North Branch, Minn: Sunrise River Press; 2001:317–334.

48. Greiner M, Nickerson G, Rosenberg S. State policy context for school-based health centers: with special focus on development of mental health and dental health services. Rosenberg & Associates; 2001. Available at: http://www.health-inschools.org/sh/policypaper.asp. Accessed September 14, 2005.

49. Kohn LT, Corrigan JM, Donaldson MS, eds. *To Err is Human: Building a Safer Health System.* Washington, DC: National Academy Press; 2000.

50. Institute of Medicine Committee on Quality of Health Care in America. *Crossing the Quality Chasm: A New Health System for the 21st Century.* Washington, DC: National Academy Press; 2001.

51. Center for Health and Health Care in Schools. AISD/Children's Student Health Services 2000–01: risk management. Available at: http://www.healthinschools.org/sh/risk2.htm. Accessed July 28, 2004.

52. Center for Health and Health Care in Schools. A continuous quality improvement tool for school-based health centers. Available at: http://www.healthinschools.org/cqi_tool.asp. Accessed September 14, 2005.

53. Koppelman J, Lear JG. The new child health insurance expansions: how will school-based health centers fit in? *J Sch Health.* 1998;68:441–446.

54. Koppelman J, Lear JG. Partnering with school-based health centers: Connecticut's Medicaid managed care experience. *Manag Care Medicaid.* 1999;5(2):4–5.

55. Taras H, Nader P, Swinger H, Fontanesi J. The school health innovative programs: integrating school health and managed care in San Diego. *J Sch Health.* 1998;68:22–25.

56. Seattle Public Schools, 1996–1997 budget.

57. Gam S. Testimony before the US Senate Finance Committee, June 17, 1999.

58. Thomas A. School psychology 2000: Average salary data. *NASP Communiqué.* 2000;28(6). Available at: http://www.nasponline.org/publications/cq286salary.htm. Accessed September 14, 2005.

59. Bureau of Labor Statistics. Occupational Employment Statistics Survey. Career InfoNet; 2002. Available at: http://www.acinet.org/acinet/occ_rep.asp?soccode=211012&stfips=06. Accessed July 28, 2004.

60. US General Accounting Office. *Medicaid in Schools: Poor Oversight and Improper Payments Compromise Potential Benefit.* Washington, DC: US General Accounting Office; 2000.

61. Morone J, Kilbreth EH, Langwell KM. Back to school: a health care strategy for youth. *Health Aff.* 2001;20:122–136.

62. Building the infrastructure for comprehensive school heath programs. In: Institute of Medicine. *Schools and Health: Our Nation's Investment.* Allensworth DD, Lawson E, Nicholson L, Wyche JH, eds. Washington, DC: National Academy Press, 1997:chap 5.

63. US Department of Health and Human Services. *School-Based Health Services: Issues to Be Addressed by the Health Security Act and Other Federal Legislation* [report of the School Health Services Analytic Project Panel]. Washington, DC: US Department of Health and Human Services; June 28, 1994.

64. Massachusetts Department of Public Health. School health services; 2002. Available at: http://www.state.ma.us/dph/fch/schoolhealth/index.htm. Accessed December 18, 2003.

65. Center for Health and Health Care in Schools. AISD/Children's Student Health Services 2000–01. Available at: http://www.healthinschools.org/sh/aisd.asp. Accessed December 18, 2003.

66. Memorandum from the director of the Medicaid Bureau to all regional administrators. Update on Medicaid program requirements for services provided in schools, December 22, 1993.

67. Health Care for All. *Medicaid and School Health: A Technical Assistance Guide.* Washington, DC: US Department of Health and Human Services; 1997.

68. Under the IDEA legislation, school districts must prepare an individualized education program (IEP) for each eligible child. The IEP must specify all special education and related services needed. The school districts are obligated by federal statute and court rulings to provide these services. In addition to federal grant support for special education, Medicaid programs may pay for those related services that are specified in the federal Medicaid statute and determined to be medically necessary by the state Medicaid agency.

69. Koppelman J, Lear JG. *From the Margins to the Mainstream: Institutionalizing School-Based Health Centers.* Washington, DC: Making the Grade Program Office; 2000.

Historical Perspectives

Reprints of Key Reports and Articles

CHAPTER 2

The Delivery of Primary Health Care in American Public Schools, 1890–1980

Michael Kort, 1984

ublic officials responsible for child welfare are expressing concern about the health of the nation's children and are suggesting that the public schools be utilized more intensively to help correct
this situation. The expansion of the schools' role in health care is being
considered for several reasons. Families have been failing to monitor
the health of their children adequately, as demonstrated by the reduction in immunization levels. Planners also want to target scarce revenue on populations within locations where the impact and payoff
will be the greatest.[1,2] It also is being asserted that the lack of medical
care contributes directly to learning disabilities.

Screening, immunization, and similar preventive measures fall
within parameters associated with school health. However, there is a
body of thought stressing the desirability of delivering direct primary
care in the schools, and there are several school districts where this

This chapter originally appeared as Kort M. The delivery of primary health
care in American public schools, 1890–1980. *J Sch Health*. 1984;54
(11):453–457. Copyright ©1984. Reprinted with permission. American
School Health Association, Kent, Ohio.

currently is being done in a comprehensive manner. The delivery of primary care, of course, is a highly controversial issue because of its implications regarding the relationship between public and private medicine in this country. This article will consider the development of the role of the school in health care and how that role became limited to familiar parameters. It also will focus on the tradition of direct treatment in the schools, which while extremely limited and often dormant, never totally died. Current programs representing a renewal of this tendency will be noted.

ORIGINS OF SCHOOL HEALTH SERVICES

The concept of having health services in American public schools dates from the origins of the public school system itself. William A. Alcott, Concord, MA, suggested in 1840 that "our schools ought to have regular physicians, as much as our houses of industry, our almshouses, or our penitentiaries." The Report of the Sanitary Commission of Massachusetts, written in 1850 by Lemuel Shattuck, suggested that schools could be used to promote health if students were mobilized under the teachers' supervision for monthly self-inspections. In 1872, the Elmira, NY, Board of Education employed a "sanitary superintendent" to cope with the prevalence of smallpox among the school population. The duties included frequent examinations of school children, exclusion of the unvaccinated, and supervision of sanitary conditions.[3] The Elmira program seems to have been a precursor rather than a stimulus or model, as it was more than 20 years before other American cities followed suit.

During the 19th Century, Europe forged ahead of the United States in public school health programs, providing the models for this nation to follow. An 1833 French law mandated that public school authorities be responsible for the sanitation of school buildings. In 1837, French kindergarten supervisors were watching over the health of their classes. A Paris law of 1842–1843 required that a physician inspect the premises and students of every boys' and girls' school.[2] Physicians were hired for public school staffs in Sweden in 1868, Germany in 1869, Russia in 1871, and Austria in 1873. Brussels was the first European city to organize a regular inspection system in 1874. All schools were inspected by a physician every three months. Later the inspection staff included vision specialists and dentists.[4] The example spread relatively quickly, with similar programs being implemented in Paris in 1879, Antwerp in 1882, Moscow in 1888, Leipzig and London in 1891, and Wiesbaden in 1896. The Wiesbaden program probably was the most successful and comprehensive of these and provided the model for copies throughout most of Germany by 1898. By 1899 the movement reached Romania, where a new law ordered annual inspections of all school children. The Medical Inspection Act, the forerunner of the present school health services in Great Britain, was passed in 1908.[3]

The use of American public schools to improve the health of children began after compulsory education brought together large numbers of children with acute infectious diseases in unsanitary and poorly heated and ventilated buildings, creating conditions ideal for the spread of those diseases.[5] The earliest school health efforts were initiated in the 1890s and developed into formal programs during the next two decades. School programs developed against a background of more general progress in the field of public health. With school health supervision, public health programs included the collection and analysis of statistics, control of common disease, infant and child hygiene, sanitation, food and milk control, public health nursing, and public heath education.[6] Among the programs most closely related to school health were the milk stations established by charitable organizations to control typhoid fever. These stations developed into well-child clinics and eventually treated children up to age six.[7]

EARLY AMERICAN EFFORTS

The earliest school-based efforts focused on communicable disease prevention. This focus reflected the problems arising from numerous epidemics and virtually no mass immunization. Jacobziner characterized the effort as an "inspection and screening service."[8] Public health departments appointed medical inspectors to make sanitary inspections both of school buildings and children. New York City appointed the nation's first school medical officer in 1892. Two years later, Boston launched the first citywide system of medical inspection by appointing 50 physicians as "medical visitors" to make daily inspections of the schools and examine all children suspected of having a communicable disease. Boston provided the model for programs in Chicago in 1895, New York City in 1897, and Philadelphia in 1898. Annual medical inspections for school children for eyes, ears, nose and throat were mandated statewide in Vermont in 1904. In 1906, Massachusetts required medical examinations in its public schools.[3] By 1910 medical inspections were required in more than 300 city school systems.[4] In New York, the medical inspectors visited public and other free schools in Manhattan each morning for about one hour to examine children referred to them by school personnel. Those who were sick were barred from school until the danger of transmitting the disease was over.[5]

By 1902, inspecting physicians in New York had intensified their efforts to control contagious eye and skin infections by inspecting all children. The success of this medical inspection raised new problems. Sick children were excused from school, but many from poorer homes never received treatment and therefore were unable to return to the classroom. In addition, the physicians were uncovering large numbers of noncontagious defects that remained untreated.[5]

School Nurses

Transient physician inspectors soon were supplemented by a more permanent presence—the school nurse—after a demonstration program in New York City dramatically reduced absenteeism due to disease. The nurse for the program, one of Lillian Wald's Henry Street nurses, worked directly with parents to assure that the children received proper care. Within a few years, nurses were in Los Angeles and Philadelphia (1903), Boston (1905), and Pueblo, CO, schools. By 1911, 102 cities employed 415 school nurses and the New York City staff had expanded to 176 nurses by 1918.[3]

An unusual program was initiated in 1905 in Los Angeles when the Los Angeles Tenth District PTA began maintaining a bed at a local hospital. This bed became the kernel of a system of clinics. A health care clinic, donated by the O. T. Johnson family, was opened in 1916. Three more health centers and two dental clinics followed between 1916 and 1928.[9,10]

During these early years, the parameters of school health services were not fixed. As immunization and other medical advances reduced the threat from communicable diseases, more attention was given to physical defects discovered during the first phase of inspections. In 1905, New York City advanced from its "inspection and screening service" to what Jacobziner calls a "case finding service." Each child was checked for defects. Nurses screened in the classrooms and physicians saw children referred to them. Children requiring treatment were referred to outside services, either private physicians or public clinics.[8]

Dental care, often including restorative treatment, was another major addition to pre-World War I school health services. In 1903, Reading, PA, hired a dentist to perform examinations; the next decade saw dental programs launched in Cleveland, Cincinnati, New York City, and Philadelphia. After Bridgeport, CT, hired 10 dental hygienists to clean teeth in 1914, that practice spread across the country.[11] Aside from a dental program that featured dental clinics in school buildings, New York City schools also had clinics for eye, ear, and orthopedic defects; between 1912 and 1915 free clinics removed tonsils and adenoids.[5]

Post–World War I Growth

After World War I, many school districts adopted a more activist posture regarding school health. This action was in part due to the shock of the number of correctable physical defects revealed by the draft, but other factors also were at work. As American society changed, the nation's philosophy of education changed. The traditional school in a predominantly rural and relatively homogenous 19th Century America had been viewed by educators as mandated to do little more than promote intellectual development. By the turn of the century, America was becoming an urban industrial society. A rapidly increasing population was becoming far more heterogeneous as millions of immigrants from Eastern European and Mediterranean countries were congregating in the cities in cultural and national ghettos. Within these industrial slums, the children of native-born classes combined with the immigrant children to form a vast pool of children for whom traditional schooling was inadequate. Progressives insisted that education needed radical reform. The curriculum had to be expanded to include areas previously considered unnecessary or properly left to other institutions. The progressives pointed to the change in family life, the withdrawal of the father and sometimes the mother from the home to the workplace, and the general corrosive effect of urbanization on family life.

Reformers cited the new need of the schools to take on the job of transmitting American culture to immigrant children. Vocational training was considered necessary because the old apprenticeship system had become outmoded. All of this was part of the progressive view of education as being a preparation for life which necessitated a broad approach going far beyond the "three Rs."[12] This new thrust in education took place against a broader background of social reform committed to eliminating a range of social ills, from poor housing and unsafe working conditions to juvenile delinquency and child labor.[6]

An essential part of the new educational reforms, therefore, was concerned with health. This concern was stressed both by the Progressive Education Association and the National Education Association (NEA). In 1918, the NEA listed its seven main objectives of education; among these "seven cardinal principles" was health.[13]

With the growth of public health and the new philosophy of education, a broad range of forces were potential promoters of school health services. These broader societal phenomena included medical and scientific progress, the development of the behavioral sciences, the impact of the physical defects revealed during World War I, and concern and leadership from a variety of organizations and individuals. By the 1920s, health programs would be firmly established in the nation's schools. Almost every state enacted laws concerning health and physical education between 1918 and 1921. By 1923, 84 of the 86 cities surveyed by the American Child Health Association had nursing services in their schools.[3] In 1920, school health services were discussed at a White House conference on child welfare. In 1925, the National Congress of Parents and Teachers promoted a campaign to get parents to send their children to school healthy. In 1927, the American Association of School Physicians, which later became the American School Health Association, was founded.[14] During the 1920s, cities like Los Angeles, Cleveland, Houston, Denver, and San Diego all had formal programs with a medical director.[15]

Establishing Basic School Health Care Policies

It was during the 1920s and the early 1930s that the basic policies determining the responsibilities of the school in health care for the next several decades were established. Schools examined students and implemented immunization programs, but the concept of delivering systematic treatment in the schools was rejected. School health services became limited largely to health inspection, assessment, and first aid.

Two factors seem to have been central to this development. The first was the prevailing concept of preventive medicine during that period. Health care was to be administered by physicians in private practice. Preventive services, including those in the schools, were seen as supplementing not substituting for or competing with the private sector. These services would not treat patients and therefore did not require the necessary facilities. Regulations governing school health institutionalized this outlook. School health almost inevitably mirrored the overall strict separation between preventive and curative services—with the latter remaining in private hands—which characterized the era in which it took shape.[7]

The second factor was the very act of locating medical services in public schools. This factor automatically set in motion forces that would restrict those services. Eisner and Callon[7] point out that school health programs have a special character that makes them harder than other preventive programs to incorporate into comprehensive services. Unlike the well-child conferences, school health programs are in institutions where education is the major objective.

The issue is one of priorities. The educator's mandate is to educate. The health professional in the schools focuses almost exclusively on health, while the educator is concerned with many activities considered more important than routine health matters. The first priority of the health professional is finding children with handicapping conditions and unsuspected health problems. School administrators are more concerned with emergency care, and the portion of their health service budgets devoted to minor first aid often surprises health professionals. Both school administrators and health professionals are concerned with medical problems that affect learning ability and behavior but, compared to these classroom concerns, the discovery of routine medical conditions are low priority objectives to educators.[7]

Given the divergence of priorities between educators and public health professionals, a key factor in determining the fate of school health services has been who is in charge of them. The debate began in the 1920s and has continued, with educators claiming the virtue of efficient administration and health departments insisting that health services should be operated by health personnel.[16] Whatever the merits of the latter rationale, boards of education have tended to control school health services. A series of surveys conducted since the 1920s reveals that boards of education generally have administered about 70% of all school health services, with the figure generally higher in large cities where most students are located.[17]

The effect of this administrative pattern is reinforced by law. In most states, statutes guiding health services generally permit health appraisal, emergency care, and the counseling of students.[18] This pattern is reflected in the role of school nurses. Nurses were originally charged with detecting and controlling contagious diseases. They were the key link between the medical inspectors and school children. During the 1920s, 1930s, and 1940s, the emphasis on health education led nurses to try to incorporate this area into their responsibilities. Later, with the emphasis on the familial origins of many children's problems, school nurses were enlisted in the efforts of educational, medical, and community agencies to pool their resources; but, in fact, school nurses generally have delivered first aid and performed various clerical functions.[19]

The period from the 1920s through the mid-1960s consequently saw the atrophy of the treatment component of school health services. A Subcommittee on School Medical Services of the 1930 White House Conference on Child Health and Protection called for the elimination of treatment in the school and a "conscious attempt by school physicians and supervisors of nurses to make more contact with practicing physicians."[20] In dentistry, the 1940s witnessed the change from restorative work in the schools to concentration on dental health education and health inspection.[15] In 1948, the proposed National School Health Bill, designed to give federal grant-in-aid to school health, was defeated in part due to the opposition of important sectors of the medical profession that feared the bill would provide funds for medical treatment of children other than those unable to pay.

In explaining its opposition to portions of the bill during hearings in the Senate, the American Academy of Pediatrics referred to its 1939 position favoring the use of federal or state funds for maternal and child welfare and the care of children from indigent groups in the population. The Senate version of the bill, the Academy's director warned, did not contain a means test; and the Academy feared federal bureaucrats administering the program would provide medical treatment for those financially able to take care of themselves. He suggested that treatment only be provided "on a basis that is equitable in view of the need for services."[21] At a special meeting, the Academy's Executive Board added that "any treatment proposed in any bill should remain within the jurisdiction of private physicians."[22] The National School Health bill was defeated. In 1953, the *New York State Journal of Medicine* reported that school health services in New York City did not offer medical treatment; all problems were referred to other agencies or private doctors.[23]

Dental Care

However, the sweep was not quite complete, at least in the area of dental care. Though school dentistry has focused on prevention rather than on restoration since the 1940s, a tradition of school-based dentistry has always existed, largely on an *ad hoc* basis. Many programs were one-chair operations that were poorly equipped, located, and financed, and staffed by part-time personnel. The overall quality of the restorative treatment they provided was subject to criticism.[24]

Nonetheless, a 1961 national survey located almost 400 schools out of 3,266 responding to 9,500 questionnaires sent out that provided fillings for at least some of their students in various types of school-based clinics.[25] In New York City, the *Journal of the American Dental Association* reported in 1951, the Department of Health operated 137 dental clinics, some of which were in schools.[26] The Denver public schools financed a clinic for indigent children for more than 46 years until discontinuing it for budgetary reasons in 1971.[27] Cleveland's pioneering program continued to offer restorative care, at least to indigent children.[28]

School-based restorative dentistry efforts at times developed into comprehensive programs. Between 1930 and 1944, all of the school children in Chisholm, MN, received dental care, including restorative treatment.[29] Extensive programs run by the Public Health Service existed in Woonsocket, RI, and Richmond, IN, between 1946 and 1952.[30–32] Wolfe County, KY, a depressed rural area of Appalachia, was the site of a five-year program of incremental care for school children between 1967 and 1972.[33] Other school-based programs have existed in Michigan, Tennessee, and Georgia. The Michigan program was initiated in 1973 and designed to continue for four years.[34] An ambitious program known as the Chattanooga Project provided comprehensive dental care at no charge to children from indigent families in a 13-county region of southeastern Tennessee and northwestern Georgia. It operated from 1968 to 1975 and treated children aged five to 15.[35]

However, these dental programs represented the exception rather than the rule. As school health programs developed during the 1940s and 1950s, treatment continued to be deemphasized. This change is clearly illustrated by the very terms in vogue to define school health services. In 1964, a publication of the Joint Committee on Problems in Education of the NEA and AMA listed six functions: appraising pupil health, health counseling and follow-up, prevention and control of communicable diseases, emergency care, services related to environmental sanitation, and protecting the health of school personnel.[3] This definition, in which nothing more than emergency care is mentioned, is typical of the prevailing opinion in the 1950s and 1960s.[36,37]

TODAY'S PROGRAMS

While the consensus remained that schools should not offer medical treatment, it was clear that many children were not getting the attention they required. This need was the major focus of the pioneering Astoria Study conducted in New York City during the 1940s.[8] World War II revealed that problems discovered after World War I remained unsolved. In 1945, representatives of federal health and education agencies and other professional associations concluded that the health assessments for World War II continued to reveal physical and mental health conditions that could have been corrected during childhood. The conference established a Committee on the School-Age Child, which in 1951 published a report reiterating the 1945 concerns.[38] In the mid-1950s, Alfred Yankauer questioned the value of periodic school physical examinations, concluding that they often revealed known but uncorrected defects.[39,40]

The 1960s was the beginning of a response to these problems, as part of the generally increased social commitment of the Kennedy and Johnson administrations. A new comprehensive pattern of public health care began to develop. Many federal health service grants became available and a variety of new programs implemented. In the specific field of school health, Title I of the Elementary and Secondary Education Act (1966) provided federal funds for expanded school health and other related services in schools with large disadvantaged populations. The bulk of these funds went for food for children and salaries of school nurses and doctors.[41] Between 1971 and 1974, 23 demonstration projects received $10 million. These projects included medical and dental screening, nutrition, and social and mental health services for children from low income families. In 1974, Title I's intent was restated to provide priority to educational purposes and "only secondarily" for health purposes. As of 1977, there was $25 million available for health-related services through Title I.[5]

The 1967 amendments to Title 19 (Medicaid) of the Social Security Act authorized the Early Periodic Screening, Detection, and Treatment (EPSDT) program to provide continuous health care for welfare children. Twelve million children were eligible, but as of 1978 only 20% had received benefits under the program, which included a standard health test, immunization, well-child health supervision, and dental care services. Among the problems were the federal government's inability to enforce the laws, the states' inability to develop adequate management and management information systems, and a lack of consensus among health professionals about what is appropriate preventive care for children.[42]

With these programs, which fall within traditional school health service parameters, significant innovative efforts were initiated in various parts of the country during the 1970s. Pioneering school health programs now exist in Cambridge, MA, Galveston, TX, Hartford, CT, and Posen-Robins (Chicago), IL. The Cambridge, Hartford, and Posen-Robins programs represent a revival of the early sporadic efforts to provide direct treatment to children in the public schools. In Cambridge, five school-based health centers provide primary pediatric care to about 50% of the city's elementary school children. The Hartford program delivers primary medical and dental care in one of two schools in the program, while the Posen-Robins project uses both school-based clinics staffed by nurse practitioners and, for more serious cases, two local hospitals.[41,43]

The Robert Wood Johnson Foundation funded four other programs during the 1970s to improve school-based school services by using school nurse practitioners. The grants totaled $4.8 million for a five-year period beginning in July 1978. The projects were in low income areas in Colorado, North Dakota, New York, and Utah.[44] The foundation also supported the National Preventive Dentistry Demonstration program. Administered by the American Fund for Dental Health, it provided school-based preventive services to about 25,000 children at 10 sites across the country during a $5\frac{1}{2}$-year period (1976–1982).[45] Meanwhile, several attempts at innovation were made within a framework that does not include direct treatment. Among them were the University of Rochester programs in Penfield, NY,[46,47] and subsequently in an entire school district in Monroe County, NY[48]; the Harlem Hospital Center's program in two ghetto elementary schools[49]; and a large examination facility serving Jersey City, NJ.[50] Attempts to upgrade programs through the use of nurse practitioners occurred in school districts from coast to coast.[41,51-53]

Another important tendency was the utilization of school-based self-applied fluoride programs. In the wake of studies conducted at home and abroad, the growth of these programs during the 1970s was dramatic. At the beginning of the decade, school dental programs consisted primarily of education; by 1980, almost one-quarter of the nation's elementary school districts offered self-applied fluoride programs.[54]

THE CHALLENGE OF THE FUTURE

As the 1970s ended, several proposals for expanding the scope and efficiency of school-based health services surfaced. These proposals included a report by the New York State Board of Regents and several proposals from the federal government. However, developments since 1980 make it difficult to predict to what extent the nation's school health services will be modified. There is a growing feeling that the schools already are overburdened and unable to fulfill their current responsibilities. Working in an era of restrictive budgets at every level of government further complicates matters. However, a long-term perspective reveals that many functions formerly performed by the American family are now provided by other institutions, the schools being prominent among them. It is clear that the challenge will be to find formulas that reconcile expanded needs with scarce resources to maximize the benefit to this nation's children.

Notes

1. Breslow L, Haggerty R, Henderson M, et al. *Preventive Medicine USA— Theory, Practice, and Application of Prevention in Personal Health Services.* Task force report sponsored by the National Institute of Health and the American College of Preventive Medicine. New York, NY: Prodist; 1976.

2. Green LW. *Determining the Impact and Effectiveness of Health Education as It Relates to Federal Policy.* Prepared for the Office of the Deputy Assistant for Planning and Evaluation/Health, US Department of Health, Education and Welfare; April 30, 1976.

3. Wilson CE. *School Health Services.* Washington, DC: Joint Committee on Health Problems in Schools of the National Education Association and the American Medical Association; 1964.

4. Anderson CL, Creswell WH. *School Health Practices.* St Louis, Mo: Mosby; 1976.

5. Lynch A. Evaluating school health programs. *Proc Acad Political Sci.* 1977;32(3):90–91.

6. Rosen G. *Preventive Medicine in the United States.* New York, NY: Prodist; 1977.

7. Eisner V, Callon LB. *Dimensions of School Health.* Springfield, Ill: Thomas; 1971.

8. Jacobziner J. The Astoria Plan. *J Pediatr.* 1951;38:221.

9. Los Angeles Tenth District PTA. *You and the Tenth District PTA* [brochure]. Los Angeles, Calif: Tenth District PTA.

10. Los Angeles Tenth District PTA. *Los Angeles Tenth District Parent Teacher Health Centers* [brochure]. Los Angeles, Calif: Tenth District PTA.

11. Stoll FA. *Dental Health Education.* Philadelphia, Pa.: Lea & Febiger; 1977.

12. Best JH, Sidwell RT, eds. *The American Legacy of Learning: Readings in the History of Education.* New York, NY: Lippincott; 1967.

13. Gross CH, Chandler CC, eds. *A History of American Education Through Readings.* Boston, Mass: Heath; 1964.

14. Haag JH. *School Health Programs.* New York, NY: Holt, Rinehart and Winston; 1958.

15. Randall HB. School health in the seventies: a decade against disease. *J Sch Health.* 1971;41:125.

16. Wisnik SH. Administrative jurisdiction of school health services. *Am J Public Health.* 1951;41:819–821.

17. Wolf JM, Pritham HC. Administration of school health services. *JAMA.* 1965;193:195–198.

18. Jenne FH, Greene WH. *Turner's School Health and Education.* St Louis, Mo: Mosby; 1976.

19. Regan PA. A historical study of the school nurse role. *J Sch Health.* 1976;46:518–520.

20. Mitchell HE. School medical service in perspective. *Pediatrics.* 1965;65:1013.

21. U.S. Congress, Senate. Hearings before a subcommittee of the Committee on Labor and Welfare, 80th Congress, 2nd Session, on S1290; 1948.

22. Pease MC. *A History of the American Academy of Pediatrics: June 1930–June 1951.* New York, NY: American Academy of Pediatrics; 1951.

23. Culbert RW, Jacobziner J. Health service to school children in New York City. *New York State J Med.* 1953;53(1):47–50.

24. Dunning JM. *Dental Care for Everyone.* Cambridge, Mass: Harvard University Press; 1976.

25. Dollar ML, Sandell PJ. Dental programs in schools. *J Sch Health.* 1961;31:11–12.

26. Strusser H, Sandler HC. Dental health education and the follow-up program in elementary and junior high schools of New York City. *J Am Dent Assoc.* 1951;42(2):43–47.

27. Division of Health Services, Denver Public Schools. *48th Report (1970–1971).* Denver, Colo: Denver Public Schools; 1971.

28. Kessler HE. Cleveland's comprehensive public school dental program and fluoridation report. *J Sch Health.* 1969;39:372–373.

29. Jordan WA. Why the need of dental clinics in the public schools. *Dental Cosmos.* 1936;78:1283–1287.

30. Law FE, Johnson CE, Knutson JW. Studies on dental care services for school children. *Public Health Rep.* 1953;68:1192–1198.

31. Waterman GE, Knutson JW. Studies on dental care services for children—third and fourth treatment service, Richmond, Ind. *Public Health Rep.* 1954;64:247–254.

32. Galagan DJ, Law FE, Waterman GE, Spritz GS. Dental health status of children five years after completing school care programs. *Public Health Rep.* 1964;79:445–454.

33. Heise AL, Mullins MR, Hill CJ, Crawford JH, Meeting the dental treatment needs of indigent rural children. *Health Serv Rep.* 1973;88:591–593.

34. Bargramian RA, Graves RC, Mohondas B. A combined approach to preventing dental caries in schoolchildren: caries reduction after one year. *J Am Dent Assoc.* 1974;93:789.

35. Doherty N, Vivian S. Expenditures for the dental care of indigent children in the Chattanooga Project, 1971–1975. *J Public Health Dent.* 1977;37:209–216.

36. Byrd O, comp. *School Health Sourcebook.* Stanford, Calif: Stanford University Press; 1955.

37. Smolensky J, Bonveshio LR. *Principles of School Health.* Boston, Mass: Heath; 1966.

38. Hutchins VL. New policies in school health. *J Sch Health.* 1977;47:428–430.

39. Yankauer A, Lawrence RA. A study of periodic school medical exams. *Am J Public Health.* 1955;45:77–78.

40. Yankauer A. Child health supervision: is it worth it? *Pediatrics.* 1973;52:272–277.

41. Cronin GE, Young WM. *400 Navels: The Future of School Health in America.* Bloomington, Ind: Phi Delta Kappa; 1979.

42. Chang A, Goldstein H, Thomas K, Wallace HM. The early periodic screening, detection, and treatment program: status of progress and implementation in 51 states and territories. *J Sch Health.* 1979;49:454–457.

43. Nader PR, ed. *Options for School Health.* Germantown, Md: Aspen Systems Corp; 1978.

44. The Robert Wood Johnson Foundation. Program summary: school health services program [mimeographed].

45. Jenny J. Alternatives mode for improving dental health status. *Dent Hygiene.* 1977;51:507.

46. McAnarney E, Nader PR, Coleman RF, Goldstein S, Friedman SB. The pediatrician in an innovative public school health program. *Clin Pediatr.* 1971;10(2):86–90.

47. Nader PR, Friedman SB. Community schools and pediatrics: philosophy of a collaborative approach to school health. *Clin Pediatr.* 1971;10(2):90–93.
48. Novak S, Rokowitz R, Zastowry T, Stebbins W, Burns C. In-school residence training for management of school problems. *New York J Med.* 1978;78:1109–1110.
49. Rogers C. Innovative school nursing in Harlem: a custom-made program. *Am J Nurs.* 1977;77:1464–1471.
50. *Jersey City Health Center* [brochure] and phone conversation with the director of the Jersey City Health Center, January 4, 1979.
51. Lynch A. There is no health in school health. *J Sch Health.* 1977;47:410–413.
52. Eddy R. Changing trends in school health services. *Thrust for Ed Leadersh.* 1977;2(4):17.
53. Lampe JM. A new approach to the delivery of health care to school children as instituted by the Denver, Colorado, public schools. *J Sch Health.* 1972;42:272–275.
54. Silversin J, Coombs JA, Drolette ME. Achievements of the seventies: self-applied fluorides. *J Public Health Dent.* 1980;40(3).

CHAPTER 3

The Public School and Social Services

Reassessing the Progressive Legacy

Michael W. Sedlak, Steven Schlossman, 1985

To those of us in our mid-thirties, the public schools have been a target of savage criticism from virtually the day we entered the elementary grades in the early 1950s. From Arthur Bestor to Jonathan Kozol to David Gardner and the National Commission on Excellence in Education, the schools, as Diane Ravitch has recently shown, have almost perpetually been on the defensive.[1-4]

Recent critics of the public schools generally make two assumptions that seem questionable to us: first, that the school is a highly permeable institution that changes often and easily in response to shifting demands made upon it; and, second, that the school has genuinely incorporated the diverse social service and curricular innovations championed since the Great Society era. The schools have been victimized long enough, the critics charge, by the ambitions and fuzzy-headedness of educators

The chapter originally appeared as Sedlak MW, Schlossman S. The public school and social services: reassessing the progressive legacy. *Educ Theory*. 1985;35(4):371–383. Copyright © 1985. Reprinted with permission from the Board of Trustees of the University of Illinois at Urbana-Champaign and by the editor of *Education Theory*.

who envision the school as repository for an endless stream of services justified in the name of "child welfare" or "community uplift." Since the Great Society era, they allege, the schools' intellectual mission has been diluted by the incorporation of numerous ill-conceived social service and curricular innovations that sap limited economic resources and do little to enhance students' academic achievement. Dispense with the curricular fluff and extraneous services that schools recently had foisted on them, the critics suggest, and public education will again be capable— both intellectually and financially—of returning America to international educational preeminence.

No doubt, as the critics aver, school routines during the past two decades were often disrupted by the plethora of government and court-initiated efforts to require new social service and curricular additions. Nonetheless, two basic points regarding these innovations deserve consideration. First, contrary to what is often implied, the Great Society reforms generally did not represent a major break with, or an alien, radical addition to, past educational thought. The reforms built conspicuously on the American "progressive" educational tradition which, from the early twentieth century onward, has challenged schools to educate the "whole child" and to provide lower-class minority students with health, welfare, and counseling services to speed their integration into the majority culture. Second, however momentarily or cumulatively disruptive the Great Society initiatives were to established school routines, very few of them actually found a secure place in public schooling. Far more successfully than one might surmise from the antagonistic rhetoric, the schools largely fended off these "friendly intruders," accepting them only intermittently or when they could be subsidized by outside funds. In sum, if there are serious deficiencies in our schools today, the blame would appear, in our judgment, to lie elsewhere, largely with the fragmentation and dilution of content knowledge within the academic program.[5–8]

These observations on the recent past raise an intriguing historical question about an earlier, equally famous period of educational reform in the early-twentieth-century Progressive Era: Why have recent efforts to expand the social service functions of schools stirred so much controversy yet received so little permanent acceptance, whereas, according to conventional historical wisdom, Progressive efforts to expand the schools' social service mission were so remarkably successful?

In the remainder of this essay, we review the origins and results of select early-twentieth-century efforts to transform public schools into multipurpose social service institutions. We argue that the "progressive" influence was a good deal less pervasive than we have been accustomed to believe, whether with regard to the organization of classroom instruction, as Larry Cuban has recently suggested, or with regard to the addition of social services and nonacademic coursework.[9–11] Most of the "progressive" agenda died aborning, was most imperfectly realized, or has only recently shown signs of coming to fruition. *While the schools have been willing to "house" the social services, they have effectively resisted "adopting" them.* As long as some external source of financial support could be found, schools provided space and time for the services. When such assistance evaporated, so did the services; or, at best, their scope was severely restricted, and their missions were dramatically narrowed. From our perspective, the failure of recent reform efforts was basically continuous with the long-term historical pattern. The social services' ties to the schools remain fragile, at best; their claims to recognition have been effectively subordinated to the prerogatives of the regular academic constituencies.

We examine first what happened to some (though, obviously, not all) of the best-known social service and nonacademic curricular innovations that the early-twentieth-century "progressives" sought to incorporate into the public schools. Having challenged the traditional view of their impact, we outline our own position regarding the abiding significance of the "progressive" legacy.[12]

THE PROGRESSIVE VISION AND MODERN REALITIES

The principal concern of the "progressives" were the first- and second-generation immigrant, working-class children who entered the schools in unprecedented numbers during the early twentieth century. The overriding rationale for virtually all "progressive" innovations was to attract such children to school and hold them as long as possible. "Progressives" introduced free school lunches, for example, to achieve this goal. Hungry or malnourished children made poor scholars, were susceptible to disease, and consequently were likely to be absent from school, the "progressives" claimed. "The brain cannot gnaw on problems while the stomach is gnawing on its empty self," observed one proponent. By World War I, public schools in approximately one hundred cities were serving meals to needy children.[13(p304)]

While the statistics were superficially impressive, most school systems had in fact done nothing to feed poor children, and those that had were far from accepting it as a legitimate function. Nearly everywhere school lunches were introduced only because volunteer and charity organizations—notably women's groups—subsidized or paid entirely for the venture. While school meals appear to have been well received by the children's parents, opposition to them was widespread, especially to the concept of public subsidy. School lunches, critics charged, represented an opening wedge to socialism in local government. Lunches were not firmly rooted in schools until federal legislation institutionalized such programs in 1946, and it was another three decades before economic eligibility standards were introduced during the 1970s to target the public subsidy toward needy children. In short, this key "progressive" innovation has been accepted by local school districts only to the extent it has been funded externally—by voluntary organizations during the Progressive era and by the federal government following World War II.[10,13,14]

Like the school lunch, the "vacation school" was introduced by women's organizations in order to expand the school's holding power and influence over poor immigrant youth. While the rationale was obviously in part to keep children who were out of school out of mischief, their sponsors emphatically stressed broader pedagogic aims. Vacation schools were not merely to be summer extensions of the regular school year but, rather, to serve as "pedagogic experiment stations" which would eventually "exert a positive influence upon regular school methods." "The idea of taking care of the children and keeping them off the streets in the hot summer is, to be sure, a philanthropic one, but is not the primary object of the vacation school," cautioned one advocate.[13(pp221–222)]

In their earliest years, particularly before 1910 when they were wholly subsidized by private organizations, vacation schools did indeed function as educational experiments. To encourage "learning by doing," field trips were common, as were expressive activities via story-telling and play-acting and the cultivation of physical dexterity via manual training. The schools were enormously popular among immigrant children and parents: an appealing alternative to the more rigid regular school curriculum.

In actuality, however, few eligible youth participated in vacation schools. While private initiative did stimulate municipal authorities to sponsor vacation schools, space remained limited, and parents in slum neighborhoods were forced to fight bitterly to gain entry for their children. Moreover, once government began to subsidize the venture, the vacation schools underwent a radical change of purpose. The original conception of a pedagogic experiment station gradually gave way to the modern notion of "summer school," where children from all socioeconomic backgrounds attend regular academic classes in order to repeat failed subjects or to pursue advanced study.[13] To be sure, the original vacation school idea was not without influence on the regular curriculum: field trips, museum visits, manual exercises, and plays were occasionally incorporated into the regular program. But, as John Goodlad has made clear, they remain in an incidental and subservient role to conventional methods of classroom instruction.

Vacation schools were only part of a larger "progressive" vision for dramatically extending the role of public schools by transforming them into "social centers." In the infelicitous but popular phrase of the day, the object was to make "wider use of the school plant."[15] Children and adults were to use the school building during late afternoons and evenings to pursue various noninstructional activities: for example, holding meetings of parent and community organizations, informally using gym and music facilities, and leisurely reading books and newspapers. The social center movement represented a bold response to the charge that schools had become too professionalized and bureaucratized, too distant from neighborhood adults whose children attended them. The public school, advocates maintained, could build community spirit and a sense of common purpose in even the poorest neighborhoods, but only if parents felt that the school belonged to them.

Because the social center idea meant different things in different communities, it is hard to determine precisely how the idea was implemented. What does seem clear, however, is that except for brief periods in only a handful of cities, the notion of easy access to the schools by adult civic groups to promote their individual goals was short-circuited by school boards who feared subsidizing the activities of radical political groups. It was one thing to make way for the Ladies' Literacy Club or the PTA and quite another to invite the local Socialist Club or labor union. The fear that the school would be used for political and, later, for religious purposes narrowed the initial goals of the social center movement: from an informal "people's club" to which diverse community groups had easy and equal access to a place for organizing recreational activities for youth and formal educational extension programs for adults.[13,16,17] While there is precious little information currently available on how public schools are used after regular classes end, it is clear that the goals of transforming ghetto schools into vital social centers and agents of neighborhood uplift, and of persuading parents that the schools belong to them, remain as elusive and disputed today as during the early twentieth century.

If the lunch, vacation school, and social center campaigns never gained substantial local support, what of other innovations that sought to provide more direct services to children via the school? Were these more widely implemented—in a form recognizable to their designers? Did they bloat local school budgets and responsibilities to the point where they detracted significantly from the central academic program?

No metaphor was more pervasive in the campaign to integrate social services into the schools than that of "prevention." The "progressives" believed that school-based programs could forestall the onset of all varieties of unwanted behavior and conditions among children and youth. The three most publicized efforts along these lines lay in the use of schools to avoid vocational maladjustment, to prevent juvenile delinquency, and to prevent illness and correct physical defects among the school-age population.

"Progressive" educators unanimously endorsed the introduction of vocational guidance counseling, which they considered one of the most scientifically grounded school social services. It would be hard to overstate their aspirations and expectations for guidance counseling as an essential educational responsibility. Through a variety of recently developed psychological tests that assessed students' aptitudes, interests, and basic character, counselors were to help adolescents choose their career paths as early as possible (certainly by the beginning of high school). With such guidance, students could efficiently utilize available school resources to realize their appropriate vocational destinies. Uncertainty about ultimate life goals, the guidance advocates believed, was utterly unnecessary: it led to student unhappiness and wasted precious manpower resources. "The training of a racehorse, and the care of sheep and chickens have been carried to the highest degree of perfection that intelligent planning can attain," observed Frank Parsons, the movement's leading spokesman. "But the education of a child, the choice of his employment, are left very largely to the current haphazard plan—the struggle for existence, and the survival of the fittest."[18(p18)] Vocational guidance would eliminate this personal and societal inefficiency, he promised, and focus the school on preparing children from all socioeconomic backgrounds for appropriate adult roles.

Most high schools and many junior high schools did, in fact, introduce vocational guidance in the early 1900s, especially when voluntary organizations were willing to train teachers to advise students and provide speakers on local employment trends and opportunities. Despite such efforts, however, counseling's leading advocates were dissatisfied with their field. Much of the problem lay with the rudimentary scientific tools in which the counselor placed so much faith: they were hardly sophisticated enough to assess basic personality traits, nor was it clear that the traits assessed were relevant to specific course offerings or to occupational success or failure. Moreover, guidance counselors were never able to gain the trust of students, parents, teachers, or prospective employers as brokers of future occupational choice. Before World War II they had, by and large, given up the pretense of preparing students for vocations and limited their role to, first, advising academically talented students about essential college preparatory courses and, second, insuring that less academically inclined students graduated with a diploma of some kind. Beginning in the 1940s they became increasingly more concerned with students' emotional than vocational development and often mediated between teachers and troublesome students. The roles that guidance counselors have played in keeping schools functioning should of course not be minimized, but it is clear that their functions were much narrower than the "progressives" had envisioned and that they never exerted more than a marginal influence in shaping student career choices.[16,19]

In a sense, virtually every social service and curricular innovation that the "progressives" sponsored was conceived as a means to prevent delinquency. To increase the school's holding power by making education more attractive and meaningful was, perforce, to eliminate the mainsprings of juvenile misbehavior. Thus, they often justified vocational education, vocational guidance, and special classes for emotionally and physically handicapped children as tools for delinquency prevention. But during the 1910s and 1920s, many went well beyond these generalized approaches to delinquency prevention and developed both a more elaborate rationale and specific instruments for early intervention into the lives of potentially troublesome youth.

"Progressives" challenged the public schools to assume primary diagnostic and treatment responsibilities for dependent, neglected, and delinquent children. Despite the best of intentions, many educational reformers argued, juvenile courts inevitably stigmatized youngsters, many of whom had committed only petty legal infractions or had been dragged into court by angry parents. To serve these children, argued Thomas Eliot, the prominent educational sociologist, the tasks of schools had to be reconceived to include "all special efforts to educate or re-educate the unusual or maladjusted—from the superior to the imbecile, from the too docile to the neurotic or delinquent."[20(p601)] Eliot and his fellow "progressives" were confident that such a comprehensive vision could be attained with the addition of a new cadre of specialists to the schools, including psychologists, psychiatrists, counselors, special education teachers, and especially social workers. These specialties claimed to possess the scientific expertise to diagnose the underlying causes of misbehavior, to instruct teachers on how to cope with "acting-out" children in the classroom, and to bring troublesome youth gradually into conformity with the social expectations and educational goals of the school.[21]

What became of the "progressives'" agenda for using the schools to prevent delinquency? In a word, little. None of the specialized professionals or programs to prevent delinquency ever came close to realizing promoters' aims. To the extent they survive, their purposes have been severely narrowed or modified over the past half century.

Consider, for example, the school social worker, who was known in the early twentieth century as the visiting teacher. Pioneered by the settlement houses in New York and Boston, the position of visiting teacher gradually gained public sponsorship during the 1910s as a score of large cities added social workers to their schools. The movement was boosted dramatically during the 1920s when the Commonwealth Fund subsidized a corps of highly trained visiting teachers in thirty communities to demonstrate their potential contribution to delinquency prevention. Trained to apply the latest techniques of social casework (which during the 1920s began to take on a psychiatric cast) to children experiencing difficulties in school that might *portend* delinquency, she endeavored "to look for what is wrong with the child *socially*."[22(p168)] That is, she sought to identify problems in the child's social relations at home, in the community, or in the classroom and school that explained his behavior pattern and to eliminate those problems via active intervention with the child, his parents and teachers, or anyone else who could conceivably help.

Working with problem children, however, was only part of the visiting teacher's role. Even more important in the "progressives'" view was her mission to "socialize" the regular school staff, that is, to sensitize teachers to the varied causes of children's "maladjustment" and to serve as the children's advocate with teachers and other public authorities. Ultimately the visiting teacher was to infuse all adult-child encounters with the social worker's perspective on child development.[23,23]

Despite foundation leadership, few cities ever deployed school social workers in sufficient numbers to begin to meet the problems they were assigned. Moreover, their roles were sharply constrained. Rather than doing therapeutic interventions with children and parents in their homes and communities and educating teachers on how to incorporate casework principles into the classroom setting, most visiting teachers were more or less indistinguishable from the school attendance force in focusing their energies on rounding up truants and persuading them to return to school. Following World War II, school social workers turned their attention from their original urban, lower-class clientele to middle-class and suburban youth with emotional problems that seemed more amenable to their psychiatric casework skills—a more responsive, comfortable clientele in many respects. Although some school social workers briefly revived an advocacy role on behalf of lower-class students when federal monies were available to support such activities in the 1960s, their role in recent years has again been circumscribed. Today many school social workers are frustrated administrators of externally funded programs who often have to refer students to private organizations that provide primary therapeutic care through purchase-of-service contracts.[10,25]

The notion that schools should absorb the juvenile court's responsibilities, although bandied about in educational circles, never really got off the ground, in part due to the strenuous objections of probation officers who would be thrown out of jobs, but even more because it became clear by the late 1930s that diagnosing and treating delinquency—whether by educators, social workers, counselors, or psychiatrists—was trickier than had initially been assumed. While educators and noneducators alike continue to observe that the school is ideally situated to play a major role in societal efforts to stem the growth of crime, the fact is that the "progressive" vision has been largely supplanted by a diametrically opposite portrait. The tendency today is to view the basic organization of public education as contributing directly to the production of juvenile delinquents and to portray the school more as a superb site for juveniles to practice crime than as a locale for its prevention. Thomas Eliot and his "progressive" colleagues are surely turning over in their graves.[26–28]

The prevention motif in "progressive" educational circles was most fully elaborated in the "school health" or "educational hygiene" movement. The movement began in the late nineteenth century in two loosely connected efforts to check contagious diseases and improve school architecture and construction. Led mainly by public health officials, these efforts brought doctors into the schools to inspect for contagious diseases, quarantine carriers, and provide vaccinations and prescribe new standards of ventilation, lighting, and sanitation in new school buildings. What most interests us is the next stage of the school health movement, that which began around 1910 and was led mainly by educators.[13,29,30] To portray its thrust quickly, we need only examine the work of Lewis Terman, the psychologist, who, before he became world famous for the IQ test, was coauthor of the leading text on educational hygiene used in teacher-training institutions.

Educators, Terman argued, must vastly extend the role of medical personnel in the schools to diagnose and treat physical defects and all "incipient deviations from the normal" that undermined children's health and ability to function optimally in school. "We are coming to believe," he argued in classically expansive "progressive" terms, "that it is legitimate to levy upon the school for any contribution it is capable of making to human welfare. . . . The school . . . must be made to preserve the child from all kinds of morbidity, repair his existent deformities, combat his unfavorable heredity and the bad conditions of his environment; in a word, fortify his constitution and render him physically and mentally fit for the struggle of life.[31(pp10–11)]

To fulfill their preventive mission, Terman urged that school health departments must also reach into students' homes to determine why physical defects and illness were so prevalent and educate parents in optimal health care practices. The school "must know more of the child's habits, what time he goes to bed, how long he sleeps, how much he works, how much he studies at home, what he eats, what he drinks, where and under what conditions he sleeps, and what the house environment is in every particular that concerns the child's health."[32(p10)] In a good statement of the overall "progressive" agenda for introducing social services into the schools, Terman concluded: "The public school has not fulfilled its duty when the child alone is educated within its walls. The school must be the educational center, the social center, and the hygiene center of the community in which it is located—a hub from which will radiate influences for social betterment in many lives."[32(p11)]

Terman proposed two major institutional innovations to fulfill this "progressive" vision: the school nurse and the school clinic. The term school nurse was misleading, for her principal responsibilities—even more than the visiting teacher's—extended into students' homes. Without the school nurse, Terman argued, doctors' examinations of children were ineffective, because there was no mechanism for follow-up. Children removed from school because of scabies, impetigo, pediculosis, and other relatively minor, treatable diseases often remained absent for extended periods without ever receiving treatment and in the process, of course, infected their fellow students after school hours. The school nurse broke this cycle of neglect.

Terman went further in lauding the influence of school nurses, especially among "the more ignorant foreign-born population." She became, he emphasized, "first and last a social worker. . . . She instructs ignorant but fond mothers in the best methods of feeding, clothing, and caring for their children. . . . In many a family she becomes a spiritual adviser, not only pointing out inadequate sanitation which keeps them sick, but also educating them on the folly of cut-throat chattel mortgages, unnecessary furniture purchased at ruinous prices on the installment, the short-sighted policy of taking children prematurely out of school to work, etc."[32(pp54–55)] As this typically expansive description suggests, the "progressives" conceived the school nurse as something of an all-purpose health, social, and moral advisor to immigrant parents whose children showed up in school with untreated illnesses, ailments, or physical defects.

To Terman and other "progressive" educators, the nurse was only a first step in transforming the school into a potent agency for conserving and upgrading children's health. The second essential step was the introduction of school medical clinics, which had already demonstrated in England and elsewhere that dramatic improvements could be effected in children's health and school attendance with only a minimal financial investment. The principal objections came from doctors who charged the "progressive" educators with advocating a form of socialism in the schools. Terman had no patience with this complaint. "Disease is to be conceived as an evil to be eradicated, not as a resource to be conserved for the benefit of any profession," he asserted. "The policy of free medical and dental clinics supported by public taxation differs in no respect from the universally accepted principles of public education. . . . there is nothing more radical in the principle of free medical and dental treatment than in the American scheme of public education and free textbooks."[32(pp118–120)]

What happened to the "progressive" vision of the school nurse and the school clinic? Briefly, while the school nurse did early become an integral part of most urban schools, the range of her duties was narrowly circumscribed, and she became, in essence, exactly what the name "school nurse" implied—a semiprofessional who confined her supervision of children's health to school grounds, exercised minimal discretion in diagnosing or treating children's minor ills, and had little systematic contact with children's homes in order to perform a larger educational mission in preventive medicine. In no sense did she serve as a health social worker, nor did she become, as Terman assumed she naturally would, a major educational force in increasing teachers' awareness of children's health needs. To be sure, the school nurse has been a key addition to school staff and became important especially in containing panic when emergencies occur, but the "progressive" vision of her role in preventive medicine never came close to being realized.

The school clinic was largely an abortive reform idea, especially after World War I when the AMA successfully launched an aggressive campaign to ostracize all doctors whose activities might threaten the sanctity of fee-for-service medicine, whether via school clinics, health maintenance organizations, or other alternatives to the conventional family physician.[33,34] For the school clinic idea was substituted the private doctor's note attesting that the child had been properly vaccinated and was in sufficiently good health to attend school. Though there have been a number of recent creative efforts to revitalize the school clinic—notably a series of demonstration experiments funded by the Robert Wood Johnson Foundation[35,36]—the prospects for reorganizing the delivery of medical services to children via the schools seem slight indeed.[37–43]

If the schools never became major dispensers of health services, what of the various health-related curricular innovations that the "progressive" educators championed, notably in general health instruction, sex education, and safety education? Regarding health instruction, the field experienced something of a heyday in the 1920s, following the publication of the famous *Cardinal Principles* report, which listed health first and foremost as *the* object of public education. This decade saw significant cooperation between physicians and educators in developing new health curricula, under the leadership of Thomas Dennison Wood of Columbia's Teachers College and Phillip Van Ingen of the American Child Health Association. Prior health instruction in the schools had a bad reputation, they believed, because it was confined to conveying arid information on the human body and moralistic principles of health maintenance, particularly regarding the consumption of alcohol, drugs, or other stimulants. By contrast, they proposed wholly new curricula which stressed not abstract principles but concrete health habits for children to learn via stories, rhymes, songs, and plays featuring such characters as Cho Cho the Health Clown and the Health Fairy.[44,45]

Enthusiasm surrounding these innovations in the interwar years was great, but it is not certain how widely they were implemented. What does seem clear is that the emphasis on cultivating "health habits" was not as pedagogically effective in altering children's health behavior as its originators had hoped, nor did the use of such characters as Cho Cho the Health Clown do much to enhance the reputation of health instruction as a legitimate part of the curriculum. Moreover, the increasing tendency in the upper grades to assign health instruction to gym instructors, who often lacked training in or professional commitment to the field, further undermined the status and practice of health education. Whether the major efforts made by health education professionals during the past decade to revitalize their field will succeed in winning over students and teachers, remains to be seen.[46–54] What is clear is that the "progressive" goal of having, in Lewis Terman's words, "health motives and practices . . . permeate the whole school life and work" never came to pass.[44(p201)]

"Progressive" educators were unanimous in insisting that schools teach students at all grade levels proper ideas and attitudes toward sex, whether as a separate subject, part of general health education, or integrated into some other course such as biology. The changing cultural context made such instruction essential, for in the early twentieth century as never before, sex had become an accepted part of public discussion. "A wave of hysteria seems to have invaded the country," wrote one commentator. "Our former reticence on matters of sex is giving way to a frankness that would even startle Paris."[55] What the "progressives" hoped to do was to counteract the sexual titillation purveyed in the media by developing new curricula that would innocently convey up-to-date scientific knowledge on sex to children while, at the same time, imbuing sex with older spiritual meanings.[56,57]

For obvious reasons, the "progressives" did not propose dramatizations or imaginary characters—no Cho Cho the Sex Clown—because there was no need to stimulate students' interest in the subject. In fact, about the only open sexual discussion most educators would tolerate involved the mating of plants. Thus, from the first the "progressives" were in a bind on sex education; they could not figure out how to apply their famous "learning by doing" principle to this subject. The schools did their best for several decades to avoid the subject entirely or so to merge it into general discussions of procreation in the plant and animal worlds that the distinctly human aspects of sexual activity and emotion escaped attention. Only in the past decade—in large part to help students deal with the sexual revolution of our own time and with the growing incidence of teenage pregnancy—have educators seriously attempted to realize the "progressive" vision of making the schools major forces in shaping students' sexual attitudes and behavior. What remains to be seen is whether these recent innovations will have any demonstrable impact, whether sex education can survive a "back-to-basics" educational philosophy, and whether parents and school boards will implement widely or tolerate very long the realistic approaches to sex education that are now widely available for instructional purposes.[10,58]

The notion of safety education derived initially from efforts by labor and industry to curtail industrial accidents and to create workmen's compensation legislation in the 1910s. Educators took up the call around World War I. The essential rationale derived from three main sources: first, the fact that potentially dangerous electrical and mechanical devices were becoming more and more part of everyday life; second, the development of reasonably accurate statistics on accident fatalities, which highlighted the prominence of automobile accidents and accidents in the home as the principal safety hazards; and, third, the belief that safety education formed an essential part of a more general "increased respect for human life . . . of every humble man and woman and child" in the Progressive era, as evidenced by the advent of tenement house legislation, preventive medicine, well-baby clinics, and the like.[59(p3)]

The "progressives" made a good case for safety education—good enough to get the NSSE to commit a four-hundred-page yearbook to it in 1926—but the question remained as to what to teach and how to teach the subject. Like the health educators, safety education advocates created lengthy lists of do's and don'ts regarding safety habits for children to learn via dramatic presentations; the Safety Fairy joined the Health Fairy in appealing to children's imaginations. Except for introducing regular fire drills and junior safety patrols, however, most school systems appear not to have paid the "progressive" educators much heed. Not until after World War II did safety education truly catch on in the schools, and it did so in a more narrow and didactic way than its advocates had anticipated. Rather than teaching about general and specific dangers in the home, community, and workplace, safety education came to focus almost entirely on after-school instruction in driver education. And a primary reason the schools latched onto this phase of safety education was that it took up no space in the curriculum, catered mainly to upper-income students and schools, and was funded almost entirely by external sources.[10,60] Whether present-day concern about chemical and nuclear health hazards will revitalize and update the broader vision of safety education that the "progressives" had in mind remains to be seen.

PHYSICAL EDUCATION AND COMPETITIVE SPORTS: THE NOTABLE EXCEPTION

As we have tried to make clear, the "progressive" vision of the school as an all-purpose social service institution did not come close to being implemented. Several of the proposed innovations were largely abortive, while those that were institutionalized either had much narrower ends and means than the "progressives" envisioned or survived only because external funding subsidized the venture. Any notion that local public schools have willingly embraced a wide variety of nonacademic social service and curricular innovations seems unwarranted.

Except in one area, that is. The one undisputed triumph of the "progressive" agenda for enlarging the social service functions of the school lay in making organized recreation and team-based, competitive athletics curricular staples. Prior to the twentieth century, the schools did not consider it their responsibility to organize or provide a site for children or adolescents to play. Play was a home responsibility, supplemented to a certain extent by the offerings of the YMCA and public parks. But in the late nineteenth century a radically different notion of the importance of play in young children's social and intellectual growth emerged among educational psychologists. This was soon followed by a well-orchestrated campaign to introduce elaborate athletic competitions into the schools, on the grounds that they taught adolescents ethical values such as obedience to rules, group loyalty, and the virtues of collective effort that were essential for citizenship in an increasingly urban and interdependent world.

Led by such formidable advocates as Luther Gulick and Joseph Lee, and boosted enormously by revelations from the World War I draft that Americans were surprisingly unfit physically, the so-called "play movement" met with remarkable success in the early part of the century. One school system after another felt obliged to build playgrounds and gyms, teach physical education, and sponsor organized, competitive athletic teams.[61,62]

Today physical education and school sports remain so central to the organization of public schools that it is difficult to appreciate what a revolution their introduction marked in the development of the nonacademic curriculum. To be sure, the "progressives" would not wholly approve of the current organization of school-based recreational activities. They would decry the highly competitive nature of interschool athletic contests, the disproportionate funding which subsidizes these activities as opposed to increasing mass student participation in organized, intraschool athletic events, and the relative inattention paid to introducing students to lifelong recreational activities. Nonetheless, the legitimization of physical education and school sports as integral components of modern public education contrasts sharply with many other innovations that "progressives" sought but failed to introduce into the public schools.

THE PROGRESSIVE LEGACY

From this brief overview, it is clear that we, like Larry Cuban and John Goodlad, are impressed with the historical continuity of schooling since the early twentieth century and caution against overemphasizing how much schools have changed in response to the pleas of educational reformers. We believe that historians (including the "revisionists") have overstated the "progressives'" influence, primarily because they have paid closer attention to rhetoric than to implementation and because they have implicitly exaggerated the permeability of the school as an organization.

Nonetheless, we are not arguing that the gym is the only lasting monument to the "progressive" dream of transforming the school into a multiservice institution. The "progressive" vision has, in our judgment, exerted a long-term, if largely indirect influence in gaining a hearing for three noble ideals in American education—ideals that, our judgment, too often get slighted when the case for public schooling is argued solely on the grounds of a "back-to-basics" philosophy. These "progressive" ideals can be simply stated and linked to the innovations whose history we have reviewed.

First is the principle that the school ought to transcend its institutional boundaries and become an instrument of local community service, identity, and pride. In promoting vacation schools, the use of schools as social centers, and competitive athletics, the "progressives" provided a special vision of the schools' role in a democratic society that had no counterpart elsewhere in the world. In our judgment, this vision still holds potential—although largely unrealized, except for the boosters of school sports—for revitalizing a sense of place and purpose in what Daniel Boorstin has termed our modern-day, faceless, "anywhere communities"[63] and for enhancing what Goodlad has called each community's "sense of ownership" over its schools.[7(p276)]

Second is the principle that American public schools are obligated to individualize needs assessment, instruction, and services, especially for students who are disruptive or who simply do not fit conveniently into the mainstream curriculum. In advocating new roles for school social workers, teachers of children with diverse handicaps, and guidance counselors, the "progressives" sought to give meaning to the educational experiences of children who had previously been ignored or kicked out of school. By proclaiming the school's responsibility to deal with "misfit" children, the "progressives," we believe, fundamentally humanized the mission of public education and transcended the "shape up or ship out" philosophy that had traditionally guided school promotion and exclusion policies.

Third and finally, there is the principle that to be effective, schools must strive to teach the "whole child"; that they dare not ignore a student's physical, social, emotional, or moral development under the pretext of being solely responsible for cultivating his mind. The advocates of school-based social service and nonacademic curricular offerings have eloquently articulated this principle for the past eighty years, whether in the cause of the school lunch, the school nurse and school clinic, the school social worker, or the gym teacher. To abandon this principle as a guide to what services schools can or ought to provide their students would, in our judgment, represent a reversion to nineteenth-century faculty psychology and a retrogression in interpreting the role of public education in shaping the lives and opportunities of most children in a democratic society.

When all is said and done, then, we believe that while the "progressives" did much less to transform the schools than has long been assumed, they introduced several vital principles of twentieth-century educational thought that remain as bold today as eighty years ago. From the "progressive" standpoint, the problem may not be that the schools have aspired to do too much, but that they have done too little.[64]

Notes

1. Bestor A. *Educational Wastelands.* Urbana, Ill: University of Illinois Press; 1953.
2. Kozol J. *Death at an Early Age.* Boston, Mass: Houghton Mifflin; 1967.
3. National Commission on Excellence in Education; Gardner DP, chair. *A Nation at Risk.* Washington, DC: US Department of Education; 1983.
4. Ravitch D. *The Troubled Crusade.* New York, NY: Basic Books; 1983.
5. Sizer T. *Horace's Compromise.* Boston, Mass: Houghton Mifflin; 1984.
6. Cusick P. *The Egalitarian Ideal and the American High School.* White Plains, NY: Longman; 1983.
7. Goodlad J. *A Place Called School.* New York, NY: McGraw-Hill; 1984.
8. Boyer E. *High School.* New York, NY: Harper & Row; 1983.
9. Cuban L. *How Teachers Taught.* White Plains, NY: Longman; 1984.
10. Sedlak MW, Church R. *A History of Social Services Delivered to Youth, 1880–1977.* Washington, DC: National Institute of Education; 1982.
11. While we believe, from an implementation perspective, that the "progressive" influence has been overstated, we are certainly not arguing that early-twentieth-century educational reformers had no impact on the structure and scope of modern schooling. Historians have captured in vivid detail the important shifts in governance that occurred during the Progressive era, particularly the emergence of centralized control vested in the hands of professionally trained administrators. Similarly, the redefinition of equality of educational opportunity shared by many "progressives" dramatically altered the composition of the student population, particularly at the secondary level. Nonetheless, it is essential to recognize that many of the proposed "progressive" reforms were not implemented widely, or expeditiously, or even in a form that their earliest advocates would have recognized or approved.

12. We exclude two basic categories of activities from the social services and nonacademic coursework we examine in this essay: vocational training and the nonathletic extracurriculum. We regard vocational education as a direct alternative to the basic academic track and therefore as fundamentally different from other specific social services and curricular additions. We acknowledge that for some children in some communities vocational classes probably functioned in a manner akin to a "social service." Nationally, however, they constituted a distinct educational track. While we consider the secondary historical literature inadequate to reconstruct the precise evolution of programs, scattered data suggest that after the initiation of vocational classes in the late nineteenth and early twentieth centuries, both their internal development and their expansion and contraction vis-à-vis the academic curriculum were shaped largely by external funding priorities (particularly the categorical and definitional shifts encouraged and enforced by the Smith-Hughes Act). This pattern of development confirms our general argument about the key role played by outside sponsors in sustaining nonacademic curricula.

Although we examine physical education and competitive sports, we exclude from systematic consideration such extracurricular activities as school assemblies, student government, and special-interest clubs. Our impression, however, is that the actual operation of the entire extracurricular movement confirms rather than contradicts our central arguments. Many extracurricular activities, including athletic, government, musical, theater, and journalistic programs, had consequences diametrically opposed to those endorsed by their "progressive" proponents. Extracurricular activities that reformers supported to build social solidarity, a shared vision of common interests, and a spirit of selfless cooperation appear to have been used by adolescents primarily to reinforce existing social and economic inequalities and to differentiate and distinguish themselves from the larger student body. Competition rather than cooperation was at the heart of the extracurricular movement as it actually operated in schools. This outcome contrasted sharply with the "progressive" vision.

13. Reese W. *Case Studies of Social Services in the Schools of Selected Cities.* Washington, DC: National Institute of Education; 1981.

14. Steiner G. *The Children's Cause.* Washington, DC: Brookings Institution; 1976.

15. Perry C. *Wider Use of the School Plant.* New York, NY: Charities Publication Committee; 1910.

16. Spring J. *Education and the Rise of the Corporate State.* Boston, Mass: Beacon Press; 1972.

17. Stevens E. Social centers, politics, and social efficiency in the Progressive Era. *Hist Educ Q.* 1972;12:16–33.
18. Rudy W. *Schools in an Age of Mass Culture.* Englewood Cliffs, NJ: Prentice Hall; 1965.
19. Stephens WR. *Social Reform and the Origins of Vocational Guidance.* Washington, DC: National Vocational Guidance Association; 1970.
20. Eliot T. Should courts do case work? *Survey.* 1928;60:601.
21. Schlossman S. End of innocence: science and the transformation of progressive juvenile justice, 1899–1917. *Hist Ed.*1978;7:207–218.
22. Richman J. A social need of the public school. *Forum.* 1910;43:168.
23. Cohen S. The mental hygiene movement, the Commonwealth Fund, and public education, 1921–1937. In: Benjamin G, ed. *Private Philanthropy and Public Elementary and Secondary Education.* North Tarrytown, NY: Rockefeller Archive Center; 1979:33–46.
24. Shea C. *The Ideology of Mental Health and the Emergence of the Therapeutic Liberal State: The American Mental Hygiene Movement, 1900–1930* [dissertation]. Urbana, Ill: University of Illinois; 1980.
25. Costin L. A historical review of school social work. *Soc Casework.* 1969;50:439–453.
26. Polk K. Schools and the delinquency experience. *Crim Just Behav.* 1975;2:315–337.
27. Toby J. Crime in the schools. In: Wilson J, ed. *Crime and Public Policy.* San Francisco, Calif: Institute for Contemporary Studies; 1983:69–88.
28. Sedlak MW. Schooling as a response to crime. In: Lewis D, ed. *Reactions to Crime.* Beverly Hills, Calif: Sage; 1981:205–226.
29. Lynch A. Evaluating school health programs. In: Levin A, ed. *Health Services.* New York, NY: Academy of Political Science; 1977:89–92.
30. Lindsay E. *Origins and Development of the School Health Movement in the United States* [dissertation]. Stanford, Calif: Stanford University; 1943.
31. Terman L, Almack J. *The Hygiene of the School Child.* Boston, Mass: Houghton Mifflin; 1929.
32. Hoag E, Terman L. *Health Work in the Schools.* Boston, Mass: Houghton Mifflin; 1914.
33. Starr P. *The Social Transformation of American Medicine.* New York, NY: Basic Books; 1982.
34. Duffy J. The American medical profession and public health: from support to ambivalence. *Bull Hist Med.* 1979;153:1–22.
35. The Robert Wood Johnson Foundation. *Selected National Initiatives to Improve Health Care: A Decade of Experience.* Princeton, NJ: The Robert Wood Johnson Foundation; 1982.

36. Cronin GE, Young WM. *400 Navels: The Future of School Health in America.* Bloomington, Ind: Phi Delta Kappa; 1979.

37. White E. Are you ready to provide the health services demanded of the public schools? *Am Sch Bd J.* 1981;168:25–28.

38. Newton J. Primary health care in a school setting. *J Sch Health.* 1979;49:54.

39. Newman IM. Integrating health services and health education: seeking a balance. *J Sch Health.* 1982;52:498–501.

40. Newman IM, Newman E, Martin GL. School health services: what costs? What benefits? *J Sch Health.* 1981;51:423–427.

41. Cowen EL, Lorion RP. Changing roles for the school mental health professional. *J Sch Psychol.* 1976;14:131–137.

42. Steinberg MA, Chandler GE. Developing coordination of services between a mental health center and a public school system. *J Sch Psychol.* 1976;14:355–361.

43. Ross DC, Meinster MO, Gingrich LJ. A program for expanding the mental health function of the school nurse. *J Sch Health.* 1978;48:157–159.

44. Means R. *A History of Health Education.* Philadelphia, Pa: Lea and Febiger; 1962.

45. Van Ingen P. *The Story of the American Child Health Association.* New York, NY: American Child Health Association; 1935.

46. Kolbe LJ. What can we expect from school health education? *J Sch Health.* 1982;52:145–150.

47. Stone D. School health education: some future challenges. *J Sch Health.* 1979;49:227–228.

48. Simonds S. Health education today: issues and challenges. *J Sch Health.* 1977;47:584–593.

49. Lynch A. There is no health in school health. *J Sch Health.* 1977; 46:410–413.

50. Kreuter M, Green L. Evaluation of school health education: identifying purpose, keeping perspective. *J Sch Health.* 1978;48:228–235.

51. Balog J. The concept of health and the role of health education. *J Sch Health.* 1981;51:461–464.

52. Thornburg E. Why the lack of health education programs in the middle school? *Contemp Educ.* 1981;52:160–162.

53. Du Shaw M, Hansen S. Current status of statewide health education programs in Michigan. *J Sch Health.* 1983;53:472–475.

54. Finn P. Alcohol education in the school curriculum: the single-discipline vs. the interdisciplinary approach. *J Alc/Drug Educ.* 1979;24:41–57.

55. Sex o'clock in America. *Curr Opin.* 1913;55:113.

56. Strong B. Ideas of the early sex education movement in America, 1890–1920. *Hist Educ Q.* 1972;12:129–161.

57. Schlossman S, Wallach S. The crime of precocious sexuality: female juvenile delinquency in the Progressive Era. *Harvard Educ Rev.* 1978;46:65–94.

58. Rienzo B. The status of sex education: an overview and recommendations. *Phi Delta Kappan.* 1981;63:192–193.

59. National Society for the Study of Education. *The Present Status of Safety Education* [25th yearbook]. Bloomington, Ill: Public School Publishing Co; 1926.

60. Cushman W, Meyerhoff R. Driver education update. *Today's Educ.* February–March 1979:74–78.

61. Cavallo D. *Muscles and Morals.* Philadelphia, Pa: University of Pennsylvania Press; 1981.

62. Knapp R, Hartsoe C. *Play for America.* Arlington, Va: National Recreation and Park Association; 1979.

63. Boorstin D. *The Americans: The Democratic Experience.* New York, NY: Random House; 1973.

64. Tyack D. The high school as a social service agency: historical perspectives on current policy issues. *Educ Eval Policy Anal.* 1975;1:45–57.

CHAPTER 4

An Evaluation of the Effectiveness of the Astoria Plan for Medical Service in Two New York City Elementary Schools

Alfred Yankauer, 1947

Selective Service rejection and "defect" statistics in the two World Wars have caused expressions of opinion to the effect that "the health level of the American people has not improved to the same degree as mortality in recent years."[1] It has also been stated that these findings reveal "many neglected physical and mental inadequacies which could and should have been prevented and corrected in childhood."[2] Such statements reflect upon the educational and medical supervision which the child receives in school, and raise the question as to how these services could be improved.

In New York City the elementary school health services operate on the basis of recommendations made by the Astoria Demonstration Study.[3] These recommendations, known as the Astoria plan, were

---

adopted in the fall of 1940. They center around continuity of record keeping and a yearly conference of teacher and nurse in which the health status of each pupil is reviewed. Children with questionable health problems or problems which cannot be handled directly by the teacher or nurse are referred to the school physician for examination. Routine health examinations by the school physician are performed only on children entering elementary school who have not been examined by an outside agency. Throughout the remainder of elementary school the child is examined by the school physician only if "selected" at a teacher-nurse conference.

Certain questions have arisen with respect to the operation of the Astoria plan in the light of Selective Service findings. Are there sick or handicapped children attending regular classes who have not received medical care or proper school placement simply because routine examinations have not been performed, and teacher or nurse is not sufficiently aware of disease symptoms or signs? If a careful initial examination is performed, can the system of teacher observation be trusted to bring to light children in need of care? What would be the value of additional routine examination by grade, with and without the presence of the parent at the examination?

Since the Astoria plan has operated for a period of six years, the health of children now in the sixth grade of New York schools should be some indication of the plan's effectiveness, provided a sufficiently large and representative sample were examined. Such an examination should also disclose snags in the operation of the plan itself and point the way toward an answer to some of the questions raised in the preceding paragraphs.

MATERIAL

Two elementary schools in the Kips Bay–Yorkville health district were selected for study. The 100-acre area from which these schools draw their pupils presents some significant features. On the one hand, the physical environment and conditions of life are poor, and the economic status of the population is approximately 25 per cent below that of the city-wide average.[4] On the other hand, a medical center, a health center, a settlement house, and a large dental clinic are located within the area, and two other large medical establishments are within short walking distance. Thus adequate free or low-cost health, medical, and dental services are easily accessible outside of the school. In addition, considerable mass health education has been carried on in this district, and it has served as a city-wide training center for school physicians.

There were 149 pupils in the sixth grade classes of these two schools, of whom 114 (58 boys and 56 girls) constitute the subjects of this study. All children were white, and the majority were of Czecho-slovakian, German, or Italian ethnic background. Ages ranged from 11 to 13, the majority falling 6 months on either side of the 12th birth-day. In 108 cases the mother was present at the interview, and in the remainder a responsible adult member of the family was present. Seventy-seven (68 per cent) of these children had been examined by the school physician on entry to elementary school. The remainder had been examined at that time by private physicians or hospital clin-ics, and the results incorporated into the school medical records.

Thirty-five of the 149 children in the two schools are not included in this survey. Of these, 23 were not given appointments because they had entered the school system after 1941, or because of parental inability or unwillingness to attend the examination, and 12 were given appointments which were broken. The school medical records and teacher judgments of these 35 children did not differ from those of the rest of the group, and it is not felt that their exclusion is of significance.

In New York City schools special classes exist for children with pro-nounced defective vision and with orthopedic handicaps or cardiac disabilities which prevent their attending regular classes. In addition, Health Improvement Classes are maintained for children to whom the unmodified school regime might be detrimental for a variety of med-ical reasons. Since the children examined were all attending regular classes, it is obvious that the group is a selected one, and it can be assumed that major physical disabilities have been eliminated from it.

METHOD

The parent was interviewed in the presence of the child, every effort being made to elicit a spontaneous anamnesis. Health problems and attitudes, the effects of previous medical contacts, the nature of fam-ily life in the home, and of parent-child relationships during the inter-view were particularly sought. Material contained in the school medical records was utilized for questioning. Elements of a routine pediatric history which remained uncovered after all leads had been followed were then reviewed directly. The interview was followed by a complete physical examination of the child, which included the eye-grounds. Approximately 40 minutes were devoted to the combined interview and examination.

Weights and heights, Snellen chart tests of visual acuity, and group 4-A audiometer tests for hearing loss were taken from teacher recordings on the school medical records. Sahli hemoglobin determinations were performed on each child, and urines were tested for abnormalities of the sediment and the presence of sugar and albumin.

Positive findings reflecting the physical and mental health of the child were recorded. In cases of suspected physical disease, referrals were made for further diagnostic assistance. Direct review of clinic records, interview with attending physician, or written reports from outside sources were utilized in arriving at diagnostic decisions. An estimate of whether a "defect" could have been noted prior to the current examination was made on the basis of existing records and direct questioning of the parent.

When an entire class had been examined, the teacher was consulted and asked to select children who seemed disturbed in personal and group relationships, and this information was incorporated into the findings.

It should be emphasized that the method used in obtaining data is considerably more exhaustive than the usual school health examination.

RESULTS

1. Physical Health

Results of medical appraisal expressed in terms of physical defects are tabulated in Table 4.1. It will be noted that the majority are minor in nature or receiving adequate medical care. Defective teeth and nutritional deficiencies were not individually evaluated because it was felt that they require methods more accurate than those employed in this survey. However, all children examined had received some form of dental care; no gross dental neglect was evident; unqualified signs of nutritional deficiency or undernutrition were not observed. Body posture was not evaluated because of its non-specificity. However, no organic postural defects were observed, and symptoms ascribable to "poor posture" were not manifest. Minor skin diseases (pediculosis, epidermophytosis, acne, etc.) are not included in the tabulation.

It is estimated that 18 (75 per cent) of the 24 defects unknown to the school could have been brought to school or parental attention

Table 4.1 Distribution of Physical Defects in 114 Sixth Grade School Children.

Physical Defect	Known to School		Unknown to School	
	Under Care	Not Under Care	Under Care	Not Under Care
Visual: 44 (57%)				
Refractory error	34	5	—	—
Traumatic cataract	1	—	—	—
Heterophoira (+20/30 vision)	2	—	—	2
Surgical: 9 (12%)				
Phimosis	—	—	—	4
Lipoma (8 cm. in diameter)	—	—	—	1
Epigastric hernia (symptomatic)	—	—	—	1
Paraumbilical hernia (symptomatic)	—	1	—	—
Inguinal hernia	—	—	—	1
Anomaly of scrotum (fusion to thigh)	—	—	1	—
Cardiac: 8 (10%)				
Congential acyanotic HD	1	—	—	—
Possible HD	2	—	—	2
Potential HD	1	—	1	1
Orthopedic: 6 (8%)				
Pronated feet (asymptomatic)	—	—	2	3
Forearm contracture (post-trauma)	1	—	—	—
Allergic: 4 (5%)				
Asthma (mild)	2	—	—	—
Rhinitis (mild)	1	—	—	1
Miscellaneous: 6 (8%)				
Hearing loss (less than 20 dcb)	—	—	1	—
Pituitary dwarfism (?)	1	—	—	—
Petit mal (?)	1	—	—	—
Albuminuria (cause undetermined)	—	—	—	1
Anemia (probably nutritional)	—	—	—	2
Totals: 77	47	6	5	19
Percentage totals: 100%	61%	8%	6%	25%

prior to the current examination if elements of the Astoria plan had functioned as intended: 13 at the time of initial examination and 5 at the time of teacher-nurse conference.

Parental resistance accounted for 2 of the 6 defects known to the school but not under care, and the remaining 4 were overlooked at the teacher-nurse conference.

Of the 19 defects unknown to the school and not under care, 15 (79 per cent) could have been discovered at the present time by physical examination alone. Parental presence was necessary for the detection of 1, and laboratory procedures for the detection of 3.

VISION. No child with corrected vision of 20/50 or worse in the better eye was observed in this group. Thirty-nine children (20 boys and 19 girls), an incidence of 34 per cent of the total group examined, had uncorrected vision of 20/40 or worse in one or both eyes. They were all fitted with glasses and (with the 5 exceptions noted in Table 1) had had their glasses checked within the past twelve months. There were 6 children with heterophoria and a vision of 20/30 or better in both eyes. Two of them were known to the school and under care. The remaining 4 were unknown and not under care; 2 of these 4 were thought to need care after an ophthalmologic work-up and are listed in the table.

TONSILS AND ADENOIDS. No children were observed in whom tonsillectomy or adenoidectomy seemed to be indicated on the basis of frequent sore throats, otitis media, cervical adenitis, hearing impairment, or nasal obstruction. Tonsillectomy and adenoidectomy had been advised in 26 children (31 per cent of the group) on examination in the first grade 6 years previously. Only 14 of the 26 had been operated upon. No significant differences in general health and frequency of respiratory infections could be observed between the tonsillectomized and the non-tonsillectomized groups.

HEART. Only one case of definite organic heart disease was present in this group. This was a congenital acyanotic cardiac, Class 1-B,[5] known to the school and under care. It is considered that this case would have been overlooked on routine physical examination since it presented no unusual signs. There was no child with a definite history of a rheumatic episode or signs of clear-cut heart disease. There were 16 children in whom the possibility of heart disease arose but in whom a diagnosis of organic disease could not be made. In 6 cases there was a history of rheumatic fever in parent or sibling but no evidence of disease in the subject. In 3 cases an apical or left sternal systolic murmur heard on examination was considered of no significance after a cardiologic work-up. The remaining 7 cases were classified as "possible" or "potential" heart disease, using criteria of the New York Heart Association,[5] after cardiologic work-up, including fluoroscopy, had been performed.

HEMOGLOBIN The mean Sahli hemoglobin of the group was 13.3 gm., with a standard deviation from the mean of 0.3 gm. There were 8 children with values of 12.0 gm. and 2 children with values of 11.0 gm. These 2 children had no symptoms or signs of anemia and appeared to be in good health. They were not of Mediterranean origin, and it is considered that their anemias were of nutritional origin.

URINALYSIS Only one significant urinary abnormality was found. This was a non-orthostatic albuminuria with a negative sediment. In spite of further work-up its etiology is still undetermined at the present time. There were 10 cases of orthostatic or benign albuminuria (an incidence of 9 per cent). Repeated clean-voided specimens were negative in the case of 4 girls who had shown 6 or more wbc/hpf. There were 2 children who had past histories of acute glomerular nephritis but showed no evidence of disease at the time of examination.

2. Mental Health

An impression of disturbing factors in the child's home environment and emotional life was sensed in 44 children (26 boys and 18 girls). This comprises 38 per cent of the total group. Thirty-three of these children showed some evidence of disturbance in their classroom work and associations as observed by the teacher. Of this group, 10 were considered so disturbed that formation of mature patterns of thought and a constructive approach to adult reality situations were seriously interfered with, and the probability of future psychosomatic problems correspondingly enhanced.

All of these 10 children were known to the school in the sense that their present and past teachers were aware of and had recorded their deviant behavior. However, its significance was not always appreciated by them. Five of the 10 children had been selected for examination by the school physician. Five had been taken frequently to purely medical agencies because of somatic complaints, and one child had received intermittent psychiatric help through a social agency.

Brief protocols of 3 typical cases are presented to show how these impressions were gained.

CHARLES H., age $11\frac{1}{2}$, is a moderately obese, quiet child whose father believes that he must stay out of fights and roughneck associations and "go his own way without making any trouble." Therefore he goes to the park with his mother after school hours and plays by himself. He has never been away from home nor will his mother consider sending him. She is certain that she will only have to take him home again as she did with his thin (enuretic until the age of 15) older brother who has recently been rejected by the Army because of "high blood pressure." During the examination the boy is abused by his mother because of an undershirt which is not spotless (yet by no means unclean), and he is praised for being such a neat, clean child who is always careful of his appearance. His obesity is easily accounted for by the quantity and quality of what he is reported to eat. Almost in the same breath he is derided for not adhering to a low-carbohydrate regime prescribed by a physician, yet reminded with pride how eager his mother is to fulfil his expressed food desires. He is practically badgered into saying that he has everything he wants. It is difficult to get him to talk in his mother's presence, but he expresses no overt desire to change his way of life. Yet he frowns and appears upset when his mother is talking, seeming particularly disturbed when she discusses his brother's camp experience. His teacher states that he is silent, shy, and studious in class, and always holds himself apart from the group. His mother accompanies him to and from school every day and he is regarded as something of a curious phenomenon by his classmates.

EILEEN S., age $11\frac{3}{12}$, is a thin, hirsute, overactive child who has been taken to many clinics and private physicians by her stout, anxious mother because of her "poor appetite," "nervousness," vomiting, headaches, and a variety of other complaints. She has been studied thoroughly and hospitalized on two occasions. No appreciable benefit has resulted. Her mother states spontaneously that she has spoiled her child and probably that is the whole trouble, but this thought is something she tends to dismiss with a smile as unimportant. Eileen prefers to spend her spare time reading or helping around the house. The reason she gives for not participating in extracurricular group activities is that she is "afraid of getting nits." Her teacher has observed that she finds it difficult to remain on friendly terms with other children in the class and frequently quarrels with them. She is a very conscientious, aggressive, and competitive scholar. She worries a great deal about the caliber and quality of her school work which is, in fact, quite superior.

WALTER P., age $12\frac{3}{12}$, a thin, drooping child of a widowed mother, sucks his thumb and occasionally wets his bed. He has little contact with children his own age except in the classroom and seems to prefer the society of adults. His mother feels that he would only get beaten up by bigger and rougher boys and that this is a commendable preference anyway. He spends a great deal of time with paternal relatives where, as the only child, he is deluged with presents, compliments, and attention. On examination he is extremely tense and cannot be drawn to talk at all. He is quite embarrassed at having to disrobe. His teacher has noted that he is very unpopular with his classmates. He annoys and teases them but runs away in fright when he is attacked, frequently coming to her whining and crying over a quarrel he himself has instigated.

COMMENT

Remarkably little evidence of physical ill health was observed in the group of children examined. The majority of physical defects or adverse conditions found were known to the school and under care. Most of those not falling into this category could have been brought to parental attention earlier if a more complete initial school examination had been performed. The Astoria plan functioned satisfactorily in these two schools.

However, these observations are necessarily limited to the district in which he survey was made. Its characteristics have already been pointed out, and it is entirely possible that, in an area where medical facilities are less easily accessible, different conditions prevail among the school children. For this reason a similar study is contemplated in schools located in a district whose socio-economic level is on a par with that of Kips Bay–Yorkville, but in which medical and health facilities outside of the school are not as adequate.

If viewed solely as a screening mechanism for the detection of physical defects, the presence of the parent at the current examination was unnecessary. However, such a conclusion is overbalanced by the demonstrated value of the parent's presence in obtaining further study and care for defects[3,9] as well as by other factors which will be discussed.

Recent trends of thought in the field of school health[7,10] have emphasized the fallibility of shaping school medical services solely to prevent and correct physical defects. The importance of educating parent and child to seek early medical assistance, of promoting a positive attitude toward the maintenance of health, and of dispelling inherent fears of doctors and disease by making the examination a desirable educational experience, has been stressed. The presence of the parent and the provision of adequate physician time are essential if this is to be accomplished in the elementary school.

Judging from the findings detailed in the section on mental health, the more time and care that is taken in the interview, the more psychic and behavior problems will be unearthed. Limitations of time and technic precluded a more accurate evaluation of the degree and significance of psychic disturbance in the individual child. Yet these findings as a whole are significant. They emphasize that this is a major field for study and direction in school health work. This is particularly true if psychic disturbances in childhood are viewed broadly as the generating forces in adult personality types and many forms of psychosomatic disorders, as well as of "mental disease" in a narrower sense.

In New York City the Bureau of Child Guidance of the Department of Education is set up to care for emotionally disturbed children and to work with teachers, and there are a number of hospital clinics and social agencies to which these children can be referred. Yet all these facilities are overburdened with work and able to reach only a small fraction of those needing their care. The necessity for expanding these facilities and for pediatricians and general practitioners to absorb some of their load is obvious.

For many years mental hygienists and some educators have felt that the adult and group contacts of the child in the classroom could be utilized to prevent a further ingraining of neurotic patterns of thought and perhaps to correct these patterns.[6] Yet before such an approach can be realized, major changes in the school curriculum and administration, in the size of classes, and in the qualifications of teachers are called for.[6] Public action effecting such changes should be vigorously supported by the medical and public health professions. They are part of a constructive answer to the challenge which the draft statistics presented, that of "seeking and correcting in childhood the roots of many adult diseases."[8]

SUMMARY

1. A health interview and examination of 114 sixth grade children is reported. The children attended two New York City elementary schools which have operated for 6 years under the Astoria plan of school medical service.

2. Only minor uncared for physical defects were observed, but there were a significant number of children in whom the seeds of future mental disturbance were sensed.

3. Most of the uncared for physical defects could have been picked up if a more complete examination had been performed on entry to elementary school.

4. The Astoria plan of school health service functioned satisfactorily in the schools surveyed.

5. The need for further study and care of emotional disturbances among school children and some of the implications of this need have been discussed.

Notes

1. St J Perrott G. Selected service rejection statistics and some of their implications. *Am J Public Health*. 1946;36:336–342.
2. Health needs of school-age children and recommendations for implementation. *School Life*. November 1945:7–14.
3. Nyswander DN. *Solving School Health Problems*. New York, NY: Commonwealth Fund; 1942.
4. Neighborhood Health Development, Inc. Health Center Districts, New York City, *Statistical Handbook*. 4th ed. New York, NY: Neighborhood Health Development, Inc.; 1944.
5. New York Heart Association. *Nomenclature and Criteria for Diagnosis of Diseases of the Heart*, 4th ed. New York, NY: New York Heart Association; 1945.
6. Ryan WC. Mental Health *Through Education*. New York, NY: Commonwealth Fund; 1938.
7. Baumgartner L. Some phases of school-health services. *Am J Public Health*. 1946;36:629–635.
8. Ciocco A. Physical growth in childhood and military fitness. *Am J Public Health*. 1945;35:927–933.
9. Walker WF, Randolph CR. *School Health Services*. New York, NY: Commonwealth Fund; 1941.
10. Health Education Council. *Suggested School Health Policies. Report of the National Committee on School Health Policies*. New York, NY: Health Education Council; 1946.

SECTION THREE

School Nursing

Reprints of Key Reports and Articles

.

CHAPTER 5

School Health Nursing
Framework for the Future, Part I

Carol C. Costante, 2001

School health nursing is a specialty that has been ahead of its time. For nearly a century, school nurses (a.k.a. school health nurses) in the United States have provided many of the same services that currently coincide with societal priorities. That is, they have always delivered components of primary health care and preventive services in a client-friendly community setting, in a cost-effective and accessible manner, and in a way that supports the full educational inclusion of a diverse populace.

Presently, school nursing (a.k.a., school health nursing) benefits from the public's emerging discovery and appreciation of its practice. Although this has not always been the case, school nursing is generally enjoying support from many different constituencies, and these proponents seem to be growing both in numbers and in interest. The opportunities for school nursing are many, and they are available now. If

Table 5.1 Professional Challenges in School Health Nursing.

- Role ambiguity
- Variable, ill-defined system of services
- Orphan status
- A maturing knowledge base
- Insufficient research
- Nonuniform educational and employment standards
- Unstable and inadequate funding

school nurses seize these opportunities, they can create a brighter future for American children while realizing their professional potential.

As the new millennium begins, school nursing is at the crossroads of its future. By virtue of predominantly external societal influences, school nursing finds itself in the most advantageous position it has ever been to become fully integrated into the health care delivery and education systems. The 21st century holds the greatest possibility for school nursing to escape the mantle of its historically invisible practice.

Although this relative prestige is a boon to school health nursing, it also creates demands, expectations, and opportunities that the specialty has never experienced. If school nursing can demonstrate its ability to meet diverse child health care needs effectively and efficiently, the way will be paved for assuming its rightful place as the most appropriate entry point for school-age children into the health care delivery system. Simultaneously, if health and learning are visibly and consistently connected, the stage will be set for full partnership with the educational community. If school nurses do not take full advantage of the opportunities now afforded, they risk their potential influence within the health and educational arenas, and as a distinct nursing specialty. Given its past and present accomplishments in the light of overwhelming obstacles, certainly the specialty of school nursing and its practitioners are up to the challenge.

The formidable internal and external issues that school health nursing faces as a specialty are barriers to achieving this full partnership status. The challenge the specialty faces is to crystallize its nebulous professional and practice issues while influencing the societal forces that have the potential to control its course. If school health nursing can adequately mobilize its forces within the specialty, the forces from without will not be empowered to mold its direction unilaterally or capriciously.

In the process of moving beyond the founding stages of its past, school nursing should strive to preserve the basic nature of its mission

Table 5.2   Issues Affecting the Future of School Health Nursing.

Program Support

- Funding
- Research
- Computerized health information

Partnerships

- Education and school reform
- Coordinated school health programs
- Telehealth
- Managed care
- School-based/school-linked health centers
- Alternative models
- Legal and ethical conflicts

Professional and Practice Issues

- Role definition
- Competencies
- Evidence-based practice
- Preparation and continuing education
- Certification
- Subspecialization
- Perilous health practices in schools
- Assistive personnel and delegation
- Nursing as a related service
- Genetic information

Program Management

- Human resources
- Staffing levels and ratios
- Supervision and management

while embracing the future with fresh zeal. The most difficult task will not be to accept new ideas, but to forget old ones that are no longer pertinent or appropriate in a changing world. For example, effectively addressing the new morbidities in children (e.g., violence, substance use, suicide, homelessness, pregnancy, and sexually transmitted diseases) within family structures that are diverse and may be unstable, dysfunctional, or less than supportive requires new, highly developed skills. Early intervention programs for developmentally delayed children from birth to age 3 under the Individuals with Disabilities Education Act (IDEA) also illustrate the need for increased involvement of school nurses with broad-based abilities. Failing to change can cause a profession to be left behind or replaced by more dynamic entities.

Undoubtedly, whatever made school nursing successful in the past will not necessarily continue to promote its advancement in the future because experience is becoming less relevant in an era in which data and information drive societal decision making. School nursing needs to cast aside irrelevant paradigms and unsubstantiated assumptions as it strives to become a force with which to be reckoned. The future challenges related to school health nursing are interconnected and frequently overlap, rather than being separate and distinct issues, because they affect professional practice and services for students.

PROGRAM SUPPORT

Funding

Essential to the advancement of any public service program is dependable funding. Without a reliable financial base, school health nursing services will remain subject to budgets and political priorities. Nationally, school nursing services are currently funded in a variety of community sensitive, often undependable, multisourced ways. These funding streams include general local and state revenues; categorical funds (e.g., Title One and Special Education); federal participation programs (e.g., Medicaid and the Child Health Insurance Program); and third-party payers, partnerships, and grants.

School nursing programs of the highest caliber seem to be in communities where both health and education agencies are philosophically and budgetarily committed to the mission of school health. Deficient funding can lead to inequities among school districts, making children the victims of disparities in health services programs. To resolve this dilemma, there must first exist a sincere belief that health is fundamental to the educational process. The bureaucratic, legal, and cultural barriers between the health and education systems need to be dissolved so school nursing services are allowed to be all that they can be. Subsequently, as programs flourish with more secure funding streams, they will be able to help communities maximize the full capacity of its youngest citizens. Aren't *all* children entitled to these opportunities?

Society increasingly has placed health care obligations onto schools, but it has neglected to ensure adequate funding to support these additional burdens. In designing strategies to address funding problems, education budgets should not be considered able to continue bearing the financial responsibility for school nursing programs. General child-health funds should be made available to school systems for the provision of health care services needed in schools. For example, to lessen the morbidity of asthma in the approximately five million U.S. children under the age of 18 who suffer from it,[1] why not take advantage of current asthma initiatives emanating from the White House and various funding agencies to support school-based health care services for students with asthma? Such action can confirm the impact of school nurses on child health and school attendance. Once effects are demonstrated, health and education agencies will need little convincing to recognize the value of solid school health nursing programs.

Finally, contracts with health care insurers can provide previously untapped funds to school systems. Documenting the unique health care services that school nurses can and do provide in a cost-effective manner and billing third-party insurers for these services will encourage the appropriation of more funding for school health services. State regulations may need to be instituted to facilitate optimal contracting, but stable health services programs with fundamental components in every school district can result.

Research

If school health nurses cannot prove that what they do makes a difference or show which service components are key to positive outcomes, why should school health-services programs continue to be funded? A solid research base that documents the outcomes of school health services will support a convincing impetus for dedicated funding.[2–4]

The rapidly increasing resources available for nursing research have opened numerous opportunities to study important questions and issues in promoting health and ameliorating the side effects of illness while optimizing individual health outcomes.[5] Two major national multiorganizational initiatives put forth research in school health nursing as a major priority in advancing the contributions of the profession.[6,7] Based on the initial work in 1996 of establishing a national research agenda for school health nursing,[8,9] Table 5.3 lists some of the research needed in the specialty.[3(p492)] In 1999, further refinement of the school nursing research agenda resulted in a framework to address these questions and a road map to accomplish the research.[10] Many of the pressing school nursing practice issues coincide with the top five American nursing research priorities[5]: (a) quality-of-care outcomes

Table 5.3   Sample Research Questions.

- Which school health services impact child well-being?
- What is the cost-benefit of school nursing services?
- What school nursing services contribute to education goals?
- What outcomes valued by the reforming health care delivery system are achieved through the provision of school nursing services?
- What minimum competencies should a school nurse possess?
- What personnel are needed in a comprehensive school health services program?
- What increases support for school health services?
- What factors should determine school nurse-to-student ratios?

and their measurement, (b) impact and effectiveness of nursing interventions, (c) symptom assessment and management, (d) health care delivery systems, and (e) health promotion and risk reduction.

In addition to supporting funding decisions, research also provides the essential database for verifying why health policy leaders should endorse school nursing services in programs such as health promotion and disease prevention, as well as for why legislators should recognize the vital contributions of school nurses in the implementation of IDEA, the Americans with Disabilities Act (ADA), and any future legislation. "For school nurses, the emphasis on measuring outcomes provides a particular challenge not only to show [how] their interventions positively influence the health of children, but also have an effect on educational outcomes".[11(p2)] Only by validating the effectiveness of school nursing services can school nurses possibly become revered as an important and even critical force in the delivery of both educational and health care services to school-age children. Only then will political support exist for the continuation and enhancement of school nurse–provided health services.

Computerized Health Information

The advent of information technology has been, and will continue to be, beneficial to the delivery of school health services.[12] The ability to conduct meaningful research will be enhanced by consistent use of computerized record keeping.[12] For example, school nurses can correlate student health-related problems and subsequent nursing interventions with educational indicators such as absenteeism, school performance, suspensions, and dropout rates. This data will make it possible for school health nursing programs to be evaluated in terms of their effects on both health and educational outcomes.[2,11,13]

Table 5.4   Uses for Computer Technology in School Health Services.

- Documenting nursing interventions
- Standardizing student health records
- Identifying, tracking, and evaluating student and community health needs and trends
- Measuring the outcomes of interventions
- Tracking students at risk for lower performance
- Monitoring individual growth and development
- Conducting health assessments
- Correlating student problems and subsequent interventions with education outcomes
- Evaluating school health services programs
- Delivering motivational health education
- Accessing current health information
- Learning via the Internet and CD-ROM

Given the agreement that computer technology facilitates research, data on the "what" needs to be collected and the "how" questions must be addressed sooner rather than later. Comparisons and generalized conclusions can only be drawn on equivalent data; therefore, standard data collection is fundamental to making decisions about school nursing programs and how health relates to education. The Nursing Outcomes Classification (NOC) and the Nursing Interventions Classification (NIC) probably hold the greatest promise for standardizing the "what" and "how" in school health nursing,[2,11] and the benefits will be enormous.[2,14]

The Nursing Minimum Data Set provides a formal structure for electronic data sets to support nursing interventions.[15] Once a minimum data set for school nursing, based on a common vocabulary such as NIC or NOC, is formalized, validated, and accepted by the specialty, data collection will be enhanced in a way that will support research and provide a solid framework for evidence-based practice. NASN could facilitate the use of such data sets by developing and distributing computerized database software to its members.

Tracking the health care needs of a defined population is but one example of the many uses for computerized record keeping. Such aggregate data will help identify effective prevention strategies, validate effective interventions, and diminish morbidity in a variety of health conditions, thereby improving children's health and supporting the continuity and expansion of school health services. Instituting widespread use of electronic record keeping within and across

**Table 5.5   Standardized Language as a Valuable Asset
to School Health Nursing.**

- Establishes core knowledge and standards
- Facilitates collection of meaningful data
- Provides consistent clinical focus
- Aids intraprofessional communication
- Promotes community collaboration
- Facilitates reimbursement processes
- Encourages evaluation of quality and cost
- Accommodates setting of priorities
- Provides basis for computerized record keeping
- Increases visibility for policy making

states will provide the volume of data needed to access state and federal funds and private grants that could subsequently catalyze standard electronic record keeping in school health nursing.

The evolving technology of health data on personal microchips is a health information access strategy that is being pilot tested in some long-term facilities and hospitals and in the armed forces.[16] Certainly, such "smart cards" can be invaluable in keeping track of children's medical and immunization records, but their use in schools would be controversial and inappropriate. Such technology is unnecessary in schools, and the legal issues related to delivery of health care services in a nonhealth environment, together with the fact that the recipients of care in schools are minors, would prohibit its appropriateness. Of greater applicability in schools would be universal computerized immunization banks.

PARTNERSHIPS

Education and School Reform

School nursing services do not belong in schools if they do not promote the ability of students to learn and achieve. These services are distinctly related to three of the National Education Goals. Therefore, health services must be consistently connected and implemented in response to the goals of education.[17] Health and educational goals are interdependent; educated people are healthier people, and healthy students are better learners.[18] Although there is substantial evidence that good health is basic to optimal learning, there is a dearth of data that demonstrates the positive influence of school nursing services on school achievement. Outcome measurement is key to linking school nursing services and educational outcomes, such as consistent attendance, graduation rates, and involvement in school activities. A model exists that demonstrates the effects, albeit indirect and multifaceted, of school health interventions on school performance outcomes.[19] Acting on recent stimulus related to school nursing research,[8–10] the specialty could readily use this model to solidify its interrelationship with education.

Funding follows data. Only when there is sufficient hard data to verify the connection of school nursing services to health and educational outcomes for children will school health services be mandated. "Providing concrete data on the contribution school nurses make to the health and educational outcomes of children will solidify nursing's position in the school setting—and show that school nurses do make a difference."[11]

Because the goal of school health services is to promote optimum student health so students are ready to learn, an effective way of confirming nursing's support of student success is through services, implemented by professional school nurses, that contribute to school improvement. One such example is the nurse-only provision for dispensing simple, over-the-counter medications designed to relieve minor discomfort (e.g., mild analgesics, throat lozenges, and cough drops) so students can remain in school and focus on learning. Parents usually support such programs, which can make significant contributions to improving school attendance and achievement.

Coordinated School Health Programs

A coordinated school health program (CSHP) is "an organized set of policies, procedures, and activities designed to protect and promote the health and well-being of students and school staff [that] utilizes personnel, agencies and programs, both in and out of the school building, which relate to student health and success in school."[13(p1)] Working together, the eight components—school health services; health education; healthy school environment; counseling, psychological and social services; health promotion for staff; physical education; nutrition services; and family and community involvement[20]—confirm the relevance and importance of health to educational productivity.

CSHPs epitomize the essence of partnerships in promoting optimum health for students. Even though their special services are critical to improving health outcomes for children, school nurses—along with the other providers of school-based health services—cannot and should not attempt to meet all of the health-related needs of today's students. Nonetheless, as the chief provider of school health services and by virtue of their holistic view of student needs and their multidimensional educational background, "school nurses are in a unique position to assume the leadership role in these programs."[13(p2)]

School nurses need to enlarge their perspectives to integrate their services with the other components of CSHPs as a way of multiplying their effect on students' health.[21] There are numerous federal initiatives to support and expand CSHPs, and school nurses need to be at the table when such programs are designed. The national and state school nursing organizations should expand their efforts to prepare school nurses in how to implement CSHPs and in leadership skills.

Telehealth

Telehealth, according to the American Nurses' Association,[22] is the removal of time and distance barriers for the delivery of health care services or related health care activities. For school health, this application of technology holds tremendous opportunities for the expansion of service delivery, particularly in rural areas,[23] but also in urban communities where human resources are not adequate to meet the health needs of children.[24]

In geographic areas where school nursing staff is inadequate, the teleconnection of one nurse to a cluster of schools would allow the nurse to direct and delegate services that are then provided by school-based health paraprofessionals.[3] Cameras can beam pictures from the school nurse's office to a regional medical center where a physician or nurse practitioner would be available for consultation, medical diagnosis, and treatment orders.[25] School nurses also could expand their assessment abilities and scope of practice through the use of medical monitoring devices that would be connected to attending physicians.

Grant funding of school-based pilot sites that model public and private partnerships could ignite a new dimension of school health nursing services in underserved communities. To improve the affordability of telehealth, legislation is needed to expand current federal reimbursement rules, amend federal and state regulations that escalate technology transmission costs, and expand access to federal monies.[25] Other remaining challenges relative to nursing are multistate licensure,[12,26] client confidentiality, and malpractice issues.

Managed Care

As managed care emerges as a dominant health care delivery model in the United States, an unparalleled opportunity exists for school nursing to gain prominence as a significant player. In a restructured health care system, there is no rational reason not to use school nurses to extend primary care services. As Denehy stated:[11(p4)]

> The profession of nursing is now retooling to meet the demands of the health care system in the new millennium. An important priority is to clearly articulate what contributions nursing makes to the health of the nation. For school nurses the time has come when attention needs to focus on how outcomes of care will be measured in the school setting.

It is possible for school health programs coordinated and delivered by qualified, professional school nurses to become the primary portal into the health care delivery system for school-age children.[3] Society can no longer afford to view school health-services programs as an extravagance or as unrelated to the health care delivery continuum inasmuch as schools serve the vast majority of youngsters from 5 to 18 years of age, as well as those with special educational needs from birth to 21 years of age. The potential for school health services programs to meet most of the prevention, screening, early intervention, health coordination, and referral needs of children is an idea whose time has come. Of the 467 objectives in *Healthy People 2010*,[27] one half can be realized by or through school health programs; school nursing services can affect five of the six goals the surgeon general has outlined for the country.[28] The managed-care arena should not be perceived as a threat to school health professionals; rather, it actually offers school-based services an opportunity for distinction in the emerging health care delivery system. "School nurses possess the education and expert knowledge needed to promote the successful delivery of managed care services."[29(p6)] School health nursing programs already provide many preventive and primary health care services in a cost-effective manner. Managed care organizations (MCOs), of which preventive health care is the cornerstone as they strive to contain health care costs while it keeps members healthy,[30] should be responsive to partnering with school nurses to provide population-based, health-related services to all school children.

Table 5.6   Advantages of Partnerships Between Managed Care Organizations and School Health Nursing Services.

Advantages to Schools
- Improved documentation
- Focus on outcome measures
- Enhanced value of individual student plans
- Cost of school nursing services are determined
- Schools can be spotlighted for prevention
- Revenue for school-delivered health services

Advantages to Managed Care Organizations
- Cost-effective, timely delivery of services
- Accessible site for preventive and primary care
- Case management by closely linked persons
- Risk assessments of vulnerable populations
- Identification of potential members
- Management of cultural barriers
- Efficient care to the Medicaid population

Advantages to the Health System and Consumers
- Improved communication among providers
- Shared protocols and standards of care
- Continuity of care
- Elimination of duplicative services
- Reduced health care costs
- Community schools can become sites of service
- Accessibility to care for school-age clients
- Removal of transportation as a barrier
- School services become part of health care system

For mutually beneficial relationships to develop, MCOs and school nurses need to be willing to learn about each other (e.g., their structure, mission, goals, values, language, personnel, services, funding, and quality assurance mechanisms).[29] School health nurses must actively promote their unique services to the managed care system by substantiating their child health outcomes. At the same time, MCOs are charged with developing trust and operating within the structure of the existing school health services program rather than attempting to capture the school-based market for itself with irresistible propositions. An alliance can result in contracted arrangements that can be profitable for both groups while improving health care services for children.[3(p493)]

School-Based and School-Linked Health Centers

School-based health centers (SBHCs) are usually initiated in areas where many children are uninsured or are without access to health care. Theoretically, federal and state Child Health Insurance Programs should capture these children in need, making school-based centers potentially unnecessary. Nevertheless, at present this model of primary health care delivery continues to move forward[31] mainly because of its accessibility and cost effectiveness, its reduction of absenteeism, and its consumer friendliness. The destiny of SBHCs will be determined by the future direction of community health care delivery systems.[32] For the SBHC model to remain practicable, states need to furnish the legal structure for them to access third-party health care funds and to establish a secure role in the managed care arena.[32] In addition, their relationship with schools and existing school health services needs to be more clearly defined, and issues such as confidentiality, revenue sharing, 24-hour coverage, quality assurance, and access to records need to be resolved.

School nurses should view SBHCs as an opportunity to expand health care services to students. Their participation in these programs is essential and an extension of traditional school health services. In terms of the interrelationship between school nurses and primary care providers, consideration should be given to the primacy of the school nurses' role due in part to their extensive knowledge of the school, its students, and their families and to the indispensable structure they provide through triaging, referral, and follow-up.

Relationships with public and private community agencies is important to assure that existing resources are used to serve greater numbers of children.[33] Such relationships also can result in the establishment of school-linked primary health care services (SLHCs). These off-campus services have formalized ties to schools in a way that seeks to serve students and families in a client-friendly manner but are less financially burdensome to schools and have fewer interactive issues to resolve than the SBHC model. Nonetheless, the school nurse is key to their success, and many of the same issues relating to SBHC–school collaborations need to be resolved before SLHCs can move forward.

Alternative Models

Some state statutes mandate joint responsibility of both state and local health and education agencies for the provision of school health services. Funding is inadequate for school health services; therefore, states that have not cemented such a health–education collaboration are forging innovative partnerships with other community public and private entities to expand health services. This has become prevalent in areas where hospitals have expanded their community service outreach into schools while concurrently curtailing inpatient services. At their best, partnerships can expand the delivery of health services to school-age children where it has been nonexistent or inadequate, but the school health nursing program stands the best chance of melding with the school community if its ultimate control remains with the education agency. If the trend toward partnerships continues in response to expanding student and program needs, certain legal and management issues must be clarified, such as confidentiality and access to records, employment and personnel, maintenance of program control, and liability.

Some educational policy makers interested in reducing school budgets believe that private entities acting as the sole providers of school health services is a desirable resource for reducing health-related barriers to learning. According to Adelman,[33] privatization of school health services ignores the value of school-owned and operated programs and the importance of restructuring these resources as part of school reform. He postulated that such attitudes may cause school personnel to feel that their contributions are discounted and their jobs in jeopardy. They may also undermine school–community collaborations.

Privately funded school-based services can be favorable if children receive services they have been previously denied or if school health services programs facing elimination can be kept intact. Nonetheless, the potentially significant hazards to contracting school health services with private groups need to be evaluated. Private entities may bid for the contract at unrealistically low rates initially and then precipitously increase fees. In addition, personnel working for private, non–Board of Education entities risk alienation as essential school team members or as vital partners in the educational system. Opportunities for collaboration and positively influencing day-to-day experiences of children and faculty diminish as services and providers are more remote and less integrated. Privatization would cease to be an issue if budget appropriations for school health programs were corrected. For school nursing, the challenge in alternative school health services models will be to integrate these models into its professional ranks and meet the needs of the expanding numbers of school nurses from varied employment settings.

Legal and Ethical Conflicts

Legal and ethical conflicts between the educational and school health communities arise because their missions are disparate and the laws and regulations governing their programs are often divergent.[26,34,35] As a result, professional nursing standards and the duty to protect the client are sometimes jeopardized. One of the most conflicting issues for school nurses is confidentiality of health information. School staff often believe they have a right and responsibility to know all about a student's personal health issues, whereas school nurses are committed to protecting each individual student's privacy related to health information.

Pending federal legislation has the potential to designate school health records as medical records. This would undoubtedly help protect confidentiality of health records in schools but would necessitate a radical change of attitude, as well as regulations governing school records. Protection of personal health information is an issue that goes hand in hand with delivering health services in an environment with an educational mission. Using the consensus guidelines from the major educational and school health organizations,[36] the challenge remains for state and local jurisdiction personnel to develop practical strategies that will assist school professionals in seeking appropriate consultation and making well-reasoned decisions when faced with quandaries in practice.

An important strategy that would safeguard confidentiality while promoting a greater understanding is the use of functional language, that is, terminology that focuses on the abilities and limitations of students in the classroom, regardless of medical diagnosis or educational label.[37] When health and educational personnel have an equivalent understanding of students' strengths and needs while still maintaining their unique professional perspectives, they are probably using functional descriptors. For example, describing a student's inability to attend to tasks and his or her impulsiveness and distractibility not only preserves confidentiality, but is far more useful than using a single diagnostic category to identify strategies to help a student with attention deficit hyperactivity disorder (ADHD) experience success in school.

Used in schools, functional language would belong exclusively to neither health nor education and would be readily understood by both. It is a universal language that transcends professional goals, missions and rhetoric, somewhat analogous to the cross-cultural effect that music can have on a global community. Functional terminology can promote trust between health and education providers and foster mutual respect for each other's expertise, providing a sound basis for a comprehensive and coordinated approach to meeting student needs. Focusing on functional abilities and needs facilitates the differentiation of educational and health-related strategies, as well as protecting privacy by removing the need to use medical and psychiatric diagnoses. This shifts the focus to learning strengths and needs, preventing students from being labeled and compartmentalized and improving communication and collaboration among staff.[3] To encourage the use of functional language, both professions will need to make significant operational revisions at the national level within professional associations and at the university preparation level.

Part II of this article [see Chapter 6] will focus on professional, practice, and management issues and on specific strategies for the future as school health nurses embrace the opportunities and challenges facing them in the new millennium.

Notes

1. American Academy of Allergy, Asthma, and Immunology, Pediatric Asthma Committee. *Pediatric Asthma: Promoting Best Practice. Guide for Managing Asthma in Children.* Milwaukee, Wis: American Academy of Allergy, Asthma, and Immunology; 1999.

2. Cavendish R, Lunney M, Kraynyak B, Richardson K. National survey to identify the nursing interventions used in school settings. *J Sch Nurs.* 1999;15:14–21.

3. Costante CC. Future challenges for school health services and the law: a manager's perspective. In: Schwab NC, Gelfman MHB, eds. *Legal Issues in School Health Services: A Resource for School Administrators, School Attorneys, and School Nurses.* North Branch, Minn: Sunrise River Press; 2001:489–506.

4. Proctor SE. The texture of practice: a plea for more qualitative research. *J Sch Nurs.* 1998;145:2.

5. Hinshaw AS. Nursing knowledge for the 21st century: opportunities and challenges. *J Nurs Scholarsh.* 200;322:117–123.

6. Brainerd E. School health nursing services progress review: a report of 1996 national meeting. *J Sch Health.* 1998;68:12–21.

7. National Nursing Coalition for School Health. School health nursing services: exploring national issues and priorities. *J Sch Health.* 1995;65:369–389.

8. Bradley B. Establishing a research agenda for school nursing. *J Sch Nurs.* 1998;141:4–13.

9. Costante CC, Wessel GL. School nursing research: are you ready to get involved? *J Sch Health.* 1997;67:315.

10. National Center for School Health Nursing. Health of America's children at school: developing a research agenda. In: Brainerd E, ed. *Proceedings of the Invitational Summit Meeting, Elkridge, Md, March 1999.* Washington, DC: American Nurses Foundation; 2000.

11. Denehy J. Measuring the outcomes of school nursing practice. *J Sch Nurs.* 2000;161:2–4.

12. Bergren MD. Electronic records and technology. In: Schwab NC, Gelfman MHB, eds. *Legal Issues in School Health Services: A Resource for School Administrators, School Attorneys, and School Nurses.* North Branch, Minn: Sunrise River Press; 2001:317–334.

13. National Association of School Nurses. *Coordinated School Health Programs* [position statement]. Scarborough, Maine: National Association of School Nurses; 1999.

14. Hootman J. Nursing diagnosis: a language of nursing, a language of powerful communication. *J Sch Nurs.* 1996;124:19–23.

15. National Association of School Nurses. *Nursing Minimum Data Set for School Nursing Practice* [position statement]. Scarborough, Maine: National Association of School Nurses; 1999.

16. Scott A. Smart cards: patient data is just a swipe away. *Adv Nurses.* 2000;217:8–10, 39.

17. Costante CC. Supporting student success: school nurses make a difference. *J Sch Nurs.* 1996;123:4–6.

18. Deutsch C. Common cause: School health and school reform. *Educ Leadersh.* 2000;576:8–12.

19. Devaney B, Schochet P, Thornton C, Fasciano N, Gavin A. *Evaluating the Effects of School Health Intervention on School Performance.* Princeton, NJ: Mathematica Policy Research; 1997.

20. Tyson H. *A Load off the Teachers' Backs.* Newton, Mass: Education Development Center; 1999.

21. Duncan P, Igoe JB. School health services. In: Marx E, Wooley SF, with Northrop D, eds. *Health Is Academic: A Guide to Coordinated School Health Programs.* New York: Teachers College Press; 1998:169–194.

22. American Nurses' Association. Telehealth: A tool for nursing practice. *Nurs Trends Issues.* 1997;2(4).

23. Pinkowish MD. The Internet in medicine: an update. *Patient Care.* January 15, 1999;30–54.

24. Whitten PS, Cook DJ. School-based telemedicine: using technology to bring health care to inner-city children. *J Telemed Telecare.* 1999; 5(suppl 1):S23–S25.

25. Lessard JA, Knox R. Telehealth in a rural school-based health center. *J Sch Nurs.* 2000;162:38–41.

26. Pohlman KJ. Legal framework and accountability for school nursing practice. In: Schwab NC, Gelfman MHB, eds. *Legal Issues in School Health Services: A Resource for School Administrators, School Attorneys, and School Nurses.* North Branch, Minn: Sunrise River Press; 2001:95–121.

27. US Department of Health and Human Services. *Healthy People 2010: Understanding and Improving Health.* Washington, DC: Public Health Service; 2000.

28. Novarra T. Surgeon general makes mental health top priority. *Nurs Spectrum.* 2000;9(6DC):15.

29. Gaffrey N, Bergren MD. School health services and managed care: a unique partnership for child health. *J Sch Nurs.* 1998;144:5–22.

30. Bensing K. Arbitrating the managed care showdown. *Adv Nurses.* 2000;212:31.

31. Wooley SF, Eberst RM, Bradley BJ. Creative collaborations with health providers. *Educ Leadersh.* 2000;576:25–28.

32. Igoe JB. An overview of school health services. *National Association of Secondary School Principals Bulletin,* November 1998;14–26.

33. Adelman HS. School counseling, psychological, and social services. In: Marx E, Wooley SF, Northrop D, eds. *Health Is Academic: A Guide to Coordinated School Health Programs.* New York, NY: Teachers College Press; 1998:142–168.

34. Institute of Medicine. *Schools and Health: Our Nation's Investment.* Allensworth DD, Lawson E, Nicholson L, Wyche JH, eds. Washington, DC: National Academy Press; 1997.

35. Schwab NC, Gelfman MHB, Cohn SD. Fundamentals of US law. In: Schwab NC, Gelfman MHB, eds. *Legal Issues in School Health Services: A Resource for School Administrators, School Attorneys, and School Nurses.* North Branch, Minn: Sunrise River Press; 2001:55–79.

36. National Task Force on Confidential Student Health Information. *Guidelines for Protecting Confidential Student Health Information.* Kent, Ohio: American School Health Association; 2000.

37. Schwab NC, Panetierri MJ, Bergren MD. *Guidelines for School Nursing Documentation: Standards, Issues, and Models.* Scarborough, Maine: National Association of School Nurses; 1998.

CHAPTER 6

School Health Nursing

Framework for the Future, Part II

Carol C. Costante, 2001

—◆◆◆—

This is the second in a two-part look at the trends and issues affecting the future of school health nursing. The relative support and favor that school nursing is enjoying at this time provides a fertile and potentially nurturing environment in which to advance the specialty into a powerful force in both the health and education communities. The improved well-being and success of America's students is dependent, in part, on school nurses accepting the challenge to develop appropriate innovative interventions while discarding outmoded and ineffective tenets. This direction will permit school nursing to use its current stature to transform the challenging aspects of its professional world. Part I of this series [see Chapter 5] addressed the societal environment in which school health nursing finds itself, as well as the mainly externally determined issues of developing

This chapter originally appeared as Costante CC. School health nursing: framework for the future, part II. *J Sch Nurs.* 2001;17(2):64–72. Copyright © 2001. Reprinted with permission from the National Association of School Nurses.

program support and partnerships that will help to sustain a thriving future. Part II deals with predominantly internal professional, practice, and management issues and offers strategies for enriching the specialty of school nursing in the 21st century.

PROFESSIONAL AND PRACTICE ISSUES

Role Definition

The missing mortar in school nursing's foundation is the lack of consensus among its practitioners in defining and standardizing a unique set of services. This problem is in part due to the historical precedence that school nurses have set by providing any and all health-related services that children need in the school setting. As a result, school nursing services as a program suffer from role-identity confusion.[1]

Role definition is strategic to advancing service delivery and producing quantifiable outcomes of those services. Fundamental to substantiating outcomes is systematizing the scope and nature of nursing practice. Unless a profession knows what services it can provide and those it provides better than anyone else, it cannot market those services. Unequivocally, the school nursing specialty needs to decide what it can and should provide that will remove health-related barriers to school achievement. Core services may include such things as health promotion and disease prevention, early identification and intervention, health care referral and care coordination, and health education and counseling.

Once the core services are determined, school nurses need to agree to focus on the identified set of services and not revert to earlier modes of operation, such as doing whatever is needed by the school community without regard for the connection of the service to positive student outcomes. In this era of cost containment, lack of clarity in professional service delivery can contribute to replacement of nurses by less costly and less educated personnel such as nursing assistants or health aides.[2] When a profession's focus is unclear, its services can appear unnecessary, which in turn makes it vulnerable to extinction when tight monetary conditions prevail.

This is, of course, a fine distinction to maintain. If school nurses do not do whatever is needed, are they even more likely to be considered expendable? On the contrary, if the specialty promotes outcome-based services and regularly evaluates its objectives in response to a changing society, it can transcend externally determined expectations. Role refine-

Table 6.1   The Value of Practice-Based Competencies.

- Structure a foundation for services
- Establish legal performance standards
- Provide the basis for accountability
- Form a framework for quality assurance
- Help systematize professional preparation
- Create universal expectations
- Support accurate performance evaluation

ment will also help develop the legal framework required to more accurately and universally establish scope of practice and liability. In terms of legislation, it will assist in decisions about what are appropriate expectations for school nursing services, such as in the provision of related services under the Individuals with Disabilities Education Act.[3]

Competencies

Determining what a practitioner must know and do to effect desired outcomes provides compelling benefits.[4(p497)] Practice-based competencies[5] need to be rooted in research and are best attained by professional nursing organizations with the help of academia. Enacting competency-based undergraduate and advanced education for school nurses will result in "better qualified nurses seeking employment in school settings, increased numbers of nurses interested in school nursing, greater understanding of school nursing by all nurses, and improved collaboration among all nurses on health care issues involving children."[6(p38)] Promoting practice-based competencies should become a focus for the National Association of School Nursing.

Evidence-Based Practice

School nursing has historically relied almost exclusively on assumptions, that is, on doing what seemed best or what clients preferred. This deference to client preference has extended to the educational community as evidenced by school nurses' allowing educators to decide how school health professionals should practice. To advance the specialty of school nursing in this century, it must become aligned with the impetus in both the health and educational communities toward outcome-based practice. Such direction will move school health nursing toward evidence-based practice.

Evidence-based practice is the "integration of individual clinical expertise with the best available external clinical evidence from systematic research."[7(p317)] that helps improve the quality of health care and enhances clinical judgement. In a restructured health care environment, practitioners can no longer rely solely on opinion processes, clinical experience, or physiological rationale.[7]

Nursing, coordinated by the American Nurses' Association (ANA), has been studying nursing-sensitive quality indicators (QIs) since 1994 to capture the essence of nursing care. "Like bandages on the Invisible Man, QIs help give shape to the seemingly transparent aspects of what nurses do."[8(p7)] The factors being documented by the ANA apply to establishing a link between acute inpatient nursing interventions and outcomes for patients. These data elements form a vivid image of the impact of nursing and provide data to verify what makes a positive difference for patients. School health nurses could use the same model for building a verified bank of data to strengthen the specialty.

Consistently using standardized language in defining patient problems, interventions, and outcomes will support the measurement of school nurses' contributions to child health outcomes. In the course of proving the worth of school nursing services, a range of interventions need to be studied so that practice and funding decisions are based on what really makes a difference. This will also assist in the effective use of personnel. For example, do the results of school-based vision and hearing screening programs positively affect students' learning? It is known that vision and hearing greatly facilitate the learning process, and we have research to substantiate the cost-effectiveness of school-based screening programs.[9] Nonetheless, the question is whether the yield from vision and hearing screening is sufficient to make a difference in the student population. Another concern is whether a professional nurse needs to provide this service. Can equally valid results be

Table 6.2   The Benefits of Quality Indicators for School Nursing.

- Prove the worth of school nurses
- Define core services
- Establish direction for the specialty
- Help role clarification
- Confirm the needed staffing mix for school health services
- Assist in marketing the specialty

obtained by technicians trained and supervised to do this type of repetitive work? Using personnel appropriately must be considered when providing services so that funding is used judiciously and school nurses are utilizing their clinical expertise in ways that make a difference for children. The need for evidence-based practice is a major reason to focus our efforts on research.

Preparation and Continuing Education

The variety of entry levels into nursing with their concomitant range of competencies not only causes public confusion, but is a considerable detriment to the advancement of the profession. In addition to the general confusion related to registered nurses with diplomas, associate degrees, baccalaureate degrees, and master's degrees, their dissimilar educational content and performance outcomes make it professionally and legally impossible to demand the same standards and accountability from nurses with different levels of preparation.[4,10] This hampers the process of role delineation, and leads to disparity in services to children.

State mandates for only one entry level into school nursing could change the face of the specialty. The autonomous nature of the skills and the clinical judgment required in unstructured and demanding situations require that a baccalaureate degree should be the minimum entry-level requirement into school nursing.[11,12] This requirement is comparable to or less than expectations of other school professionals and would help to address other problematic areas, such as salary parity and the perceived value of school health services.[4] Because of the independent nature of its practice, baccalaureate preparation is even more critical to school nursing than it is to other areas in nursing.

Even though school nursing is recognized as a complex practice specialty with a wide scope of practice demanding specific skills and a broad knowledge base,[1,11,13] master's degree preparation should not be held as a requirement for entry-level school nurses. For those in management, supervisory, or consultant positions, however, it should be an unconditional requisite. In addition, this advanced educational preparation is desirable where the school nurse is the only health provider for a community and delegates the delivery of most services to paraprofessionals.

Although advanced assessment skills and critical thinking are essential in school nursing, a master's-prepared nurse practitioner is not necessary, or even desired, for all schools.[4,13] The skills and knowledge of nurse practitioners are most appropriate and cost-effective in school-based health centers.

Pragmatically speaking, neither education nor health budgets can support master's-prepared school nurses in every school in America, nor are there enough nurses with this preparation even if finances were not an issue. Equity of school nurse qualifications across all schools and states at a minimum of a bachelor's degree should be the first priority along with making qualified school nurses available to every student in the country. Once this is attained, moving toward master's preparation of school nurses is both justified and desirable.

School nurses need to be "bilingual," that is, they must be well versed in both the disciplines of health and education and have special expertise regarding the role of health on student learning.[14] It is incumbent upon the school nurse to speak the language of education for health services to be meaningful to the educational process. To assist in this process, knowledge beyond the baccalaureate level about health and education, about issues such as family systems, principles of education, community health, special education, and health education, is necessary to function optimally in the role of school nurse.[1,4,6,11,13] This also promotes full integration into the school faculty, which is fundamental to school health services being regarded as equal to other services provided by schools.

Advanced education should not only be expected, but required of school nurses just as it is of teachers. Professionals working in the same institution and toward complementary goals should have similar educational expectations. If teachers are required to obtain a master's degree within a certain number of years, then that also should be the expectation for school nurses. The acquisition of post-baccalaureate education models a respect for learning that assures a workforce that functions on a higher plane and also provides adequate leadership and mentoring for new nurses. Furthermore, to maintain currency, non-credit continuing education should be the norm for anyone practicing in the health care field.

State and national school nursing organizations should promote baccalaureate preparation and collaborate with institutions of higher education to provide RN to BS programs. States also should support existing qualified associate degree and diploma nurses while establishing the baccalaureate degree as the requirement for entry into practice.

Certification

Professional certification of school nurses endorses the core knowledge for competent practice[1,4,10,11,15] and promotes safe, quality services for students beyond those assured by state RN licensure. National certification establishes a minimum clinical practice level in the specialty of school nursing based on nationally agreed-upon standards. State teacher certification or licensure for school nurses as determined by State Departments of Education designates employment standards beyond the baccalaureate degree that meet state-specific requirements. Currently, 27 states stipulate some form of state certification or licensure, and others are in the process of standardizing expectations of school nurses.

Importantly, states that institute certification requirements demonstrate a commitment of value; this is a standard to which all states should strive. Furthermore, where state certification is mandated, requirements for preparation are usually higher and salaries are more substantial. In addition to promoting professional certification, state school nurse organizations should actively encourage their state legislatures to demand state-based certification for school health services providers to minimize the disparity of services across the state and ensure that all students have access to services from equally prepared practitioners.

Subspecialization

Even though school nursing is a recognized specialty in nursing, it is in many ways a generalist practice because the school nurse is often responsible for health care delivery to all students served by the school district, as well as school staff. Schools are microcosms of communities. Because the school nurse's role is expanding in response to health-related societal needs, subspecialty practice within school nursing should be considered. Possible subspecialties include early intervention, adolescent health, and substance abuse prevention and identification.

Children would profit from subspecialization in school nursing. As with other broad-based health specialties, it is difficult if not impossible to keep current with rapid advances in the health care field, making it difficult to deliver up-to-date, evidence-based care for children of all age levels with a variety of health concerns. If children were served by nurses specializing in their particular issues, the service delivered would be both safer and more current and tailored to their individual needs.[4]

Barriers to subspecialization include the increased number of health providers that would be required and the funding necessary to support them. Although the benefits are obvious, the corresponding costs cannot and should not be borne by education budgets. Key to this future vision are availability of basic school health programs for all children, major restructuring of the health care delivery system, and secure funding that would recognize and utilize schools as sites for the provision of health care services.

Perilous Health Practices in Schools

More intense responsibility for the welfare of children is being placed on schools, and this responsibility includes health-related services. The health care procedures and monitoring needed by some students during the school day may be provided by education personnel if health professionals are not available in schools. Expecting educators to provide skilled health care services is analogous to demanding that nurses implement the language arts curriculum. More important, it is unsafe for students. Such modes of operation may also constitute practicing nursing without a license, which carries legal sanctions.

The lack of health professionals to assess student needs, to develop individualized health care plans, and to evaluate the outcomes of the care does not justify the delegation of professional functions to unlicensed staff. These functions are critical to recognizing and meeting students' health care needs. Without this nursing care, diminished health and learning may result.

The number of students requiring prescribed medications during the school day continues to accelerate. A change also has occurred in the types of medications administered, including potent psychotropic, inhaled, and percutaneous drugs. Clinical judgments need to be made on a continual basis about the effects of these medications, and therefore safety is of prime importance.[16] In schools where laypersons routinely administer oral medications, nurses need adequate time to supervise those who have been trained to administer medications. Only a few states mandate the administration of medications by nurses, but other states should do likewise to promote children's safety.

To eliminate inappropriate and hazardous health practices in schools, professional education and school nursing organizations, as well as parent teacher organizations, must oppose these practices. Providing sufficient funding for school nursing programs will aid in the reduction or elimination of inappropriate staffing patterns and unsafe practices. State statutes mandating the use of school health professionals for medication administration and health care procedures should be required.

Assistive Personnel and Delegation

Along with professional nurses, the number of assistive personnel, including lay volunteers, school staff, health aides, licensed practical nurses and non–state-certified RNs, will continue to increase in response to the growing health-related needs of students. In general, the use of assistive personnel can supplement the delivery of health services but can be counterproductive if allowed to replace professional health care providers. For the safe delivery of care to students, the qualifications and use of assistive personnel can be dictated by local policy but ultimately should be state regulated.[15] The issue of assistive personnel is closely aligned with nursing delegation of health care activities. State Nurse Practice Acts address the issue of delegation, but its application in schools is frequently either absent or nebulous.[17,18] To assure the safe provision of health care to children, states need to clearly regulate nursing delegation to unlicensed assistive personnel in schools. Moreover, these regulations need to be enforced. Even where they are clearly stipulated in the law, compliance frequently is not monitored, and those acting contrary to the law are not held accountable. The topic of delegation is one that demands ongoing explanation to school personnel in ways that speak to the issues of safety and liability.

School Nursing as a Related Service

Students with special health care needs are becoming more prevalent, and this trend shows no sign of retreating. With continuous advances in health care, school nurses must keep pace with the depth and breadth of services that this specific population requires so that no student is denied full access to learning. Schools have certain legal responsibilities to students requiring health care services in order to access appropriate education services.[3,19] This obligation extends to educational programming that occurs beyond the schoolhouse, including cooperative learning experiences and full-day or overnight field trips. If the need for a nurse is included in a 504 Plan or Individual Education Plan, the school is obligated to provide one.[20]

Despite the fact that a full-time registered nurse is in the school, some students' health needs may not be safely met by a nurse who has simultaneous responsibility for hundreds of other students. The U.S. Supreme Court ruled [in *Cedar Rapids* v. *Garret*] that schools must provide any school nursing services that a student requires to access special education services, including one-on-one nursing services.[21] In its decision, the court has interpreted IDEA [Individuals with Disabilities Information Act] in a clear and direct manner that supports the elimination of any nursing-related barriers to the education of disabled students. Under the leadership of the National Association of School Nurses (NASN), the task of school nursing during the future reauthorizations of IDEA is to strengthen the language to specifically include school nurses in the list of providers and to elaborate their role with students who have special health care needs.

In all issues related to ensuring school nursing as a related service, what must be avoided is the tendency to dilute the existing school nursing staff to meet the complex and continuous health needs of medically complex students. This has the potential of diminishing preventive, health promotion, early identification, and early intervention services to other students. Although the Supreme Court was originally petitioned to rule on the *Garret* case relative to nursing services under IDEA, its decision also provides clear support for nursing as a related service under Section 504 of the Rehabilitation Act of 1973 for any student who needs it. The court's ruling has the potential of eliminating the discrepancy of services that now exists among schools, school districts, and even states by eliminating obstacles to the educational process that can be minimized by the provision of appropriate school nursing services. Parents and schools need to be made aware of their rights under the law to obtain school health nursing services for all qualified students.

Federal laws clearly require there should be no barriers to education experiences based on disability,[3,19] but funding does not accompany these laws. Either new laws must be enacted or new revenue sources identified to fund the existing mandates. Preferably, the latter will occur because the outcomes for disabled students are markedly enhanced when they are included to the fullest extent reasonable.

Genetic Information

The recent definition of the human genome compels the profession of nursing to grapple with its implications for clinical practice. As genetic testing becomes more common, schools will inevitably become involved in issues related to genetic information. According to Fibison,[22] some questions include:

- Is there an advocacy role for the school nurse in protecting the student's right not to know in situations where parents want presymptomatic or carrier testing?
- What future role should school nursing play once genes are identified for adult onset disorders when effective early intervention has been proven to prolong health?
- Should screening programs be instituted in schools?
- How will genetic information be used to meet the goals of optimal learning for students?

For example, the results of current research on the genetic influences of behavior may lead to earlier, more accurate diagnoses, as well as more effective interventions for conditions such as Attention Deficit/Hyperactivity Disorder (ADHD). Researchers are exploring

Table 6.3   School Nurses' Roles Relative to Genetic Information.

- Promote its wise and careful use by and in schools
- Prevent abuse of genetic information
- Respond to questions from the community
- Direct others to appropriate resources
- Preserve confidentiality of health information
- Prevent stigmatization of identified students

genes associated with the susceptibility for ADHD,[23] and once that gene (or genes) is identified, a genetic test likely will be developed. One can only imagine the potential benefit—as well as the potential harm—in having a genetic test to identify children at risk for ADHD; the implications are staggering. Another concern is how emerging bio-genetic information may affect the classification of children in schools. For example, how does the concept of "self-fulfilling prophecy" apply to positive testing results in the absence of signs or symptoms? According to Fibison,[22] school nurses may be able to help create solutions that reduce the potential harm to those students whose school-related behaviors differ from the norm.

PROGRAM MANAGEMENT

Human Resources

The aging nursing work force, coupled with the fact that more and better-compensated careers have been opened to women, has led to a dangerous national nursing shortage. This is a serious issue with many complex causes and no readily evident, long-term solutions. Although inpatient health care settings are most affected, there ultimately will be a trickle-down effect into the schools. Therefore, school nurses need to collaborate with their colleagues on a state level to attack this enor-mous societal and professional dilemma. School nurses can play a major role in recruiting quality candidates into nursing through their influence with middle and high school students who are exploring potential careers.

With the escalating demands for health services in schools, the need for school nurses will only increase. Strategies that would help the school nursing community to attract qualified professionals include marketing the unique advantages of the specialty, promoting com-petitive compensation for its practitioners, and collaborating with institutions of higher education to ensure that undergraduate nurs-ing education can support effective practice in schools. Many parts of the country also may need to expand or implement tiered systems of care, such as differentiating staffing based on client need and educa-tional preparation of providers. Even if school nursing services were mandated and nurses were plentiful, nurses may be unwilling to work in schools if their role on the professional school team is not valued. Until there is pay equity with other health institutions where nurses work and are regarded as essential, this will remain an issue for schools. This situation goes beyond monetary factors to those of esteem and expectations. When nurses are on an equal playing field with education peers, there is a prevailing attitude of teamwork. This issue is directly connected to an attitude that health is critical to the learning process. When health is highly regarded, compensation normally follows.

School nurses should be compensated at the same level as their education peers with comparable professional preparation. Similarly, they should have the same increased professional preparation and continuing-education requirements. Although this is generally a local regulatory issue, states need to legislate school health services as provided by professional nurses to promote access to quality health services for all students.

As the health needs of students become more challenging, preserving safe levels of health care when the usual providers are absent becomes an important consideration. Although the liability associated with the performance of substitute health personnel is usually incurred by schools, as it is for substitute teachers, questions regarding substitutes remain to be answered.[4]

1. What type of substitute health services provider is required?

2. Should substitute type be decided individually by schools or the regular school nurse?

3. What are the minimum qualifications for a substitute?

4. To what extent is the school nurse or the school system required to orient, train, and supervise substitutes?

5. What are the legal ramifications for the regular school nurse and the school if an appropriate substitute is not secured?

The monetary reimbursement for substitute school nursing services directly affects availability. What schools are willing to pay is usually so poor that attracting qualified substitute nurses is virtually impossible. Increasing the rate of pay for substitutes would be less financially burdensome than contracting with nursing agencies to supply nurses. Until schools become competitive with other institutions employing nurses, this issue will remain.

Staffing Levels and Ratios

Staffing levels engender issues related to safety, accountability, and quality assurance. Determining school health staffing is generally a local function, although a few states have dictated ratios of nurses to students just as they do for teachers to students. Until school health services programs are mandated by states, ratios are meaningless.

NASN recommended ratios based on the type of educational programming students need, and *Healthy People 2010* articulated a goal of a 1:750 ratio of school nurse to students.[25] Nonetheless, these ratios do not consider the diverse models of service delivery, the use and supervision of paraprofessionals, the expanded role of school health services, or the increasing needs of students and families met through school programs. These ratios were developed nearly 30 years ago and may not be relevant to the current educational arena in which inclusion of all students is the norm.

School health nursing needs to develop more appropriate and safer ways to determine staffing requirements. One data-driven model that shows great promise is the School Health Intensity Rating Scale, which bases the allocation of resources on the functional needs of individual students.[26] Although this model needs more research to establish reliability for school nursing practice, it has the potential of producing a framework to create realistic and equitable staffing levels based on population differences. The use of this model or other comparable models is yet another reason to support the use of functional descriptors and standardized data sets within and across schools. The complexities related to appropriate staffing are critical issues that the professional organizations need to address with local and state school systems.

Supervision and Coordination

In far too many school districts, principals or central office personnel provide the only supervision and coordination for professional and unlicensed school personnel. This practice of supervision by non-nurse administrators continues despite the fact that many state nurse practice acts require nurses to be supervised by nurses capable of judging another nurse's clinical knowledge and skill. Non-nurse supervision of unlicensed personnel who carry out nursing activities also may be unlawful. Clearly, laypersons are not capable of directing or judging clinical nursing practice. Unquestionably, principals have important contributions to the appraisal of school nurses, but their expertise relates to nonclinical issues, such as cooperation, productivity, communication skills, team participation, and collaboration. Performance evaluations of school nurses are more valid if they are joint endeavors between principals and nursing supervisors.

School systems with the most stable and progressive school health programs are those with nursing managers to provide the judgment for clinical appraisal, quality assurance, and the infrastructure required for effective service delivery.[4] Still, even where there are school nurse managers, they often face unrealistic and unsafe supervisory ratios of 50 or more to 1. This is complicated by the fact that school nurses usually are spread out across the school district. Although this is a local policy issue, the state and national school nursing organizations and state boards of nursing could be instrumental in developing state regulations related to the supervision of nursing services in schools.

CONCLUSION

School nursing programs promote both the health and educational goals for school-age children and youth. Riding the current wave of the specialty's credibility, school nurses need to capture the opportunities afforded them. Increasing demands for services, in addition to students with complex health care needs in schools, require that antiquated paradigms be modified and perspectives broadened so the provision of services remains responsive to the changing needs of today's students. School nurses can solidify their role and practice by supporting their professional organizations, marketing their services, visibly connecting their programs to health and educational outcomes, and advancing their education and clinical expertise. State and national school nurse organizations should work to empower their members by promoting education and research, taking the leadership for professional issues, and promoting state and national partnerships to advance the specialty of school nursing. In Table 6.4, Costante summarizes strategies for addressing the challenges that will face school nursing in the future.[4(p505)] By working in concert toward mutual goals, school nurses and organizational leaders will strengthen the specialty, thereby improving the health and learning of America's school-age children.

Table 6.4   Future Challenges for School Health Nursing: Strategies for Advancing the Specialty.

Program Support

- Provide stable budgetary sources
- Commit health and education agencies' monetary support
- Access existing child health funds
- Lobby for attached monies to state and federal mandates
- Create new funding streams with partnerships
- Promote the legal entitlement basis for nursing services
- Expand contracting with third-party insurers
- Eliminate barriers between health and education
- Utilize grants to expand school nursing programs
- Prove that school nursing services make a difference
- Identify nursing programs that are key to positive outcomes
- Connect school nursing to health and education outcomes
- Document cost-effectiveness of school nursing services
- Develop and implement a national research agenda
- Research and fund effective health services programs
- Support increased electronic record keeping
- Facilitate and promote standard classification systems
- Standardize a minimum data set for school nursing
- Use computerized data to conduct research
- Expand the use of technology to access information

Partnerships

- Promote health and education agencies' collaboration
- Affirm health as vital to the education process
- Show positive education outcomes from school nursing
- Advance the role of school nurses in CSH programs
- Pilot telehealth in underserved school communities
- Describe students' strengths and needs in functional terms
- Secure schools' position as health care portal for children
- Deliver programs that support student success
- Promote school nursing's child health outcomes
- Collaborate with managed care organizations (MCOs)
- Foster regulations to merge MCOs and school services
- Promote SBHCs' access to health care funds
- Solidify operations between schools and SBHCs/SLHCs
- Approach cautiously privatized school health services
- Embrace school nurses from varied employment settings
- Forge new public and private partnerships

Table 6.4 Future Challenges for School Health Nursing: Strategies for Advancing the Specialty (*Continued*).

Professional and Practice Issues

- Define and standardize a unique set of health care services
- Determine the role of school health nursing in schools
- Establish practice-based clinical competencies
- Promote evidence-based practice
- Mandate baccalaureate entry level for school nurses
- Establish school-nurse-friendly RN to BS programs
- Promote national certification for school nurses
- Institute state certification for all school nurses
- Require advanced and continuing education for nurses
- Demand masters' preparation for nurse administrators
- Make school nurses equal members of the education team
- Provide school nurses pay parity with education staff
- Equate school nurses' job requisites with educators
- Consider subspecialties within school nursing
- Define and advocate nursing's role regarding genetic information
- Require nurse-only management of health care procedures
- Increase protection of health information in schools
- Disallow replacement of nurses by assistive personnel
- Enforce nurse-only delegation of nursing activities
- Enact standards for paraprofessionals
- Regulate the use of assistive personnel
- Augment health services using assistive personnel
- Ensure nursing as a related service for eligible students

Program Management

- Mandate qualified nurses for school health services
- Promote school nurses' leadership and management skills
- Establish safe, realistic staffing and supervisory levels
- Set appropriate, needs-based nurse-to-student ratios
- Strengthen infrastructures with nurse managers
- Market school health nursing as a desirable career
- Compete with other employers for quality nurses
- Increase requirements and pay for substitute nurses
- Define legal parameters for substitute health providers
- Resolve issues related to private-duty nurses
- Ensure funding for required one-to-one nursing services

Notes

1. Wold SJ. School health services: origins and trends. In: Schwab NC, Gelfman MHB, eds. *Legal Issues in School Health Services: A Resource for School Administrators, School Attorneys, and School Nurses.* North Branch, Minn: Sunrise River Press; 2001:7–54.

2. Cavendish R, Lunney M, Kraynyak B, Richardson K. National survey to identify the nursing interventions used in school settings. *J Sch Nurs.* 1999;152:14–21.

3. Individuals with Disabilities Education Act, 20 USC §1400 et seq; regulations at 34 CFR §300 (1997).

4. Costante CC. Future challenges for school health services and the law: a manager's perspective. In: Schwab NC, Gelfman MBH, eds. *Legal Issues in School Health Services: A Resource for School Administrators, School Attorneys, and School Nurses.* North Branch, Minn: Sunrise River Press; 2001:489–506.

5. Southern Regional Education Board. *Expected Competencies for Entry-Level Positions as School Nurses.* Atlanta, Ga: Southern Regional Education Board; 2000.

6. Poster EC, Marcontel M. School nursing role and competence. *J Sch Nurs.* 1999;152:34–42.

7. Rosswurm MA, Larrabee JH. A model for change to evidence-based practice. *Image.* 1999;31:317–322.

8. Farella C. Let's show 'em what we know. *Nurs Spectrum.* 2000;10(8DC): 26–27, 29.

9. Fryer GE, Igoe JB, Miyoshi TJ. Considering school health program screening services as a cost offset: a comparison of existing reimbursements in one state. *J Sch Nurs.* 1997;132:18–21.

10. Proctor SE. The educational preparation of school nurses: implications for hiring and liability protection. In: Schwab NC, Gelfman MHB, eds. *Legal Issues in School Health Services: A Resource for School Administrators, School Attorneys, and School Nurses.* North Branch, Minn: Sunrise River Press; 2001:473–482.

11. National Association of School Nurses. *The Professional School Nurse Roles and Responsibilities: Education, Certification, and Licensure* [position statement]. Scarborough, Maine: National Association of School Nurses; 1996.

12. National Nursing Coalition for School Health. School health nursing services: exploring national issues and priorities. *J Sch Health.* 1995;65: 369–389.

13. Proctor SE. Identifying a "critical mass" of specialty content for school nursing. *J Sch Nurs.* 1998;143:2–4.

14. Costante CC. Supporting student success: school nurses make a difference. *J Sch Nurs.* 1996;123:4–6.

15. Schwab NC, Hootman J, Gelfman MHB, Gregory E, Pohlman KJ. School nursing practice: professional performance issues. In: Schwab NC, Gelfman MHB, eds. *Legal Issues in School Health Services: A Resource for School Administrators, School Attorneys, and School Nurses.* North Branch, Minn: Sunrise River Press; 2001:123–165.

16. Hootman J, Schwab NC, Gelfman MHB, Gregory E, Pohlman KJ. School nursing practice: clinical performance issues. In: Schwab NC, Gelfman MHB, eds. *Legal Issues in School Health Services: A Resource for School Administrators, School Attorneys, and School Nurses.* North Branch, Minn: Sunrise River Press; 2001:167–230.

17. National Association of School Nurses. *Delegation* [position statement]. Scarborough, Maine: National Association of School Nurses; 1995.

18. National Association of State School Nurse Consultants. *Delegation of School Health Services to Unlicensed Assistive Personnel* [position paper]. Kent, Ohio: National Association of State School Nurse Consultants; 1995.

19. Rehabilitation Act of 1973, sec 504, 29 USC §794; regulations at 34 CFR §104 (1973).

20. Gelfman MHB, Schwab NC. Discrimination in school: section 504, ADA, and title IX. In: Schwab NC, Gelfman MHB, eds. *Legal Issues in School Health Services: A Resource for School Administrators, School Attorneys, and School Nurses.* North Branch, Minn: Sunrise River Press; 2001:335–371.

21. Cedar Rapids Community School District v. Garret F. 119 SCt 992, 29 IDELR 966(US 1999).

22. Fibison W. Future directions: the genetic revolution. In: Schwab NC, Gelfman MHB, eds. *Legal Issues in School Health Services: A Resource for School Administrators, School Attorneys, and School Nurses.* North Branch, Minn: Sunrise River Press; 2001:483–488.

23. Smalley SL. Genetic influences in childhood-onset psychiatric disorders: autism and attention-deficit/hyperactivity disorder. *Am J Hum Genet.* 1997;60:1276–1282.

24. National Association of School Nurses. *Caseload Assignments* [position statement]. Scarborough, Maine: National Association of School Nurses; 1995.

26. Klahn JK, Hays BJ, Iverson CJ. The school health intensity rating scale. *J Sch Nurs.* 1998;144:23–28.

25. US Department of Health and Human Services. *Healthy People 2010: Understanding and Improving Health.* Washington, DC: Public Health Service; 2000.

CHAPTER 7

The Importance of Research to School Nurses and School Nursing Practice

Janis Hootman, 2002

⸺∿⸺ T he essence of a discipline is its body of scientific knowledge, its system of values and ethics, and its societal worth. Evidence from research helps formulate this core intelligence. Nursing's contributions to client outcomes have had limited exploration. Historically, nursing has described itself in terms of diseases and medical conditions. Florence Nightingale stated that the elements of nursing were unknown.[1] In 1981, Wold and Dagg reported that there was a deficit of school nursing research.[2] This was a time of poor economy in the United States, and without grounded evidence of what school nursing contributed to children's health, the positioning and funding of school nursing was challenged. Fortunately, with this awareness began increased participation in research by school nurses enrolled in graduate studies. Today it is a myth that there is no school nursing

Table 7.1   Standards of Professional School Nursing Practice.[4]

Standards of Care	Standards of Professional Performance
I. Assessment	I. Quality of care
II. Diagnosis	II. Performance appraisal
III. Outcome identification	III. Education
IV. Planning	IV. Collegiality
V. Implementation	V. Ethics
VI. Evaluation	VI. Collaboration
	VII. Research
	VIII. Resource utilization
	IX. Communication
	X. Program management
	XI. Health education

research. Proctor emphasized that there is not a scarcity of school nursing research but rather a gap in the focus of research.[3] The void is absent data about the effectiveness of school nursing interventions.

Increasingly schools are expected to intervene as today's youth have decreasing access to health care and changing morbidities from physical disease to behavioral conditions. Yet insufficient funding continues to plague school districts. Consequently, difficult decisions are being made about positions for school nurses. The time is ripe for policy development regarding the infrastructure and funding for school health and school nursing services. It is time for nurses to describe what they diagnose and treat in school communities and to detail the outcomes of their practice. It is essential that school nursing prioritize the studies needed to obtain sufficient information for imminent decision making and clinical application. One example of an imminent need is a study on the impact of implementing the ratio of 1 school nurse for every 750 students.

So important to clinical practice is the conduct and application of research that it is specified in the *Standards of Professional School Nursing Performance* of the National Association of School Nurses (NASN),[4] (see Table 7.1) and also in the American Nurses Association's *Standards of Clinical Nursing Practice* for the profession of nursing.[5]

Not only do these standards establish professional accountabilities, they also communicate to others the professional roles of the nurse. Every practicing school nurse needs to have a copy of these standards and review them regularly. Research is essential to the advancement of children's health and the practice of school nursing; therefore,

**Table 7.2   National Association of School Nurses (NASN) Support
for School Nursing Research.**

1994	Participated in national meeting sponsored by the National Nursing Coalition for School Health in collaboration with the Division of Adolescent and School Health. National issues and priorities for school nursing services were identified with a commitment made to delineate the school nurse's contribution to the health and education of children and to develop the infrastructure (standards of care, training, finances) that would advance the role of school nurses.[6]
1996	Participated in the School Health Nursing Services Progress Review. Progress was monitored with respect to the 1994 commitments, and goals were formulated to advance the practice of school nursing and secure funding, including conducting research about school health nursing services. Collaborated with the American School Health Association in conducting a focus group to establish a research agenda for school nursing. Twenty individuals representing clinicians, nurse educators, school health services consultants from State departments of education and health, nurse administrators, and researchers participated and proposed questions for school nursing research.[7]
1997	NASN's Research Committee sponsored a data summit to initiate strategies for adequate data collection on school nursing practice, its cost-effectiveness, and the quality and outcomes from school nursing services on student health and academic success. Attending were school nursing scholars and experts in school nursing legal issues, nursing languages, research, information technology, school nursing standards and documentation, and representatives of State departments of health and education. Recommendations were made to NASN's Standards of Practice, Research, and Conference Committees to provide training for clinicians about using standardized languages and the need for a minimum school nursing data set.
1999	Participated in the Invitational Summit Meeting to develop a school nursing research agenda. NASN initiated an endowment funding stream for school nursing research.
2000	Identified obesity and access to care as the priorities for focused research in the coming year.

NASN has made it a priority to create a supportive culture that promotes school nursing research. Table 7.2 presents a historical overview of some research efforts of NASN over the past decade.

RESEARCH AND SCHOOL NURSING PRACTICE

Research is complex in nature, involving multiple fields of knowledge, such as ethics, conceptual and theoretical frameworks, and research design. School nursing practice is likewise complex. Primarily, school nurses treat children 5 to 18 years old, a wide age span with many developmental milestones and the potential for many varied health problems. Students entitled to special education services can be enrolled through their 21st year. With the advances in medical technology, increasing numbers of students have special health care needs that must be addressed during the school day. School nursing roles vary from comprehensive direct service provider to consultant. It also requires collegiality with multiple disciplines such as education, social services, medicine, and public health as well as with families and the community at large. Consequently, school nursing practice demands a broad knowledge base to meet students' health needs and to work effectively with the multiple school and community team members.

The research needed to provide the best school nursing practice will grow in the next few years. Sharing research responsibilities with others vested in the outcomes of school health services can help manage the workload, increase the breadth and depth of investigation, and share more evenly the associated expenses. Respectful of the value from partnerships in school nursing research, in 1999 NASN participated with the National Center for School Health Nursing and the National Nursing Coalition for School Health in a Research Summit to frame a school nursing research agenda.

Who are these partners? The National Center for School Health Nursing began within the American Nurse Foundation in 1996 to advance excellence in school health nursing practice. The center's desired outcome is to optimize the health and learning of all children and youth. Initial funding of the center was provided by the Centers for Disease Control and Prevention, Division of Child and Adolescent Health (CDC/DASH). The National Nursing Coalition for School Health functions as the advisory board for the National Center for School Health Nursing. The coalition strives to promote collaboration of specialty nursing organizations whose focus is the improvement of the health and learning of the nation's children. Coalition partners include the National Association of School Nursing, American School Heath Association, National Association of State School Nurse Consultants, American Public Health Association, National Association of Pediatric Advanced Nurse Practitioners, and the American Nurses Association.

THE RESEARCH SUMMIT MEETING

The goal of the research summit meeting was to frame a research agenda that would guide school nursing in meeting the health needs of America's youth. Table 7.3 describes the most significant and preventable health threats for the nation, including its youth. NASN is aware that without a sense of direction provided by a research agenda, school nursing practice and school health policy and funding will be driven by crisis and will never attain focused work on health promotion, disease prevention, and coordination of services.

At the March 1999 meeting, 24 leaders in school nursing and nursing research met together to frame a research agenda for school nursing. Although needs and issues were identified and are described more completely below, the goal of developing a comprehensive framework was not reached. This should not discourage respect for the information that was generated at this meeting, however. The major outcome was the identification that school nurses need to be (1) informed about research, (2) supportive of research, and (3) active participants in conducting and using research. The standards of care for school nurses reinforces this accountability. Brainerd and Igoe[9] published a comprehensive report on the 1999 Research Summit.

Be Informed About Research

The *Standards of Professional School Nursing Practice: Applications in the Field* clearly frame information responsibilities regarding research.[10] School nurses must be lifelong learners. They must regularly read professional school nursing journals and other related professional literature to be informed about practice issues, including new research findings. School nurses are vulnerable for substandard or negligent practice if they are not using evidence-based information to guide their practice.

Table 7.3   Health Promotion and Disease Prevention Agenda for the United States.[8]

• Physical activity	• Mental health
• Overweight and obesity	• Injury and violence
• Tobacco use	• Environmental quality
• Substance abuse	• Immunization
• Responsible sexual behavior	• Access to health care.

In addition, it is important to be a member of professional specialty organizations, such as NASN. Membership benefits include access to current research and practice information as well as having a venue for contributing to the specialty's body of knowledge and practice standards. Other options for accessing research information include the Internet, academic programs offered through NASN, state and local conferences, continuing and university education programs, study groups with professional colleagues, and consultation with practice experts. Before school nurses can read and use research, however, they must know how to critique research reports. This skill is taught in courses on research. Such courses are generally part of the curriculum in baccalaureate and master's degree programs in nursing.

Being informed also includes having awareness of the information that came from the 1999 Research Summit discussion. Themes that emerged from the meeting were the following:

1. School nurses need to be part of research teams and must improve their research competencies to be knowledgeable contributors.

2. Partnerships are valuable to effectively conduct comprehensive school nursing research.

3. A common language and standardized data collection methods are essential to facilitate understanding and comparison of research findings.

4. Determining the outcomes of school nursing interventions must be a priority focus in forthcoming research to identify the impact of school nursing on children's health and academic success.

Be Supportive of Research

School nurses must be more than simply informed about research. The Research Summit urged school nurses to be supportive of research. This calls for a personal, proactive, professional, and philosophical framework about and involvement with research. To provide the most effective interventions for children's health and academic outcomes, school nurses must be supportive of, advocate for, and participate in studies regarding school health services and the role of school nurses in providing these services. Research must always be in the budget to facilitate quality school nursing services, improved funding appropriations, and supportive school nursing policy development. Today everyone is feeling the pinch of limited time and resources. Rather than saying "I can't make time," however, each school nurse must put a high priority on research. Ideally this includes direct individual participation through personal investigations, completion of research surveys, or facilitating investigation sites. If this is not possible, an indirect personal contribution through financial contributions or identifying study questions is showing support for school nursing research.

Be an Active Participant in Conducting and Using Research

It is in school nurses' best interest to be involved in research, or others will do the work and leave school nursing out of school health services. A core data set for school nursing will help collect similar information and facilitate a more accurate description of school nursing's body of knowledge and treatment outcomes, allowing comparisons with other care providers. NASN is in the process of developing a core of data elements. The American Nurses Association adopted a minimum data set in 1988 (see Table 7.4).[11(pp402–403)] A Nursing Minimum Data Set for School Nurses will provide the structure needed for documentation and research about school nursing services.

Table 7.4   Nursing Minimum Data Set (NMDS).

Nursing Care Elements	Client Demographic Elements	Service Elements
• Nursing diagnosis • Nursing intervention • Nursing outcome • Intensity of nursing care	• Personal identification • Date of birth • Gender • Race and ethnicity • Residence	• Unique facility or service agency number • Unique health record number of client • Unique number of principal registered nurse provider • Episode admission or encounter date • Discharge or termination date • Disposition of client • Expected payer

School nurses can participate in research by

1. Demanding that software vendors provide the minimum data elements and standardized language in their software packages.
2. Identifying research questions that need to be studied and giving input into prioritization of these studies.
3. Forwarding research suggestions and needs to national, state, and local research committees.
4. Finding resources, such as schools of nursing, graduate programs, or expert clinicians, that can provide mentorship or assistance in developing research or practice improvement projects.
5. Tabulating data.
6. Disseminating research results.
7. Submitting findings in a manuscript submitted for publication to *The Journal of School Nursing*; if necessary, seeking out a mentor or contacting the journal editor for information about how to draft a manuscript.
8. Continuously seeking updated research information and using that research to direct clinical practice.
9. Financially supporting local, state, and NASN foundations that fund school nursing research.
10. Supporting peers when they ask for assistance with special projects.

Every school nurse has a significant contribution to make to the research base needed for quality, up-to-date school nursing practice.

SCHOOL-COMMUNITY PARTNERSHIPS

The demands for school health services are increasing. Factors influencing the increase include (a) changing morbidities in youth (e.g., increasing tobacco use by children, childhood obesity, and behavioral and mood disorders), (b) challenges to health care access (e.g., increasing costs and disarray in the health care system), and (c) changing populations and correlating social and health care needs (e.g., immigrants and family structures that are impacted by divorce and remarriage). School nursing cannot be all things to everyone. Tustin advised school nurses to seek partners and leverage the power and effectiveness of collaboration.[12] This includes the work of research. Research is essential to identify effective interventions that address factors influencing student health. Education is struggling with inadequate financial resources for funding sufficient school support services, including school nursing. Community partners may be an untapped resource for increasing funding for support services and research.

School nurses need to partner with other social service and health care providers as well as educators to compile outcome research data. Kibel described the historical challenge of social and health programs in proving worth in terms of outcomes.[13] He described the complexity of health interventions, including the multiple services and goals, customized and modified service models, multiple providers, outside influences, and the need for student or parental participation. In addition, Kibel articulated the difficulty in linking these health services to outcomes in a quantifiable way. He stated that nurses are more than "fix it/cure it" providers.[13] A pill or one piece of information generally does not relieve the problems confronting today's students.

In partnerships, others may be better positioned to conduct the research, allowing school nurses to assume a greater responsibility with coordination, management, and clinical services. Other potential benefits from partnerships in conducting school nurse research include

1. A broader experiential and knowledge base to draw on when multiple disciplines are participating.

2. Increased scrutiny and evaluation of data when involving a variety of analysts having different professional interests and backgrounds.

3. Increased human resources to share the work.

4. Advocacy for sufficient resources when outside systems become better informed about students' treatment needs.

School nurses can help frame the research questions to study and facilitate access to the students and school communities. Some examples of timely research questions are the following: What is the role of the school nurse in violence prevention? What health screenings should be offered in school communities? What is the most effective model for providing immunizations to students? and Do school-based services decrease utilization of emergency care facilities?

It is important that school nurses build and participate in appropriate partnerships. Consider who is in the community that may help with the needed research implementation and its funding—an evaluation specialist in the building, a local health care system, a research program in a local university, or a philanthropic organization that funds research and best practice programs. School nurses have the experience and positioning to make partnerships happen. They have skills in relationship building, an essential ingredient in successful partnerships. School nurses are the providers of health services in schools and often function as the coordinator of the school health services program. There are an estimated 56,000 school nurses within the 88,000 schools in the United States.[14] Because school nurses have daily access to many of the 50 million U.S. children in school,[15] they are in an influential position to positively impact the health of the nation's youth. School nurses not only contribute significant information about students' health issues, they also can be leaders in their school communities for initiating changes in the milieu and services provided.

With this strategic positioning, there is accountability to support youth by connecting their health and education outcomes. Important research questions regarding this linkage include the following: What process is most effective in providing self-sufficiency learning for managing chronic conditions such as asthma, spina bifida, or diabetes? What is the most effective model for improving attendance? and What is the most important hearing assessment model to improve phonetic learning? School nurses must seek out alliances that are dedicated to doing research that promotes evidence-based practice. The goal of such alliances should be to enhance the well-being of today's youth rather than promoting special interests of individuals or groups. By speaking to the mutuality of partners' vision statements and program objectives, partners maintain a common focus for their work.[16]

As with client relationships, partnerships between agencies take active listening, support, and time. A sense of trust must develop in agency partnerships before one can expect information sharing and a request for help to be honored. Cavanaugh suggested community partners observe, listen to, and learn the host system's rules and language, go slowly, be flexible, follow through, and find a buddy.[17] Partnerships require meticulous communication skills and clear direction about such issues as the boundaries of authority and participants' roles and responsibilities. Contracts should be developed to facilitate clear communication among involved persons about process and outcome expectations. Concerns regarding informed consent, privacy, and the protection of data about students need to be addressed. Legal counsel can best guide school nurses about appropriate contractual language.

SCHOOL NURSE DOCUMENTATION

Documentation is crucial to validating the care provided by school nurses and providing data about school nursing practice. It should include information about student health issues, assessment data, nursing diagnoses, outcomes, goals, and interventions. Questions of current interest that documentation can answer include the following: What are the student health issues? What nursing interventions have the best outcomes for student health needs? and What nursing interventions promote student academic success? All school nurses must become proficient at collecting and reporting data about the health issues in school communities and developing a plan to measure the outcomes of school nursing interventions. "If you are not in the database, you don't exist" (M. Hasset, personal communication, March 7, 1998). This demands that school nurses have a standardized language or vocabulary to describe or name data and a standardized method to collect data. Without them, it is impossible to make accurate descriptions or comparisons about issues and outcomes.

The North American Nursing Diagnosis Association (NANDA) began developing the first nursing language in 1973. Nursing diagnoses are clinical judgements "about individual, family, or community responses to actual or potential health problems/life processes."[18(p245)] In 1994, NASN adopted and reaffirmed in 2000 a position statement supporting the use of NANDA's classification system to advance a uniform diagnostic terminology for school nursing practice.[20] The success of the specialty's ability to describe the health problems that school nurses diagnose and treat depends on all its clinicians using NANDA language.

Physicians know through ongoing research which procedures and medications are most effective, safe, and cost-effective for their patients. So, too, should school nurses be able to describe the interventions that are most effective, safe, and cost-effective in treating student health problems presenting at school; they should also be aware of which interventions have the greatest impact on academic success. Two newer standardized languages are also important to school nursing: the *Nursing Interventions Classification* (NIC)[20] and the *Nursing Outcomes Classification* (NOC).[21] NIC includes a wide scope of interventions used by professional nurses. NOC provides a mechanism to measure the effectiveness or outcomes of nursing interventions. Both languages standardize the descriptive data gathered about school nursing services. All three languages—NANDA, NIC, and NOC—will assist in the documentation of the nursing process to which all nurses are accountable as stated in the *Standards of Professional School Nursing Practice.* Research has identified a core list of interventions in specialty areas. The school nursing core is listed in NIC.[22(p823)] More work needs to be done to better describe the scope of school nursing practice, its complexity, and the intensity of time and services that are necessary to successfully address student health needs.

The drive for outcome data comes from many sources, including school administrators, funders, policy makers, and the health and education systems, because there are increasing demands for limited resources and high expectations for effective services. Driving questions include the following: What is working and why? What contributes to successful programs? and Are the expenditures of time and money making a difference? If school nursing cannot answer these questions, funding likely will not be invested for their services. In addition, there is an increasing demand for reliable, evidence-based information to make decisions about best practices, effective utilization of resources, and the impact of nursing services on student academic success. The NOC will help school nurses tabulate and analyze the effectiveness of nursing interventions on student health.

School nurses can and should help frame questions that may provide better outcome measures for correlating nursing interventions with academic success. Consider the following:

1. After counseling with the school nurse about asthma medication management, did the student have fewer requests to leave physical education class and have increased participation in activities?

2. After the school nurse's review with the prescribing neurologist about the medication dose, did the student experience fewer seizures and was the student able to more completely participate in class discussions and have improved math scores and reading comprehension?

3. After starting a midmorning nutrition snack program, did students have improved math and spelling scores in late morning testing?

SUMMARY

Technological advances, changing social and population conditions, and legislative mandates require schools to respond to and manage a wide range of children's special health needs. These include chronic, acute, and emergent physiological conditions as well as emotional problems. In addition, schools are expected to provide a healthy environment, disease and injury prevention services, as well as health promotion activities. Sadly, funding resources for school health services and school nursing are in competition with educational reform activities. Consequently, difficult questions about the contributions of school nursing are being asked. School nurses recognize the importance of research in providing answers about the effectiveness of its interventions on students' health and educational outcomes. NASN has made concerted efforts to provide an infrastructure for school nursing research. School nurses must be informed about, use, support, and be involved in school nursing research to strengthen their ability to respond to student health needs. All school nurses must move toward research-based practice, and they must begin today.

Notes

1. Nightingale F. *Notes on Nursing.* New York, NY: Dover; 1969. Original work published 1859.
2. Wold SJ, Dagg N. *School Nursing: A Framework for Practice.* North Branch, Minn: Sunrise River Press; 1981.
3. Proctor SE. Undergirding issues: a response to "Call to Action." In: Brainerd E, Igoe JB, eds. *Health of America's Children at School: Developing a Nursing Research Agenda.* Proceedings of the Invitational Summit Meeting, March 1999. Washington, DC: American Nurses Foundation; 2000:9–10.
4. National Association of School Nurses. *Standards of Professional School Nursing Practice.* Scarborough, Maine: National Association of School Nurses; 1998.
5. American Nurses Association. *Standards of Clinical Nursing Practice.* 2nd ed. Washington, DC: American Nurses Publishing; 1998.
6. Henry SB. A nursing informatics approach for addressing national issues and priorities for school nursing services. *J Sch Nurs.* 1997;124:39–42.
7. Bradley B. Establishing a research agenda for school nursing. *J Sch Nurs.* 1998;141:4–13.
8. US Department of Health and Human Services. *Healthy People 2010: Understanding and Improving Health.* Washington, DC: Public Health Service; 2000.
9. Brainerd E, Igoe JB, eds. *Health of America's Children at School: Developing a Nursing Research Agenda.* Proceedings of the Invitational Summit Meeting, March 1999. Washington, DC: American Nurses Foundation; 2000.

10. Lordi SL, Bradley B. *Standards of Professional School Nursing Practice: Applications in the Field.* Scarborough, Maine: National Association of School Nurses; 2000.

11. Werley HH, Lang NM, eds. *Identification of the Nursing Minimum Data Set.* New York, NY: Springer; 1988.

12. Tustin J. Building bridges. *J Sch Nurs.* 1999;15(3):6–7.

13. Kibel B. The push for outcomes: using client success stories as hard evaluation data. *Georgia Academic Journal.* Spring 1998:12–15.

14. National Center for Education Statistics. *Digest of Education Statistics.* Washington, DC: US Department of Health and Human Services; 1998.

15. Guiden M. Children's health collaboration [Web page]. Washington, DC: Center for Health and Health Care in Schools; 2000. Available at: http://www.gwu.edu/~mtg/sbhcs/collaboration.htm. Accessed December 14, 2000.

16. Hootman J, Houck GM, King MC. School health services: a review. In: Brainerd E, Igoe JB, eds. *Health of America's Children at School: Developing a Nursing Research Agenda.* Proceedings of the Invitational Summit Meeting, March 1999. Washington, DC: American Nurses Foundation; 2000:31–44.

17. Cavanaugh S. Tips for partnering with outside agencies. In-service presentation to Portland Public School and other agency staff participating in Safe Schools Project and implementation of multidisciplinary assessment teams. 2000.

18. North American Nursing Diagnosis Association. *Nursing Diagnoses: Definitions and Classification, 2001–2002.* Philadelphia, Pa: North American Nursing Diagnosis Association; 2001.

19. National Association of School Nurses. *Nursing Diagnosis* [position statement]. Scarborough, Maine: National Association of School Nurses; 2000.

20. McCloskey JC, Bulecheck GM, eds. *Nursing Interventions Classification.* 3rd ed. St Louis, MO: Mosby; 2000.

21. Johnson M, Maas M, Moorhead S, eds. *Nursing Outcomes Classification (NOC).* 2nd ed. St Louis, MO: Mosby; 2000.

Grant Report Summary from the Robert Wood Johnson Foundation

STUDY OF POTENTIAL COLLABORATIONS OF MANAGED CARE ORGANIZATIONS AND SCHOOL HEALTH SERVICES

(last updated February 2000)

This grant funded a project that examined the potential collaboration of managed care organizations and school health services. It was developed by the National Association of School Nurses (NASN), in cooperation with the American School Health Association (ASHA) and with the participation of the Academy of Pediatrics (AAP). The major activity was a symposium held in September 1997 in Alexandria, Virginia. Attended by recognized experts in the fields of school health and managed care, the symposium created a dialogue and reached a consensus that there is a mutual benefit in the collaboration of managed care and school health. An article based on the proceedings of the symposium was published in the *Journal of School Nursing* in October 1998.

School Health: Rationale, Structure, and Promise

Reprints of Key Reports and Articles

CHAPTER 8

Schools and Health:
Our Nation's Investment
Executive Summary

Institute of Medicine Committee on Comprehensive
School Health Programs in Grades K–12
Diane D. Allensworth and James H. Wyche, Cochairs, 1997

S chools have been the site for health programming in
the United States since the early colonial period. When public education became compulsory in the mid-nineteenth century, the strategic
role that schools could play in promoting and protecting health
became recognized; schools soon became the front line in the fight
against infectious disease and the hub for providing a wide range of
health and social services for children and families.

As times changed, school health programs have changed to keep
pace with the changing needs of children and adolescents. The Centers
for Disease Control and Prevention (CDC) has noted that six categories
of behavior are responsible for 70 percent of adolescent mortality and
morbidity: unintentional and intentional injuries, drug and alcohol
abuse, sexually transmitted diseases and unintended pregnancies,

---

This chapter was originally issued as a report by the Institute of Medicine.
Edited by Allensworth DD, Lawson E, Nicholson L, Wyche JH. *Schools and
health: our nation's investment. Executive summary of the report of the Committee on Comprehensive School Health Programs in Grades K–12.* Washington, DC: Institute of Medicine; 1997.

diseases associated with tobacco use, illnesses resulting from inadequate physical activity, and health problems due to inadequate dietary patterns. A significant segment of our nation's youth is at risk for dropping out of school as a consequence of a broad range of health and behavioral problems; further, many children do not have access to basic preventive and primary care.

The concept of a comprehensive school health program (CSHP) was proposed in the 1980s to address many of the health-related problems of today's children and young people.[1] CSHPs are intended to take advantage of the pivotal position of schools in reaching children and families by combining—in an integrated, systemic manner—health education, health promotion and disease prevention, and access to health-related services at the school site. CSHPs may be a promising way both to improve health and educational outcomes for students and to reduce overall health care costs by emphasizing prevention and easy access to care.

The original charge to the committee was to: (1) assess the status of CSHPs; (2) examine what factors appear to predict success (or failure) of these programs; and if appropriate, (3) identify strategies for wider implementation of such programs. This charge was refined by the committee at its first meeting to better describe the scope of work to be undertaken. The revised charge states that the committee will develop a framework for (1) determining the desirable and feasible health outcomes of CSHPs; (2) examining the relationship between health outcomes and education outcomes; (3) considering what factors are necessary in the school setting to optimize these outcomes; (4) appraising existing data on the effectiveness (including the cost-effectiveness) of CSHPs; and (5) if appropriate, recommending mechanisms for wider implementation of those school health programs that have proven to be effective.

Early in the course of the study, the committee established its own working definition of a CSHP as follows:

> A comprehensive school health program is an integrated set of planned, sequential, school-affiliated strategies, activities, and services designed to promote the optimal physical, emotional, social, and educational development of students. The program involves and is supportive of families and is determined by the local community, based on community needs, resources, standards, and requirements. It is coordinated by a multidisciplinary team and accountable to the community for program quality and effectiveness.

In developing this definition, the committee examined a variety of models and definitions of school health programs. However, whatever the program model, the committee found that there are three critical areas that should be considered in designing a CSHP.

The first critical area is the **school environment,** which includes (1) the *physical environment,* involving proper building design, lighting, ventilation, safety, cleanliness, freedom from environmental hazards that foster infection and handicaps, safe transportation policies, and having emergency plans in place; (2) the *policy and administrative environment,* consisting of policies to promote health and reduce stress, and regulations ensuring an environment free from tobacco, drugs, weapons, and violence; (3) the *psychosocial environment,* including a supportive and nurturing atmosphere, a cooperative academic setting, respect for individual differences, and involvement of families; and (4) *health promotion for staff,* in order that staff members can become positive role models and increase their commitment to student health.

The second critical area is **education,** which consists of *physical education,* which teaches the knowledge and skills necessary for lifelong physical fitness; *health education,* which addresses the physical, mental, emotional, and social dimensions of health; and *other curricular areas,* which promote healthful behavior and an awareness of health issues as part of their core instruction.

The third critical area is **services,** which includes *health services,* that depend on the needs and preferences of the community and services for students with disabilities and special health care needs; *counseling, psychological, and social services,* which promote academic success and address the emotional and mental health needs of students; and *nutrition and foodservices,* which provide nutritious meals, nutrition education, and a nutrition-promoting school environment.

Three of the most common models examined include the following:

1. **The Three-Component Model:** This is the traditional model for CSHPs. According to this model, the three essential components of a school health program are health education, health services, and a healthful environment.

2. **The Eight-Component Model:** According to this model, the eight essential components of a CSHP are health education, physical education, health services, nutrition services, health promotion for school staff, counseling and psychological services, a healthy school environment, and parent and community involvement.

3. **Full-Service Schools:** In addition to quality education, these combine a wide range of health services, mental health services, and family welfare and social services for students and their families.

The committee determined that the most frequently encountered models and definitions for school health programs had much in common and that no single model was best. CSHPs must be locally tailored—with the involvement of all critical stakeholders—to meet each community's needs, resources, perspectives, and standards.

FINDINGS, CONCLUSIONS, AND RECOMMENDATIONS

The committee examined four topics of school health in depth: education, services, infrastructure, and research and evaluation. The principal findings, conclusions, and recommendations pertaining to each area are presented in the remainder of this section.

EDUCATION
Findings and Conclusions

The status of the two curricular components of a CSHP—physical education and health education—is sometimes questioned because they were not originally mentioned in the National Education Goals as "core subjects" in which students should demonstrate competence. However, with each updated report, the National Education Goals panel has added language emphasizing the importance of physical education and health education, affirming that these two subjects should be an integral part of the school curriculum.

Physical Education

Research has confirmed a direct relationship between a physically active life-style and improved long-term health status. Therefore, the new generation of physical education programs is shifting emphasis from competitive sports to physical activity and fitness. Three recent documents—the National Standards for Physical Education, the School Health Policies and Programs Study[2] (SHPPS), and the CDC's Guidelines for School and Community Health Programs to Promote Physical Activity Among Youth—emphasize the new priorities and recommendations in physical education and collectively provide a sound basis for developing quality physical education programs in the future. The committee supports these recommendations.

Health Education

The traditional health education curriculum has been based on 10 conceptual areas identified by the School Health Education Study of the 1960s: community health, consumer health, environmental health, family life, mental and emotional health, injury prevention and safety, nutrition, personal health, prevention and control of disease, and substance use and abuse. Recently, CDC recommended that the six major contributors to adolescent mortality and morbidity mentioned earlier be priority areas of emphasis for health education because these problems are based in behaviors that can be prevented or changed. The overarching goal of the recently released National Health Education Standards is the development of health literacy—the capacity to obtain, interpret, and understand basic health information and services and the competence to use such information and services to enhance health.

Research conducted since 1970 has shown that specific health education curricula are effective, for example, those focused on categorical problems such as tobacco avoidance. Studies have shown that in order for health education to produce behavior change, effective strategies, considerable instructional time, and well-prepared teachers are required. Students' behavioral decisions are also heavily influenced by environmental variables—peers, family, schools, community, and the media. A recent cost-benefit analysis shows that school health education is cost-effective, and several recent national surveys indicate that parents and students overwhelmingly consider health education to be very important and useful.

Despite the potential effectiveness and favorable perception of health education, SHPPS found a considerable gap between what health educators consider to be desired practice and actual current practice. Typically, only one semester of health education is required at the middle or junior high level and one semester at the high school level, and the attention given to certain priority topics falls considerably short of recommended goals. Although most teachers of health education have not majored in the field, there is not an overwhelming demand for staff development. This lack of demand may be due to a lack of awareness on the part of teachers and administrators of the potential and complexities of health education or the fact that teachers with majors in other fields prefer to teach in those fields and see no value in improving their skills in health education.

Recommendations

The committee believes that three recently released documents—the National Action Plan for Comprehensive School Health Education, the National Health Education Standards, and the SHPPS report—collectively provide comprehensive recommendations and a strong framework to move health education forward in the future. Beyond this, however, several aspects of health education merit further emphasis and discussion.

The committee believes that the period prior to high school is the most crucial for shaping attitudes and behaviors. By the time students reach high school, many are already engaging in risky behaviors or may at least have formed accepting attitudes toward these behaviors.

> *The committee recommends that all students receive sequential, age-appropriate health education every year during the elementary and middle or junior high grades.*

At all grade levels, instruction should focus on achieving the performance indicators outlined in the National Health Education Standards. Early years might focus on such topics as nutrition and safety, but beginning at the late elementary or early middle school grades, instruction should shift focus to an intensive, age-appropriate emphasis on the CDC priority behaviors and should be provided by teachers who understand early adolescents and are especially prepared to deal with these sensitive and difficult topics.

> *The committee recommends that a one-semester health education course at the secondary level immediately become a minimum requirement for high school graduation. Instruction should follow the National Health Education Standards, use effective up-to-date curricula, be provided by qualified health education teachers interested in teaching the subject, and emphasize the six priority behavioral areas identified by the CDC.*

According to SHPPS, 83.9 percent of all senior high schools already require at least one semester of health education, and within this 83.9 percent, the CDC topics are frequently emphasized. Thus, such an immediate requirement is not unrealistic. Additional courses or electives in health education at the high school level would be preferable to a single semester.

The committee debated how to reconcile the call for students to receive health education every year, from kindergarten through the twelfth grade, with the reality of the crowded curriculum at the secondary level and decided that the critical issue should be whether high school students achieve the performance indicators described in the National Health Education Standards, not the amount of "seat time." Thus, the committee recommends that the "seat time" be a minimum of at least one semester, but that student health knowledge and understanding be assessed at the end of this course. If a community finds its young people falling short on this assessment, the existing course must be improved or additional courses instituted. The committee believes that some form of health education must occur every year at the secondary level but that some of this education can take place through alternative approaches, such as "booster" sessions, health modules in other courses, field trips, assemblies, school-wide campaigns, after-school peer discussion groups, and one-on-one or small group counseling for students with identified needs.

Effective elementary health education is the foundation for the future critical middle school years, and well-prepared elementary teachers are the key for providing this education.

> *The committee recommends that all elementary teachers receive substantive preparation in health education content and methodology during their preservice college training. This preparation should give elementary generalist teachers strategies for infusing health instruction into the curriculum and prepare upper elementary teachers to lay the groundwork for the intensive middle or junior high health education program.*

SERVICES
Findings and Conclusions

Although the scope of school health services varies from one school district to another, many common elements exist throughout the country. Most schools provide screenings, monitor student immunization status, and administer first aid and medication. Schools are also required to provide a wide range of health services for students with disabilities and special health care needs.

There is agreement among virtually all school districts that a core set of services is needed in schools, but the topic currently generating a great deal of discussion is the role of the school in providing access to "extended services" that go beyond traditional basic services, such as primary care, social, and family services. The committee believes that extended services should not be the sole—or even the major—responsibility of the schools; instead, the school should be considered by other community agencies and providers as a partner and a potentially effective site for provision of needed services—services that will ultimately advance the primary academic mission of the school.

Although the demands and complexity of basic school services have increased, these services are often supervised by education-based administrators who have no clinical preparation in the delivery of health services. Thus, it is important to develop closer links between the school and community health systems and to encourage greater involvement of community health care professionals in the planning and implementation of basic services. School-based health centers (SBHCs) and other extended services are a relatively new phenomenon, and research in this area is in its early stages. Studies have shown that SBHCs provide access to care for needy students and increase students' health knowledge significantly. However, it has been difficult to measure the impact of SBHCs on students' health status or high-risk behavior, such as sexual activity or drug use. This is consistent, however, with other interventions to reduce high-risk behavior—increased knowledge has little effect unless the environment and perceived norms are changed. The committee believes that access, utilization, and possibly a reduction in absenteeism may be more appropriate **measures of outcomes of effectiveness** of SBHCs than change in health status or high-risk behavior.

Recommendations

School health services should be formally planned, and the quality of services should be continuously monitored as an integral part of the community public health and primary care systems.

In the planning process, school health services should be considered an integral part of the overall community public health and primary care system. The range of services actually provided at the school site must be determined locally, based on community characteristics and needs. Special concerns should be emphasized about two areas of services that a significant proportion of students need—mental health or psychological counseling and school foodservice. The committee believes that mental health and psychological services are essential in enabling many students to achieve academically; these should be considered mainstream, not optional, services. The committee also believes that the school foodservice should serve as a learning laboratory for developing healthful eating habits and should not be driven by profit-making or forced to compete with other food options in school that may undermine nutrition goals.

Many questions remain unanswered about school services, particularly questions regarding the relative advantages, disadvantages, quality, and effectiveness of providing extended services at the school rather than at other sites in the community. Thus, the committee recommends the following:

> *Research should be conducted on school-based services, particularly on the organization, management efficacy, and cost-effectiveness of extended services.*

Additionally, the committee found that there is no current consistent school health data collection process among and between schools. Accurate data collection protocols and standards would greatly facilitate school health research of all kinds.

So that the privacy of families and adolescents be maintained, the committee recommends the following:

> *Confidentiality of health records should be given high priority by the school. Confidential health records of students should be handled and shared in the school setting in a manner that is consistent with the manner in which health records are handled in nonschool health care settings in the state.*

The lack of a consistent and adequate funding base has been a barrier to establishing school health services. Thus, the committee recommends the following:

> *Established sources of funding for school health services should continue from both public health and education funds, and new approaches must be developed.*

Strategies that have shown promise and should be explored further include billing Medicaid for services to eligible students, developing school-based insurance groupings, forming alliances with managed care organizations and other providers, instituting special taxes, and placing surcharges or special premiums on existing insurance policies.

THE CSHP INFRASTRUCTURE
Findings and Conclusions

Many parts of the infrastructure—the basic framework of policies, resources, organizational structures, and communication channels—needed to support CSHPs already exist or are emerging. However, these parts are often fragmented and uncoordinated, and resources are typically transient or limited to specific categorical activities. Leadership and coordination at all levels—national, state, local—will be crucial for programs to become established and grow.

Recommendations

At the national level, the federal Interagency Committee on School Health (ICSH) was established in 1994 to improve coordination among federal agencies, identify national needs and strategies, and serve as a national focal point for school health. The National Coordinating Committee on School Health (NCCSH), which works closely with the ICSH, brings together federal departments with approximately 40 national nongovernmental organizations to provide national leadership in school health.

> *The committee recommends that the mission of the federal Interagency Committee on School Health be revitalized so that the ICSH fulfills its potential to provide national leadership and to carry out critical new national initiatives in school health. In addition, the committee recommends that the National Coordinating Committee on School Health serve as an official advisory body to the ICSH and that individual NCCSH organizations mobilize their memberships to promote the development of a CSHP infrastructure at the state and local levels. The committee also recommends that the membership of the NCCSH be expanded to include representatives from managed care organizations, indemnity insurers, and others who will be key to resolving financial issues of CSHPs.*

The responsibilities of the national leadership should include coordinating programs and funding streams, providing technical assistance to states, and advancing the CSHP research agenda.

At the state level, the infrastructure can be anchored by a structure similar to the ICSH-NCCSH arrangement at the national level.

The committee recommends that an official state interagency coordinating council for school health be established in each state to integrate health education, physical education, health services, physical and social environment policies and practices, mental health, and other related efforts for children and families. Further, an advisory committee of representatives from relevant public and private sector agencies, including representatives from managed care organizations and indemnity insurers, should be added.

The state coordinating council should coordinate state programs and funding streams, propose appropriate state policies and legislation, and provide assistance to local districts. Establishing a regional "school health extension service," modeled after the Agricultural Extension Service offers a particularly promising approach for providing technical assistance.

To anchor the infrastructure at the community or district level, the committee recommends the following:

A formal organization with broad representation—a coordinating council for school health—should be established in every school district.

Among its duties, the district coordinating council should involve the community in conducting a needs and resource assessment, developing plans and policies, coordinating programs and resources, and providing assistance to individual schools. Communities must be prepared to confront barriers in building their CSHP infrastructure, including time and resource constraints, turf battles, indifference, or controversy over sensitive aspects of programs. An effective method for mobilizing support has been to enlist parents and other community leaders as program advocates. Compromise on small issues may be essential for the sake of advancing the larger program.

At the school level:

The committee recommends that, at the school level, individual schools should establish a school health committee and appoint a school health coordinator to oversee the school health program.

Under this leadership, schools should address the major issues facing students and/or the components of the CSHP, develop policies, coordinate activities and resources, and seek the active involvement of students and families in designing and implementing programs.

In order to implement quality comprehensive school health programs, the training and utilization of competent, properly prepared personnel should be expanded.

Specific personnel needs are described in the full report. In general, an interdisciplinary approach is needed in the preservice and inservice preparation of CSHP professionals to enable them to communicate and collaborate with each other. Educators in all disciplines—particularly administrators—need preparation in order to understand the philosophy and potential of CSHPs.

RESEARCH AND EVALUATION
Findings and Conclusions

Research and evaluation of CSHPs can be divided into three categories: basic research, outcome evaluation, and process evaluation. Basic research involves inquiry into the fundamental determinants of behavior as well as mechanisms of behavior change. A primary function of basic research is to inform the development of interventions that can then be tested in outcome evaluation trials. Outcome evaluation involves the empirical examination of interventions on targeted outcomes, based on the randomized clinical trial approach with experimental and control groups. Process evaluation determines whether a proven intervention was properly implemented and examines factors that may have contributed to the intervention's success or failure. Basic research and outcome evaluation are typically conducted by professionals from university or other research centers and are largely beyond the capacity of local education agencies. The committee believes that process evaluation is the appropriate level of evaluation in local programs.

Research and evaluation are particularly challenging for CSHPs. Since these programs comprise multiple interactive components, it is often difficult to attribute observed effects to specific components or to separate program effects from those of the family or community. Determining what outcomes are realistic and measuring outcomes in students is often problematic, especially when outcomes involve sensitive matters such as drug use or sexual behavior. Furthermore, since CSHPs are unique to a particular setting, the results of even the most rigorous evaluations may not be generalizable to other situations.

Interventions associated with the separate, individual components of CSHPs—health education, health services, and nutrition services—should be developed and tested using rigorous methods involving experimental and control groups. However, such an approach is likely to be difficult—and possibly not feasible—for studying entire comprehensive programs or determining the differential effects of individual components and combinations of components.

A fundamental issue involves determining what outcomes are appropriate and reasonable to expect from CSHPs. The committee recognizes that, although influencing health behavior and health status is an ultimate goal of a CSHP, such end points involve factors beyond the control of the school. The committee believes that the reasonable outcomes on which a CSHP should be judged are equipping students with the knowledge, attitudes, and skills necessary for healthful behavior; providing a health-promoting environment; and ensuring access to high-quality services.[3] Other outcomes—improved cardiovascular fitness or a reduction in absenteeism, drug abuse, or teen pregnancies, for example—may also be considered, but the committee believes that such measures must be interpreted with caution, since they are influenced by factors beyond the control of the school. In particular, null or negative measures for these outcomes should not necessarily lead to declaring the CSHP a failure; rather, they may imply that other sources of influence oppose and outweigh that of the CSHP or that the financial investment in the CSHP is so limited that returns are minimal.

Recommendations

In order for CSHPs to accomplish the desired goal of influencing behavior, the committee recommends the following:

> *An active research agenda on comprehensive school health programs should be pursued to fill critical knowledge gaps; increased emphasis should be placed on basic research and outcome evaluation and on the dissemination of these research and outcome findings.*

Research is needed about the effectiveness of specific intervention strategies such as skills training, normative education, or peer education; the effectiveness of specific intervention messages such as abstinence versus harm reduction; and the required intensity and duration of health services and health education programming. Evidence suggests that common underlying factors may be responsible for the clustering of health-compromising behaviors and that interventions may be more effective if they address these underlying factors in addition to intervening to change risk behaviors. Additional research is needed to understand the etiology of problem behavior clusters and to develop optimal problem behavior interventions. And finally, since the acquisition of health-related social skills—such as negotiation, decision-making, and refusal skills—is a desired end point of CSHPs, basic research is needed to develop valid measures of social skills that can then be used as proxy measures of program effectiveness. Diffusion-related research is critical to ensure that efforts of research and development lead to improved practice and a greater utilization of effective methods and programs. Therefore, high priority should be given to studying how programs are adopted, implemented, and institutionalized. The feasibility and effectiveness of techniques of integrating concepts of health into science and other school subjects should also be examined.

Since the overall effects of comprehensive school health programs are not yet known and outcome evaluations of such complex systems pose significant challenges, the committee recommends the following:

> *A major research effort should be launched to establish model comprehensive programs and to develop approaches for their study.*

Specific outcomes of overall programs should be examined, including education (improving achievement, attendance, and graduation rates), personal health (resistance to "new social morbidities," improved biological measures), mental health (less depression, stress, and violence), improved functionality, health systems (more students with a medical home; reduction in use of emergency rooms or hospitals), self-sufficiency (pursuit of higher education or job), and future health literacy and health status. Studies could examine differential impacts of programs produced by such factors as program structure, characteristics of students, and type of school and community.

A thorough understanding of the feasible and effective (including cost-effective) interventions in each separate area of a CSHP will be necessary to provide the basis for combining components to produce a comprehensive program.

> *The committee recommends that further study of each of the individual components of a CSHP—for example, health education, health services, counseling, nutrition, school environment—is needed.*

Additional studies are needed in a number of other areas. First, more data are needed about the advantages (cost and effectiveness) and disadvantages of providing health and social services in schools compared to other community sites—or compared to not providing services anywhere—as a function of community and student characteristics. This information will require overall consensus about the criteria to use for determining the quality of school health programs. It is also important to know how best to influence change in the climate and organizational structure of school districts and individual schools in order to bring about the adoption and implementation of CSHPs. Finally, there is a need for an analysis of the optimal structure, operation, and personnel needs of CSHPs.

MOVING SCHOOL HEALTH PROGRAMS INTO THE FUTURE

Schooling is the only universal entitlement for children in the United States. The committee believes that students, as a part of this entitlement, should receive the health-related programs and services necessary for them to derive maximum benefit from their education and to enable them to become healthy, productive adults. This view appears to be broadly accepted, since the committee has found that many of the components of a CSHP already exist in many schools across the country—health education, physical education, nutrition and food-service programs, basic school health services, counseling and psychological services, and policies addressing the quality of the school environment. The question then arises: What would it take to transform existing programs in typical communities into the vision of a comprehensive school health program?

First, although many components of a CSHP already exist widely, their implementation and quality require attention. New standards and recommendations have been released in many fields that have yet to reach the local level. Another serious deficiency is the apparent lack of involvement of critical community stakeholders in designing and supporting current programs. Perhaps the most difficult issue to resolve before existing programs can be considered "comprehensive" involves the role of the school in providing access to services typically considered the responsibility of the private sector, such as certain preventive and primary health care services. "Providing access" does not necessarily mean that services will be delivered at the school site; rather, it implies ensuring that all students are able to obtain and make use of needed services. Each community must devise appropriate strategies to ensure that all of its students have access to these basic preventive and primary care services.

Although there are divergent opinions about some categorical aspects of school health programs, the committee found a uniform belief that school health programs are important and valuable. Nonetheless, despite this uniform opinion, there is a wide gap between the conceptualization of programs and their implementation. Before school health programs can achieve their promise, concerted action will be needed to bridge this gap. Such action could include coordinating scattered activities; improving the quality and consistency of implementation; engaging the participation of crucial stakeholders; and providing an adequate, stable funding base.

Although dedication and cooperation will be required, the committee believes that the vision of a comprehensive school health program is attainable, and the situation is not so complicated that, even today, a local community could not begin to work toward this vision. The committee is not calling for schools to do more on their own; instead, it is asking communities to recognize and take advantage of the key role that schools can play in promoting and protecting the health and well-being of our nation's children and youth. An investment in the health and education of today's children and young people is the ultimate investment for the future.

Notes

1. The committee uses the term "health" in its broadest sense. Health is more than simply the absence of disease; health involves optimal physical, mental, social, and emotional functioning and well-being.

2. The School Health Policies and Programs Study was conducted in 1994 by the Centers for Disease Control and Prevention to examine policies and programs across multiple components of school health programs at the state, district, school, and classroom levels.

3. This is consistent with the view that for the local school, the desired level of evaluation is process evaluation. If the school is providing health curricula and services that have been shown through basic research and outcome evaluation to produce positive health outcomes, the committee suggests that the crucial question at the school level should be whether the interventions are implemented properly.

School Health Policies and Programs Study, 2000

Overview and Summary of Findings

Lloyd J. Kolbe, Laura Kann, Nancy D. Brener, 2001

~~~

Since 1987, the Centers for Disease Control and Prevention (CDC) has funded states, territories, and large urban school districts to help schools implement effective programs to prevent HIV infection. Since 1992, CDC has funded states to help schools implement broader school health programs to prevent a wide range of health problems. CDC has encouraged these states to focus especially on preventing heart disease, cancer, stroke, diabetes, and other chronic diseases by reducing tobacco use, poor nutrition, physical inactivity, and obesity among youth.

To monitor the impact of these and other efforts to improve school health programs, CDC conducted the first School Health Policies and Programs Study (SHPPS) in 1994.[1] SHPPS 1994 was the first national study to measure policies and programs at the state, district, school, and classroom levels across multiple components of the school health

This chapter originally appeared as Kolbe LJ, Kann L, Brener ND. School health policies and programs study, 2000: overview and summary of findings. *J Sch Health*. 2001;71(7):253–259. Copyright © 2001. Reprinted with permission. American School Health Association, Kent, Ohio.

program. Specifically, SHPPS 1994 assessed health education; physical education; health services; food service; and health policies prohibiting tobacco use, alcohol and other drug use, and violence. At the state and district levels, SHPPS 1994 measured policies and programs in elementary, middle/junior high, and senior high schools. At the school and classroom levels, SHPPS 1994 measured policies and programs in middle/junior and senior high schools.

In 2000, CDC conducted the second SHPPS. SHPPS 2000 has broader content and scope than the 1994 study. SHPPS 2000 is the first study to assess all eight school health program components as originally described by Allensworth and Kolbe[2]: health education, physical education and activity, health services, mental health and social services, food service, school policy and environment, faculty and staff health promotion, and family and community involvement. As in 1994, at the state and district levels, SHPPS 2000 measured policies and programs in elementary, middle/junior high, and senior high schools. At the school and classroom levels, SHPPS 2000 measured policies and programs not only in middle/junior and senior high schools, but also in elementary schools. Further, in recognition of the increasing prevalence of school-based health centers and school-linked health services,[3] SHPPS 2000 included questions specifically to assess these programs and services. SHPPS 2000 is the largest and most complete assessment of school health programs undertaken to date.

Many organizations provided extraordinary support for SHPPS 2000. In addition to delegating experts to review questionnaires, study methodology, and draft reports, the national organizations listed in Figure 9.1 provided letters of support for SHPPS 2000. These letters proved critical in obtaining clearance to conduct the study in many states, districts, and schools.

PURPOSES AND USES OF SHPPS 2000 DATA

SHPPS 2000 was designed to answer the following questions:

1. What are the characteristics of health education, physical education and activity, health services, mental health and social services, food service, school policy and environment, faculty and staff health promotion, and family and community involvement at the state, district, school, and classroom levels nationwide?

Figure 9.1
National Organization Providing Letters of Support,
School Health Policies and Programs Study, 2000.

American Association for Health Education
American Association of School Administrators
American Medical Association
American Nurses Association
American School Food Service Association
American School Health Association
Association of State and Territorial Health Officials
Council of Chief State School Officers
National Assembly on School-Based Health Care
National Association of School Nurses
National Association of State Boards of Education
National Association of State School Nurse Consultants
National Education Association
National Education Goals Panel
National Middle School Association
National Parent Teacher Association
National School Boards Association
President's Council on Physical Fitness and Sport
Society of State Directors of Health, Physical Education, and Recreation

2. Who is responsible for coordinating and delivering each component of the school health program and what kind of education and training have they received?

3. What collaboration occurs among staff from each school health program component and with staff from state and local agencies and organizations?

4. How have the characteristics of school health programs changed since 1994?

SHPPS 2000 data are being used in the following ways:

1. To measure seven *Healthy People 2010* objectives (Table 9.1, pp. 174–175)[4];

2. To help assess National Education Goals[5] that call for safe and disciplined school environments that are free of drugs and alcohol; access for all students to physical education and health education

to ensure that students are healthy and fit; and increased parental partnerships with schools to promote the social, emotional, and academic growth of children;

3. To support public and private school health program initiatives;

4. To help states determine technical assistance, professional preparation, and funding needs and priorities among their schools and districts;

5. To help parents, school board members, school administrators, teachers, and other community members determine how their own school health policies and programs compare to policies and programs nationwide; and

6. To help understand how school health policies and programs address the priority health risk behaviors that occur among students.

METHODS

State-level data were collected from all 50 states plus the District of Columbia. District-level data were collected from a nationally representative sample of public school districts and from dioceses of Catholic schools included in the school sample. School-level data were collected from a nationally representative sample of public and private elementary, middle/junior high, and senior high schools. Classroom-level data were collected from teachers of randomly-selected classes in elementary schools and randomly-selected required health and physical education courses in middle/junior and senior high schools.

Questionnaires

SHPPS 2000 questionnaires assessed health education, physical education and activity, health services, mental health and social services, food service, school policy and environment, and faculty and staff health promotion at the state, district, and school levels. In addition, SHPPS 2000 assessed health education and physical education at the classroom level. Family and community involvement in school health programs was assessed at the state, district, school, and classroom levels with questions integrated into the questionnaires for the other seven school health program components.

Data Collection and Respondents

State- and district-level data were collected by self-administered mail questionnaires completed by designated respondents for each of seven school health program components. These respondents had primary responsibility for or were the most knowledgeable about the policies or programs addressing the particular component being studied. All seven state- or district-level questionnaires (each addressing one school health program component) were mailed to the contact person in each state and district, who distributed the appropriate questionnaire to each designated respondent. Multiple attempts to gather missing data were made through mail and telephone follow-up as needed.

School-level data were collected by computer-assisted personal interviews. During recruitment, the principal or other school-level contact designated a faculty or staff respondent for each component, who had primary responsibility for or was the most knowledgeable about the particular component.

Respondents to the classroom-level computer-assisted personal interviews were teachers whose elementary-school classes or middle/junior or senior high school courses had been selected during the sampling process. All interviews were completed between January and June 2000.

Response Rates

All 51 (100%) state education agencies completed the state-level questionnaires for which they were eligible. At the district level, between 491 and 523 districts (66% to 72% of those eligible) completed the questionnaire for a particular component. At the school level, between 817 and 938 schools (66% to 71% of those eligible) completed the interview for a particular component. At the classroom level, 1,534 respondents completed the health education interview (90% of those eligible) and 1,564 completed the physical education interview (90% of those eligible).

Data Analysis

Data from state-level questionnaires are based on a census and are not weighted. District-, school-, and classroom-level data are based on representative samples and are weighted to produce national estimates.

A more detailed description of SHPPS 2000 methodology can be found in the article by Smith et al. in this special issue of the *Journal of School Health.*

SUMMARY OF FINDINGS

Eight of the remaining nine articles in this report in the *Journal of School Health* provide detailed information about state-, district-, and school-level policies and practices for each of eight school health program components. This section of this article summarizes general findings by component.

Health Education

Most states and districts require elementary, middle/junior high, and senior high schools to teach some health education and most schools require that students receive some health education. While the percentage of schools that require health education increases by grade from 33% in kindergarten to 44% in grade 5, the percentage of schools requiring health education actually decreases from 27% in grade 6 to only 2% in grade 12. Thus, during the grades when the prevalence of health risk behaviors increases among students,[6] schools progressively provide less health education.

Most states require or recommend that districts or schools follow national or state-developed health education standards or guidelines. Three-fourths of these states use the *National Health Education Standards*[7] as the basis for these requirements or recommendations. At least three-fourths of all schools require students to receive instruction on alcohol or other drug use prevention, growth and development, nutrition and dietary behavior, physical activity and fitness, and tobacco use prevention. Unfortunately, many middle/junior and senior high schools teach required health education topics in courses devoted primarily to other subjects, which decreases the coverage if not the effectiveness of instruction about important health education topics.

More than three-fourths of middle/junior and senior high schools require instruction on HIV prevention and human sexuality. Among these middle/junior and senior high schools, most teach abstinence as the most effective method to avoid pregnancy, HIV, or other sexually transmitted diseases (STD); one of five middle/junior high schools and about one-half of senior high schools teach students how to correctly use a condom.

Most states and many districts and schools have someone who oversees or coordinates health education. Many state health education coordinators have an undergraduate or graduate degree in health education or health and physical education combined. However, few required health education classes or courses have a teacher who majored or minored in health education or health and physical education combined. Fortunately, most states and districts provide staff development in health education topics to health education teachers. During the two years preceding the study, at least one-fourth of required health education classes or courses had a teacher who received staff development on accident and injury prevention (Note: Although the SHPPS 2000 questionnaires used the word "accident" because it is familiar to many people, public health officials prefer the word "injury" because it connotes the medical consequences of events that are both predictable and preventable), alcohol or other drug use prevention, CPR, emotional and mental health, first aid, HIV prevention, nutrition and dietary behaviors, tobacco use prevention, or violence prevention.

Physical Education and Activity

Most states and districts require elementary, middle/junior high, and senior high schools to teach some physical education and nearly all schools require some physical education for students. However, while only about one-half of schools require physical education in grades 1 through 5, even fewer (25%) require it in grade 8, and only 5% require it in grade 12. Few schools provide daily physical education or its equivalent for the entire school year for all grades in the school. During the grades when levels of physical activity decline among students,[6] schools progressively provide less physical education.

Most states require or recommend that districts or schools follow national or state-developed physical education standards or guidelines. Almost three-fourths of these states use the *National Standards for Physical Education*[8] as the basis for these requirements or recommendations.

About two-thirds of states and districts and most schools have someone who oversees or coordinates physical education. Many state coordinators have either an undergraduate degree, graduate degree, or both degrees in physical education or physical education and health education combined. Many physical education teachers also have either an undergraduate degree, graduate degree, or both degrees in physical education or physical education and health education combined. Only about one-half of states require teachers to earn continuing education credits on physical education topics to maintain state certification, licensure, or endorsement to teach physical education.

Almost three-fourths of elementary schools provide regularly scheduled recess in all grades kindergarten through 5. Among all schools, about one-half offer intramural activities or physical activity clubs for students and most of these schools do not provide transportation home for students who participate. Almost all middle/junior and senior high schools offer interscholastic sports.

Health Services

Most states, districts, and schools have a person who oversees or coordinates school health services. Most schools have a part-time or full-time school nurse who provides health services to students at the school, although only about one-half of schools have the recommended 1:750 nurse-to-student ratio.[4] School nurses are the primary providers of most school health services, although some schools also have a physician or health aide who helps provide health services. More than one-half of states certify school nurses and require school nurses to earn continuing education credits on school health services topics to maintain certification. Further, most states and districts offer or provide funding for staff development for school nurses.

While nearly all schools provide health services such as first aid, administration of medications, and CPR, fewer schools offer prevention services such as alcohol and other drug use prevention in one-on-one or small group discussions as part of school health services. Most states have at least one school-based health center (SBHC) where enrolled students can receive primary care, including diagnostic and treatment services. Among states with SBHCs, many provide funding for the SBHCs and most have at least one SBHC that serves as a Medicaid provider. While few states require districts or schools to provide health services to students through school-linked health centers or special arrangements with health care providers, more than one-third of districts and schools have such arrangements.

Most states and districts have adopted policies on students and faculty and staff with HIV or AIDS. These policies typically require schools to allow students with HIV or AIDS to attend class and participate in other school activities as long as they are able and require schools to allow faculty and staff with HIV or AIDS to continue working. About one-half of schools have adopted policies on students with HIV or AIDS. These policies are consistent with state and district guidelines.

Mental Health and Social Services

About one-half of states, two-thirds of districts, and three-fourths of schools have a person who oversees or coordinates mental health and social services. In addition, three-fourths of schools have a part-time or full-time guidance counselor, two-thirds of schools have a psychologist, and less than one-half of schools have a social worker who provides mental health or social services to students. Most states and districts offer or provide funding for staff development for mental health and social services staff.

Almost two-thirds of schools offer a student assistance program. More than three-fourths of schools provide crisis intervention for personal problems; identification of or counseling for mental and emotional disorders; identification of or referral for physical, sexual, or emotional abuse; and stress management services.

In many schools, mental health and social services staff collaborate with staff from other components of the school health program and with staff from various community organizations and agencies. Because of limited resources and the fragmented nature of school mental health and social services, even more collaboration is needed.

Food Service

Most states, districts, and schools have a person who oversees or coordinates school food service. Few states offer and even fewer require professional certification for school or district food service coordinators. During the two years preceding the study, more than three-fourths of states and districts provided funding for or offered staff development to district or school food service staff on food preparation, planning healthy meals, and sanitation and safety, and at least three-fourths of school food service managers received staff development on these topics.

Most schools provide students with a variety of healthy food choices in the cafeteria. However, about one-third of schools do not offer students a daily choice between two or more types of fruit or fruit juice, between two or more entrees, or between two or more vegetables. Many food preparation practices that have been recommended by nutritionists as strategies for reducing the fat, sodium, and added sugar content of school meals are not "always or almost always" implemented by most districts and schools. Most schools offer either low-fat or skim milk, but almost two-thirds of all milk ordered by schools is high in fat (i.e., whole or 2% milk).

Food is readily available at school outside the cafeteria. About one-fourth of elementary schools, two-thirds of middle/junior high schools, and almost all senior high schools have one or more vending machines at the school from which students can purchase food or beverages. The three foods and beverages most commonly available in vending machines and through school stores, canteens, or snack bars are soft drinks, sports drinks, or fruit drinks that are not 100% fruit juice; salty snacks that are not low in fat; and cookies and other baked goods that are not low in fat. Most of the schools that sell these products allow students to buy them during the lunch period.

School Policy and Environment

Although most states, districts, and schools have some elements of an ideal tobacco-use policy in place, only about two-thirds of states, districts, and schools have a comprehensive tobacco-use policy, as recommended in CDC's *Guidelines for School Health Programs to Prevent Tobacco Use and Addiction.*[9] The Guidelines recommend that schools prohibit all forms of tobacco use by students, school staff, and school visitors on school property, in school vehicles, and at school-sponsored functions away from school property.

Almost all states, districts, and schools have policies that prohibit use of alcohol and illegal drugs, physical fighting, weapon possession and use, and harassment of students by other students. Most schools "always or almost always" take some remedial action for alcohol and illegal drug use violations, while fewer schools do so for cigarette smoking and smokeless tobacco use violations. Fewer than one-half of schools "always or almost always" take some remedial action when students violate rules on fighting and weapon possession.

Most schools also prevent or reduce unintentional injuries by inspecting and providing appropriate maintenance for fire extinguishers; kitchen facilities and equipment; lighting in school buildings; school property such as halls, stairs, and regular classrooms; and school buses and other vehicles used to transport students.

Faculty and Staff Health Promotion

Prior to employment for all school faculty and staff, about one-fourth of states and one-third of districts require a physical examination and about one-half of states and districts require tuberculosis screening, but few states and districts require illegal drug use screening. About one-fourth of states require districts or schools to provide funding for or sponsor health screenings for tuberculosis and very few states require districts or schools to provide any other type of health screening. During the 12 months preceding the study, at least one of five schools offered screening for blood pressure level, hearing problems, tuberculosis, and vision problems. About one-third of schools provide an employee assistance program for faculty and staff.

Family and Community Involvement

Most activities related to family and community involvement in school health programs are addressed by district and school, rather than state, policies. Many districts and schools provide information to parents about all components of the school health program. Fewer districts and schools engage in more interactive activities with families and communities. For example, during the two years preceding the study, only about one-half of schools involved parents and community members in developing school health policies and, during the 12 months preceding the study, less than one-half of schools met with parents' organizations to discuss components of the school health program. Teachers in most required health education classes and courses reported using homework assignments or projects that involved family members.

About two-thirds of schools have one or more groups that develop policies or coordinate activities on health issues. These groups, typically called school health councils, include school staff, parents, and other interested community members.

Healthy People 2010 Objectives

SHPPS 2000 provides data to measure seven *Healthy People 2010* objectives.[4] For each objective, the 2010 target and baseline data from SHPPS 2000 are provided in Table 9.1.

Table 9.1 National Health Objectives from *Healthy People 2010* Measured by the School Health Policies and Programs Study, 2000.

Objective Number	Objective	2010 Target (%)	Baseline Data from SHPPS 2000 (%)
7-2a	Increase the proportion of middle, junior high, and senior high schools that provide school health education to prevent health problems in the following areas: unintentional injury; violence; suicide; tobacco use and addiction; alcohol and other drug use; unintended pregnancy, HIV/AIDS, and STD infection; unhealthy dietary patterns; inadequate physical activity; and environmental health.		
	Unintentional injury	70	25.4
7-2b	Violence	90	68.3
7-2c	Suicide	80	73.1
7-2d	Tobacco use and addiction	80	59.1
7-2e	Alcohol and other drug use	95	87.8
7-2f	Unintended pregnancy, HIV/AIDS, and STD infection	95	89.0
7-2g	Unhealthy dietary patterns	90	61.9
7-2h	Inadequate physical activity	95	83.5
7-2i	Environmental health	90	76.3
7-2j		80	59.9
7-4	Increase the proportion of the nation's elementary, middle, junior high, and senior high schools that have a nurse-to-student ratio of at least 1:750.	50	52.9[1]
8-20	Increase the proportion of the nation's primary and secondary schools that have official school policies ensuring the safety of students and staff from environmental hazards, such as chemicals in special classrooms, poor indoor air quality, asbestos, and exposure to pesticides.	None set[2]	94.4
15-31	Increase the proportion of public and private schools that require use of appropriate head, face, eye, and mouth protection for students participating in school-sponsored physical activities.	None set	38.7[3]

Table 9.1 National Health Objectives from *Healthy People 2010* Measured by the School Health Policies and Programs Study, 2000 (*Continued*).

Objective Number	Objective	2010 Target (%)	Baseline Data from SHPPS 2000 (%)
22-8	Increase the proportion of public and private schools that require daily physical education for all students.	Elementary schools: none set Middle/junior high schools: 25 Senior high schools: 5	8.0[4] 6.4[4] 5.8[4]
22-12	Increase the proportion of public and private schools that provide access to their physical activity spaces and facilities for all persons outside of normal school hours (i.e., before and after the school day, on weekends, and during summer and other vacations).	None set	35.2[5]
27-11	Increase smoke-free and tobacco-free environments in schools, including all school facilities, property, vehicles, and school events.	100	67.6[6]

[1]Calculated using school-provided enrollment figures and the criterion that a school had a nurse if one was present in the school for at least 30 hours per week during the 30 days preceding the study. The 1994 percentage includes only RNs, the 2000 percentage includes RNs and LPNs.

[2]Developmental objective: 2010 target not set.

[3]Defined as schools that require students to wear appropriate protective gear when engaged in physical activites in physical education, intramural activities and physical activity clubs, and interscholastic sports, among schools that offer each activity.

[4]Defined as the equivalent of at least 150 minutes per week for elementary shool students and at least 225 minutes per week for middle/junior and senior high school students for all grades in the school for the entire school year (i.e., at least 36 weeks).

[5]Defined as schools in which physical activity facilities are used for community-sponsored sports teams, classes, "open gym," or unsupervised programs for children and adults during one or more of the following times: before school, after school, evenings, weekends, or during school vacations.

[6]Defined as the percentage of schools prohibiting the use of all tobacco products by students, faculty and staff, and school visitors on school property, in school vehicles, and at school-sponsored events not on school property.

175

TRENDS OVER TIME

Between 1994 and 2000, school health policies and programs generally remained stable. For example, the percentage of states and districts requiring schools to teach alcohol and other drug use prevention, nutrition and dietary behavior, HIV prevention, accident or injury prevention, and physical activity and fitness and the percentage of schools requiring students to receive instruction on these topics remained fairly constant. Similarly, the percentage of states and districts providing staff development on these topics for health education teachers generally remained constant.

Nonetheless, a few broad changes are worth noting. For example, states, districts, and schools are placing an increased emphasis on violence prevention as evidenced by an increase in the percentage of states (from 38.5% to 60.8%) and districts (from 61.0% to 88.7%) requiring schools to teach the topic, the percentage of states (from 61.0% to 88.7%) and districts (from 34.1% to 62.1%) offering staff development for health education teachers on violence prevention, and the percentage of middle/junior and senior high schools requiring students to receive instruction on violence prevention (from 58.3% to 73.1%). We also detected an increase in the percentage of districts offering staff development for school health services staff on violence prevention (from 23.9% to 48.9%) and the percentage of middle/junior and senior high school health services coordinators who received staff development on violence prevention (from 28.9% to 57.5%). In addition, the percentage of states (from 60.0% to 98.0%) and districts (from 33.8% to 81.1%) offering staff development to schools on how to implement violence prevention policies or programs for school faculty and staff in general increased. From 1994 to 2000, the percentage of districts that required a closed campus for students increased from 45.2% to 56.0% and the percentage that prohibited students from wearing gang colors or gang attire increased from 22.0% to 53.4%. Similarly, the percentage of middle/junior and senior high schools prohibiting gang colors or gang attire increased from 44.7% to 64.5%.

Tobacco use prevention efforts in schools also increased from 1994 to 2000. For example, the percentage of districts requiring schools to teach tobacco use prevention increased from 83.2% to 92.1%, although the percentage of middle/junior and senior high schools requiring students to receive instruction on tobacco use prevention remained constant (85.6% in 1994 and 87.8% in 2000). During the same time period, the percentage of middle/junior and senior high schools having all the elements of an "ideal" tobacco use prevention policy according to CDC's *Guidelines for School Health Programs to Prevent Tobacco Use and Addiction*[9] increased from 36.5% to 63.8%. The percentage of states providing staff development on how to implement tobacco use prevention policies and programs for school faculty and staff in general increased from 64.0% to 92.0% and the percentage of districts providing the same type of staff development increased from 28.2% to 62.2%. Further, the percentage of districts providing staff development on tobacco use prevention specifically for health education teachers increased from 24.2% to 59.5% and the percentage of districts providing staff development on tobacco use prevention specifically for health services staff increased from 26.1% to 44.8%. The percentage of middle/junior and senior high school health services staff who received staff development on tobacco use prevention increased from 23.5% to 51.4%.

Between 1994 and 2000, we also detected changes in physical education policies and programs. For example, the responsibility for coordinating and directing physical education may be moving from the state to the district level, as evidenced by an at least 10 percentage point decrease in the percentage of states offering staff development on helping students develop individualized physical activity plans, administering or using fitness tests, methods to increase the amount of class time students are physically active, and encouraging family involvement and a simultaneous increase of at least 10 percentage points in the percentage of districts offering staff development on these same topics. Similarly, the percentage of states with someone to oversee or coordinate physical education decreased from 76.5% in 1994 to 68.6% in 2000 and the percentage of districts with someone to oversee or coordinate physical education increased from 51.4% to 62.2% during this same time period.

School nurses appear to be increasingly responsible for providing health services to students. From 1994 to 2000, the percentage of middle/junior and senior high schools with a part-time or full-time school nurse increased from 65.0% to 74.2% and the percentage of middle/junior and senior high schools with a nurse-to-student ratio of 1:750 or better increased from 28.2% to 52.8% (Note: the 1994 percentage includes only RNs, the 2000 percentage includes RNs and LPNs). During the same time period, the percentage of middle/junior and senior high schools with a part-time or full-time physician who provided health services to students decreased from 31.3% to 15.2%.

Three health services—case management for students with chronic health conditions, pregnancy prevention, and suicide prevention—received increasing emphasis among school health service providers. From 1994 to 2000, the percentage of both states and districts providing staff development to school health services staff on case management for students with chronic health conditions, pregnancy prevention, and suicide prevention increased at least 10 percentage points. We detected similar increases in the percentage of school health services coordinators who received staff development on case management for students with chronic health conditions, pregnancy prevention, and suicide prevention. Possibly in support of increased efforts among health services staff to prevent pregnancy and suicide, we also found efforts to prevent pregnancy and suicide had increased in health education classes and courses. For example, the percentage of states providing staff development for health education teachers on suicide prevention increased from 39.2% to 50.0%, while the percentage of districts providing staff development for health education teachers on suicide prevention (from 18.2% to 41.5%) and on pregnancy prevention (from 12.4% to 43.2%) also increased. During the same time period, the percentage of states requiring schools to teach suicide prevention increased from 37.8% to 48.0% and the percentage of districts requiring schools to teach suicide prevention (from 66.7% to 80.2%) and pregnancy prevention (from 72.1% to 83.3%) increased.

Between 1994 and 2000, we detected at least a 10 percentage point increase in the percentage of middle/junior and senior high school food service coordinators who received staff development on implementing the *Dietary Guidelines for Americans*[10] in school meals, promoting school meals, sanitation and safety, and making school meals more appealing. During the same time period, the percentage of middle/junior and senior high schools that participated in the School Breakfast Program increased from 43.2% to 60.2%. The percentage of middle/junior and senior high schools that offered brand-name fast foods (for example, Pizza Hut) increased from 16.6% to 25.4%. The fat content of milk available in schools appears to have decreased from 1994 to 2000: the percentage of middle/junior and senior high schools offering whole milk dropped from 76.7% to 54.8%, while the percentage offering 1% milk increased from 39.5% to 52.0%.

UNANSWERED QUESTIONS

Despite the breadth and scope of SHPPS 2000, some important questions about school health programs remain unanswered. For example, SHPPS 2000 did not assess the use of specific health education and physical education curricula. While we considered asking about this, we realized that without detailed information about the fidelity with which the curricula were implemented and an understanding of how multiple curricula were combined, data on this topic could be misleading. Further, SHPPS 2000 was not designed to evaluate the impact or effectiveness of specific policies, interventions, and services. More intervention research is needed to better understand "what works" across all school health program components. Because SHPPS 2000 did not collect data from students, we could not assess students' perceptions of the programs and services available to them. We realize that providers and recipients can view the same policies, programs, and services very differently. Also, SHPPS 2000 did not collect data from enough schools with SBHCs to allow any detailed assessment of their characteristics. Finally, SHPPS 2000 provides answers to only some questions about the physical environment and even fewer answers about the psychosocial culture and climate of schools. Further studies are needed to provide this important information.

FUTURE PLANS

This special issue of the *Journal of School Health* provides only initial descriptive results from SHPPS 2000. Another publication, *State-Level School Health Policies and Practices: A State-by-State Summary from the School Health Policies and Programs Study 2000,* describes state-level policies and practices across school health program components by state. In addition, a series of fact sheets has been developed to summarize highlights from SHPPS 2000 by important cross-cutting topics, such as HIV prevention, tobacco use prevention, and violence prevention. This special issue of the *Journal of School Health, State-Level School Health Policies and Practices,* and the fact sheets are available at no cost from the Division of Adolescent and School Health (DASH), National Center for Chronic Disease Prevention and Health Promotion, Centers for Disease Control and Prevention, 4770 Buford Highway, NE, MS-K33, Atlanta, GA 30341, telephone (770) 488-6160, fax (770) 488-6156. In addition, *State-Level School Health Policies and*

Practices and the fact sheets can be found on the SHPPS Web site at http://www.cdc.gov/shpps.

CDC plans to conduct further and more detailed analyses of SHPPS 2000 data. These findings will be published in other discipline-specific journals and presented at key national conferences. CDC encourages other school health researchers to conduct their own analyses of SHPPS 2000 data. All the SHPPS 2000 data sets and code books are available at no cost on the SHPPS web site. DASH staff can provide limited technical assistance for accessing and using the SHPPS 2000 data.

We hope that health and education officials, school health professionals, and others will view SHPPS 2000 as an important contribution to their understanding of the characteristics, strengths, and limitations of school health programs nationwide. The success of SHPPS 2000 will be determined less by how well it measures changes and more by how much it stimulates improvements in school health policies and programs nationwide. CDC would be pleased to work with all individuals and organizations interested in enabling schools to implement effective school health programs that help youth establish healthy lifestyles and achieve academic success.

Notes

1. School health policies and programs study: a summary report. *J Sch Health.* 1995;65:289–353.
2. Allensworth DD, Kolbe LJ. The comprehensive school health program: exploring an expanded concept. *J Sch Health.* 1987;57:409–412.
3. Institute of Medicine. *Schools and Health: Our Nation's Investment.* Allensworth DD, Lawson E, Nicholson L, Wyche JH, eds. Washington, DC: National Academy Press; 1997.
4. US Department of Health and Human Services. *Healthy People 2010: Understanding and Improving Health.* Washington, DC: Public Health Service; 2000.
5. National Education Goals Panel. *The National Education Goals Report: Building a Nation of Learners.* Washington, DC: US Department of Education; 1994.
6. Kann L, Kinchen SA, Williams BI, et al. Youth risk behavior surveillance— United States, 1999. *MMWR Surveill Summ.* 2000;49(SS-5):1–96.

7. Joint Committee on National Health Education Standards. *National Health Education Standards: Achieving Health Literacy.* Atlanta, Ga: American Cancer Society; 1995.

8. National Association for Sport and Physical Education. *Moving into the Future: National Standards for Physical Education.* Reston, Va: National Association for Sport and Physical Education; 1995.

9. Centers for Disease Control and Prevention. Guidelines for school health programs to prevent tobacco use and addiction. *MMWR.* 1994;43(RR-2):1–17.

10. US Department of Agriculture, US Department of Health and Human Services. *Nutrition and Your Health: Dietary Guidelines for Americans.* 5th ed. Washington, DC: US GPO; 2000. Home and Garden Bulletin No. 232.

CHAPTER 10

Schools as Places for Health, Mental Health, and Social Services

Joy G. Dryfoos, 1993

———

The caring professions, community leaders, parents, and young people themselves are being overwhelmed by the threat of the "big four" adolescent problems: sex, drugs, violence, and depression. In every behavioral and attitudinal survey, these items are at the top of the list of what troubles teenagers and stands in the way of their achieving healthy and safe maturity. In the past, professional attention to these problems has been conducted within entirely separate domains, with categorical programs for prevention of substance abuse, teen pregnancy, and delinquency and promotion of mental health. Each domain has its own experts, interventions, and sources of funds. These programs are isolated from one another and, with few exceptions, are operated separately from the educational system. Only recently has there been an acknowledgement that behaviors such as abusing drugs or engaging in early sexual intercourse are interrelated with and influenced by educa-

---

This chapter originally appeared as Dryfoos JG. Schools as places for health, mental health, and social services. *Teachers Coll Rec*. 1993;94(3):540–567. Copyright © 1993. Reprinted with the permission from Blackwell Publishing.

tional outcomes such as grades, attendance, retention, and graduation. In a reciprocal mode, young people who do well in effective schools are less vulnerable to the "new morbidities" while young people who are protected from problem behaviors achieve academically.[1]

Recognition of the linkages between adolescent health status and educational achievement is leading to the proliferation of new forms of institutional arrangements. Health, mental health, social services, recreation, and arts programs are being brought into schools to augment the services that school systems have put together to deal with the difficult problems arising in today's social environment. The goal of these new efforts is to create "one-stop" service centers in a convenient place where young people can attend to their many needs. The place is the school. The theory is that school is where to find most adolescents, at least before they drop out, and if middle and junior high schools are included in these interventions, almost all young people could be reached through school-based facilities.

This is neither a new nor a radical idea. About a century ago, in response to the massive impact of immigration, urbanization, and industrialization, large numbers of doctors, dentists, and nurses were brought into overcrowded city schools to screen for communicable diseases, treat caries, get rid of pediculosis, and even perform minor surgery such as tonsillectomies and tooth extractions.[2] By the 1920s, the medical profession backed away from these interventions, fearing socialized medicine. Schools hired their own nurses to check for immunization and attendance status, relied on health-education curricula to influence youth to change health behaviors, and assumed that the private sector would take care of adolescent health needs. In the early 1970s, a new generation of pediatricians initiated demonstration projects in a few cities that brought medical and dental units back into schools, but these innovative programs lasted only as long as the grants.[3]

This article describes the resurgence of a school-based services movement, bringing an array of community-health, mental-health, and social services back into schools during another period of social upheaval. The description of these centers and programs is followed by an analysis of the advantages and the limitations of these developments. Finally, a discussion of the future for one-stop adolescent health centers is presented. The focus of this article is on improving the health status of adolescents through school-based initiatives. However, this subject comprehends only one side of an equation; the other side is the restructuring of schools to make them into places in which all young people have an equal opportunity to learn. Schools cannot assume the sole responsibility for producing competent adults if they are to fulfill their primary mission—to educate. Other articles focus on that mission.[4-7]

SUPPORT FOR THE CONCEPT
OF SCHOOL-BASED PROGRAMS

Some twenty-five major reports were published between 1989 and 1991 that addressed the interconnectedness of young people's health status and their educational experience, called for a more comprehensive approach to health, and supported the placement of health-promotion and health-service programs in schools.[8] For example, two organizations representing disparate major interest groups, the American Medical Association and the National Association of State Boards of Education, issued *Code Blue: Uniting for Healthier Youth.*[9] Code Blue is the parlance used in medicine to signify a life-threatening emergency, which is how the organizations' joint commission characterized contemporary health problems of youth. Their recommendations stem from their agreement that *education and health are inextricably intertwined,* that efforts to improve school performance that ignore students' health are ill-conceived, as are health-improvement efforts that ignore the role of education. Thus the commission strongly supported the establishment of health centers in schools, attention to the school climate and issues related to achievement, and the restructuring of public and private health insurance to ensure access to services: "Families, schools, neighborhoods, the health community, and the public and private sectors will need to forge new partnerships to address the interconnected health and education problems our young people are experiencing."[9(p41)]

The Office of Technology Assessment (OTA), charged by Congress with reviewing the health status of American adolescents, recognized school-linked clinics as one of the most promising recent innovations to improve adolescent's access to health services. The report proposed as its major strategy that "Congress could support the development of centers that provide comprehensive and accessible health and related services specifically for adolescents in schools and/or communities."[10] The OTA documented that many adolescents are not covered by private health insurance, and that many adolescents in low-income families are not enrolled in the Medicaid system. The report pointed out that all adolescents face age-related barriers to access to confidential medical care because of parental-consent requirements, lack of information about services, a scarcity of providers trained to deal with adolescent issues, and, in rural areas, long distances to travel and inadequate public transportation. The OTA recommended that the federal government provide "seed money" for the development of comprehensive health centers in or near schools and funding for continuation of established programs. They added a strong caveat, noting the limited systematic evidence that school centers improve adolescent heath outcomes.

The movement toward creating service centers in schools is being driven by educators as well as health professionals. Studies of school-restructuring issues have highlighted the relationship of good health to educational achievement, and the importance of bringing health services into schools. *Turning Points,* the Carnegie Council on Adolescent Development's challenge to middle-school reform, called for the placement of a health coordinator in every school to organize the necessary resources to ensure that young adolescents would be healthy in order to learn.[11] The task force recognized, however, that the needs of some students might exceed the available resources, and therefore schools should consider options such as school-based and school-linked health centers. They envision a comprehensive services network with the school as the center, and community agencies acting as the lead coordinating organizations.

TRADITIONAL HEALTH AND SOCIAL SERVICES IN SCHOOLS

Every school system has its own board policies, and every state has different legislation covering school health. In general, our nation's 83,000 public elementary and secondary schools rely heavily on school nurses and guidance counselors.[12] School nurses typically provide vision and hearing screening, check for immunization compliance and head lice, arrange for emergency care, give students excuses to go home if they are ill or injured, and help with attendance records. Some schools still test for scoliosis (curvature of the spine), although this is no longer considered cost-effective because of low reliability of case finding and low incidence of serious problems. In most states, school nurses are not allowed to give students medication, even aspirin. Currently, there are about 45,000 school nurses, roughly one for every two schools.[13] The ratio of school nurses to students is approximately one per 1,000, but the geographic distribution is uneven and some schools have no nurses (for example, in New York City) while others exceed the desirable ratio of 1:750. According to Philip Nader, a pioneer in school-based services:

> Economic pressures on schools, a return to the basics and a lack of documentation of the value of school health services has resulted in a trend toward replacement of the professional school nurse by less qualified nurse aides or licensed practical nursing personnel, further diminishing the quality and quantity of school health services available to children.[14(p464)]

There are about 70,000 guidance counselors in public schools, about 1 per 600 students. The high school guidance counselor's primary role is to assist students in making decisions about curricular choices and applying to colleges. Because of the large number of students for whom they are responsible, they are not able to provide psychological counseling or deal with behavioral problems. The 1988 *National Education Longitudinal Study* of eighth-graders found that only 11 percent of students had talked to a school counselor or a teacher about personal problems within the previous year.[15] Some school systems employ social workers and psychologists who may work as part of the pupil personnel services team, specifically to attend to more complex problems of students and their families.

School administrators, particularly (but not only) in disadvantaged communities, are increasingly acknowledging that they cannot continue to be the "surrogate parents" for young people with overwhelming health, social, and psychological problems, needs that cannot be met by school personnel. In certain circumstances, parents are not available to help their children; they have too many problems of their own. Existing pupil personnel staff is being stretched to the limit. School systems are confronted with massive budget cuts in which school nurses and other support personnel are among the first to be eliminated. Faced with these daily crises, school administrators are much more open than in the past to allowing local health and social agencies to relocate their services in school building sites.

SCHOOL-BASED HEALTH CLINICS (SBCS)

A school-based health clinic (SBC) is a facility located in a school building or adjacent to a school building where an array of services is provided by medical and social service personnel. In general, the comprehensive package of services includes health screening, physical examinations, treatment of minor injuries and illnesses, and counseling and referral. Attention to reproductive health care and mental-health services varies according to the program. The Jackson-Hinds (Mississippi) Comprehensive Health Center's School-Based Clinics program is typical of the earliest "models," which focused more on reproductive health care than did later ones (see Appendix 1).

In 1984, only ten SBCs could be identified around the country. The first SBC at the high school level was organized in Dallas in 1970 by the Department of Pediatrics, University of Texas Health Science Center.[16] The program included family planning and a decline in the birth rate appeared during the early years of the project. The most publicized model, in St. Paul, Minnesota, was started in 1973 by the Maternity and Infant Care Program of the local medical center. When the program was first initiated in one high school clinic with a focus solely on family planning, it failed to enroll students. After the program was expanded to include comprehensive health services and placed in four sites, enrollment grew. In 1980, it was reported that birth rates had dropped significantly after the initiation of health services including family planning in four high school sites.[17] However, this research did not include a control group or account for abortions.

Between 1985 and 1991, SBCs were organized in high schools and middle schools in almost every state, primarily in urban areas. There is no exact count, but the most recent survey (1991) conducted by the Center for Population Options (CPO) started with a listing of 328 sites.[18] While a major goal of many of the earlier programs was prevention of pregnancy, more recent entries are focused on a wide range of goals, including dropout and substance-abuse prevention, mental health, and health promotion. Because of the early focus on pregnancy prevention, SBCs were dubbed "sex clinics" by the media and detractors, and until recently, this theme has dominated whatever attention school-based health service programs have received. Yet SBCs have not proven to be effective at pregnancy prevention, although they show enormous promise as centers for integrating services such as counseling and general health screening that may indirectly impact on sexual behaviors.[19]

The growth of SBCs has resulted from a variety of forces: demand arising at the community level to help schools deal with the "new morbidities"; popularity of an innovative model for working with high-risk youth; responses to requests for proposals from foundations; and stimulation by state government initiatives. A number of the new program models have been designed by adolescent-medicine physicians and public-health practitioners who want to develop a delivery system of services for adolescents.

In 1986, the Robert Wood Johnson Foundation (RWJ) initiated a grants program to establish SBCs to make health care more accessible to poor children and reduce the rates of teen pregnancy.[20] Some twenty-three health clinics were organized in schools by teaching and community hospitals, county health departments, not-for-profit agencies, and, in some cases, the school systems. However, school systems that received grants had to subcontract with community health providers rather than directly hiring health professionals. According to Lear et al.:

> The primary reason for this approach was the belief that the way to strengthen health services provided in schools is to make those services an integral part of the community's health care delivery system ... [these] health care institutions are best able to arrange medical referrals, address infection control, arrange laboratory pick-ups, protect medical confidentiality, provide medical back-up when the health centers are closed and respond to the myriad of issues that arise in the daily management of a health center.[13(p450)]

Many states provide funds to stimulate the organization of SBCs at the local level, typically through competitive health department grants. Arkansas, California, Connecticut, Delaware, Florida, Georgia, Iowa, Kentucky, Maryland, Massachusetts, Michigan, New Jersey, New York, and Oregon currently support some form of school-centered health and social services for children, youth, and families (see Appendix 2). The California State Education Department has been designated the lead agency for the new $20 million Healthy Start initiative for development of school-based health, mental-health, and social and academic support services, and a consortium of foundations has set up a new nonprofit agency to provide monitoring, evaluation, and technical assistance to California communities and schools. Most state legislation has placed restrictions on the use of state funds for the distribution of contraceptives and referral for abortion on school premises.

No single SBC model has emerged during this developmental stage. A wide array of agencies administer SBCs. According to the Center for Population Options, in 1991 three-fourths of SBCs were sponsored by public-health departments, community-health clinics, and hospitals or medical schools; 6 percent by community-based organizations and private nonprofit agencies; and 7 percent by the school district itself.[18(p2)] Because of the great variety of models and sizes, annual costs range from about $50,000 to $300,000. Most of these funds come from state health departments, Medicaid, city governments, and foundations, not from school district budgets.

The average clinic enrollment is around 700 (with a wide range) and there are about 2,000 visits per year.[21] In most schools, about 70 percent of the students register for the clinic. All schools require parental permission to enroll, with some exceptions covered by state and federal laws for emergency care, reproductive-health care, and drug and mental-health counseling. SBCs are typically staffed by nurse practitioners, social workers, clinic aides, and other specialized personnel (nutritionists, health educators, psychologists). Physicians come in part-time for scheduled examinations and treatment, and are available on call for consultations and emergencies. The clinic coordinator is frequently the nurse practitioner. If the school still has a school nurse, her services are integrated with those of the clinic operations as much as possible. Most clinics provide general and sports physicals, diagnosis and treatment of minor injuries, pregnancy tests, immunizations, laboratory tests, chronic-illness management, health education, extensive counseling, and referral. Over 90 percent prescribe medications.

A 1990 CPO report reveals that 97 percent of high-school and 73 percent of middle-school clinics provide counseling on birth-control methods.[22] About three-fourths of the high schools and half of the middle schools conduct gynecological examinations, follow up contraceptive users, and provide referrals to other agencies for methods and examinations. However, only half write prescriptions for contraceptives and only 21 percent actually dispense them. Although the clinics say they are offering these "family-planning" services, only 10–20 percent of the students report using the clinics for family planning. Not surprisingly, the clinics that offer the most comprehensive family-planning services appear to be the most heavily utilized by the students for family planning. One study of six clinics found that at only two sites were more students using contraceptives than in comparison sites without clinics, but there were no differences in pregnancy or birth rates across sites. Kirby et al. concluded that the clinic could not have an effect on pill and condom use unless much higher priority were given to pregnancy or AIDS prevention throughout the program and the school.[23] This implies much greater attention to follow-up of sexually active students to ensure compliance with contraceptive methods.

Program data show that clinic users are more likely to be female, African-American or Hispanic, and disadvantaged (eligible for free-lunch programs). However, a large number of males do use the clinics, especially for physical examinations and treatment for accidents and injuries.[24] Reports from clinic practitioners invariably mention personal counseling as the most sought after service, reflecting the stressful lives of contemporary adolescents. In some clinics, 30–40 percent of the primary diagnoses are mental-health related.[25] The presence of a nonthreatening, confidential advisor apparently opens up communication about such issues as sexual abuse, parental drug use, and fears of violence.

In summary, a movement toward the development of school-based centers has emerged during the past decade reflecting a response to the overwhelming needs of today's students for health services. It is estimated that in aggregate some 400 school-based clinics may now be serving about 300,000 students per year, a minuscule proportion of the total number of enrollees in junior and senior high schools. Nevertheless, these "pioneer" programs prove that such efforts are both possible and feasible, and, in a sense, this cohort may be the "cutting edge" for the implementation of a wide range of service programs, each individualized to the particular needs of the students, the school, and the community.

MENTAL-HEALTH CENTERS IN SCHOOLS

A key finding in surveys of students is the high incidence of depression and suicidal ideation. The OTA estimated that one out of five adolescents age ten to eighteen suffers from a diagnosable mental disorder, including depression, and that one out of four adolescents reports symptoms of emotional distress.[10(p97)] Yet few depressed students have access to mental-health care in the community, and the already overextended school psychologists and school social workers cannot possibly meet this critical need. As a result, there is a growing interest in bringing outside services into school sites.

Several different approaches are being used to bring mental-health services into schools: on-site counseling and treatment for mental-health problems by mental-health professionals; building mental-health teams to work with school personnel to develop more effective responses to high-risk children; and development and implementation of competency-building curricula in classrooms.[26–27] These three kinds of interventions have in common that they are designed, implemented, and funded by community agencies, outside of the school system, and brought into schools in the same way as SBCs, primarily through foundation grants and/or statewide funding.

While all of these models are interesting and important, I will concentrate here primarily on the emergence of centers within schools that provide actual screening, diagnosis, and treatment for psychosocial disorders. These direct-service programs are similar in organization to school-based health clinics but they start out with the specific goal of remediation of psychosocial problems. The School-Based Youth Services Program in New Brunswick (N.J.) is an example of a mental health program operated in a school by a local community mental health center (see Appendix 3, pp. 209–210).

The work of carving out this subset of activities is being refined by the School Mental Health Project at the University of California–Los Angeles, a national clearinghouse that offers training, research, and technical assistance.[26] This project works in conjunction with the Los Angeles Unified School District's School Mental Health Center and based on that experience is in the process of developing a guidebook for practitioners who want to follow a mental-health model. Howard Adelman and Linda Taylor, who direct the project, believe that the major challenge for school-based mental health centers is to identify and collaborate with what is already going on in the school district. Many schools have programs focused on substance abuse and teen pregnancy prevention, crisis intervention (suicide), violence reduction, and "self-esteem" enhancement, and other kinds of support groups. However, these efforts lack cohesiveness in theory and implementation, often stigmatize students by targeting them, and suffer from the common bureaucratic problem of poor coordination between programs. One of the most demanding roles for the mental-health center is to establish working relationships with key school staff members.

In response to the often overwhelming demand for services, mental-health practitioners (primarily social workers or clinical psychologists) have initiated a number of innovative group-counseling approaches. For example, staff at the San Fernando High School (Los Angeles) school-based center developed "Biculturation Groups" for helping students from other countries make the transition into a new school and community.[28] Three kinds of problems are dealt with: acculturating to a new environment; coping with common problems of adolescence; and dealing with pre-immigration problems such as war-related trauma or family separation.

A school-based clinic program in four junior high schools in the Washington Heights area of New York City operated by the Columbia University School of Public Health has added mental-health components to the original health model in response to the serious psychosocial problems of the students.[29] Social workers provide individual and group counseling, offer group intervention, and maintain contact with parents, teachers, and other school personnel as needed to meet the needs of the students. The social workers do comprehensive psychosocial assessments on children identified by surveys, medical staff, and school personnel for given problems and follow up with group, individual, or family counseling; home visiting; mentoring; parent workshops; or school consultation with guidance counselors or teachers. As this program has evolved, the social work staff (rather than the nurse practitioners) have assumed most of the responsibility for dealing with sexuality issues. They run groups focusing on decision-making skills, reproductive knowledge, and refusal skills. As part of this activity, they escort sexually active students to the family-planning clinics at the backup hospital. They are also responsible for following up contraceptive patients to ensure their compliance. Direct and immediate social work intervention is required in all cases of reported or suspected child abuse and psychiatric emergencies.

In addition to the development of direct mental-health services in schools, other initiatives have received considerable attention, particularly the "Comer Process." Developed in 1968 by James Comer at Yale University and currently being widely replicated, this program attempts to transfer mental-health skills to schools, where "change agents" must be created by strengthening and redefining the relationships between principals, teachers, parents, and students.[30] An essential element is the creation of a mental-health team including the school psychologist and other support personnel, who provide direct services to children and advise school staff and parents. A member of the mental-health team plays an active role on the management-oriented School Improvement Team, along with representatives of teachers, teacher aides, and parent groups.

In summary, a variety of mental-health programs are being offered in schools by community mental-health centers, university psychology and social work departments, and mental-health practitioners. A few might be classified as school-based mental health centers but most of the efforts to cope with the rising number of psychosocial problems appear to be attached to existing health clinics or other approaches. It is not possible to enumerate the number and location of schools with discrete mental-health programs (as distinguished from school psychologists and social workers who may counsel students a part of school function).

COMPREHENSIVE MULTIFACETED PROGRAMS

School-based health centers increasingly use the language of "comprehensiveness." As centers open in schools, the demand for many different services arises. As we have seen, programs that started out as pregnancy-prevention rapidly shifted to general health services, and those that provided general health services had to incorporate psychosocial counseling. As the demand for personal counseling grew, the clinics began to assume more of the aura of mental-health services.

Yet when these centers are opened in school sites, they often meet a bewildering array of categorical prevention and treatment programs. One principal of an inner-city junior high school in New York displayed a list of 200 different programs coming into his school from outside community agencies. He stated that he had no idea what they did, and would be happy to replace them with one central facility that coordinated and monitored services provided to his students.

The call for coordinated services is being heard across the land, not only in relationship to adolescent health issues, but in regard to maternal and child health, early childhood services, welfare reform, and practically every other social endeavor.[8,31,32] Most of the new plans call for the development of one-stop centers and typically these centers are in or near schools. "Teen Moms" is an example of a comprehensive model that has been in existence for some time. Those interested in alleviating the many problems connected with early teenage parenthood have long been packaging services for teenage parents that include on-site infant care along with educational remediation, parenting skills, health services, and personal counseling.[33] More recent models embrace the concepts of case management with the use of "community women" who are supposed to act as mentors and advocates. A few of these teen-parent programs are located within schools (as in Jackson, Mississippi) but most are operated by school systems as alternative schools.

New York State supports fourteen community schools charged with developing school/community collaborations that use the schools as sites for access to social, cultural, health, recreation, and other services for children, their families, and other community adults.[31(p42)] In Rochester, New York, the Chester Dewey School uses a full-time coordinator to encourage community agencies to bring in afterschool care and mentoring, and evening programs and activities for adults. The Community School Project has worked with the Department of Social Services to address the serious housing needs of the parents through workshops on tenants' rights, assisting parents to find better housing and to reduce evictions.

The national Cities in Schools (CIS) initiative has promoted the collaborative model, bringing social services into schools by placing social workers from community agencies as case managers on school sites.[1(pp214–215)] Each participating community works out its own version of this approach and there are a number of "spin-offs" that were started by the CIS process but later became independent. One large-scale undertaking in Pinal County, Arizona, the Prevention Partnership, places site directors in twelve schools along with VISTA volunteers who act as service brokers to 120 service providers in the county. This program employs a school-based management system, and referrals are made for counseling, mentoring, parenting skills, employment and welfare assistance, prenatal and preventive health services, and emergency services. The four New Futures experiments being conducted by the Annie Casey Foundation in Pittsburgh, Savannah, Dayton, and Little Rock are attempting to build "oversight collaboratives" that will bring together community leaders, schools, and community agencies to create new institutional arrangements that will alter the way services (including education) are delivered to children.[34] Preliminary reports suggest that these New Future initiatives are "slow going," with little effect on restructuring schools or changing the ways that agencies conduct their business.[35] However, researchers found enhanced dialogue between leaders in schools and community agencies with the potential for improvement in the future. Aside from educational interventions, these programs have successfully implemented supplemental new initiatives such as case management and school-based clinics.

SINGLE-PURPOSE SCHOOL-BASED PROGRAMS

Perceptions about what can be brought into schools by outside community agencies are becoming more and more inclusive. As has been pointed out, many task forces and commissions have recommended comprehensive collaborative community-wide programs. Yet some of these large-scale comprehensive programs are proving difficult to implement (e.g., New Futures) and slow to evaluate (e.g., Cities in Schools). In fact, most of the documented successful prevention programs are categorical and are operated by individuals and/or teams from single community agencies that come into schools and provide specialized counseling, treatment, and referral to outside agencies.[1]

An example in the substance-abuse prevention and treatment field is called Student Assistance. In this effort, social workers from an outside agency are assigned to schools, where they work with the principal, teachers, and other support personnel to identify high-risk students, provide individual and group counseling, facilitate referrals and follow-up, and help create a healthy and safe school climate.[36]

A similar model has proven successful in the teen-pregnancy prevention field. Counselors, usually social workers, from outside agencies are placed in schools, where they conduct individual and group counseling and referral for family planning. Each counselor has a private office in the school and confidentiality is carefully safeguarded.[37] Another school-based pregnancy prevention program, Team Outreach, incorporates a life-planning curriculum, mentoring, and counseling along with volunteer job placements in the community.[38]

The successful categorical programs feature a number of common components such as early intervention, intensive one-on-one individual attention, training in social skills and competency building, exposure to the world of work, and involvement of peers and parents.[1] Many programs that work to prevent social-behavioral problems focus on the acquisition of basic academic skills and schools are essential partners in much of the prevention activity. However, no one component is believed to work miracles. The comprehensive efforts that are currently emerging typically package most of these elements into an integrated intervention.

ADVANTAGES OF PLACING SERVICES IN SCHOOLS

Schools are rapidly becoming the locus of a wide range of collaborative efforts related to health, mental health, and social services. Although these programs are diverse in size, function, organization, and outcome, there are important common features of school-based programs for adolescents. Placing services in schools gives certain students access to care they would not otherwise be able to obtain. Most of the clinic sites are in low-income communities that do not have a large supply of private physicians, and many of the families have no medical insurance. While some qualify for Medicaid, the children in the family may not have confidential access to the Medicaid card. Almost all school-based services are free. A few charge a token fee but collections are minimal.

Adolescent-medicine physicians and public-health practitioners support the concept of school-based services because such services give them access to high-risk populations that do not ordinarily use private-sector medicine or even community-based clinics. Some SBC advocates believe that by utilizing these clinics, adolescents gain a "medical home" while in high school and learn communication skills that will help them access the medical care system in the future. It is probable that the utilization of school clinics lowers the demand on emergency rooms, where adolescents frequently go for crisis care and even general health services. Preliminary data suggest that school-based clinics may be more cost-effective than purchasing comparable care from private physicians (assuming that physicians were available).[39]

Almost all of these programs have been implemented with funds from state, foundation, local, or private sources. Very few school systems are able to finance these kinds of programs, estimated to cost about $100,000–$200,000 per year. However, school systems have contributed matching funds by making space available and providing maintenance and security. In some systems, school personnel such as school nurses and psychologists become integrated with the staff of the clinic or center.

Almost all of the programs are organized and managed by outside agencies that bring in their own funds and protocols. Experience has shown that planning a school-based clinic or center takes at least a year. The selection of the service mix results from planning by a representative committee including school staff, community agencies, parents, and students. In the most effective efforts, one staff member is designated coordinator to give full attention to developing the program, supervising staff, and negotiating between the school and provider agencies.

Evaluation of the effectiveness of school-based centers is still at an early stage. An excellent management-information system, designed by David Kaplan for the Denver school-based clinic program, is now being utilized by more than 100 programs around the country.[40] A number of unpublished papers have been presented at professional meetings, and it should be expected that these findings will soon appear in journals. While the earlier study results were quite optimistic about school-based clinic programs' potential for preventing pregnancy, they were also crude. More recent work has failed to find a consistent effect on pregnancy rates, although it seems clear that in those schools where clinics make contraception available, contraceptive use is higher. As part of their study of SBCs, Kirby and Wascek compiled data on a high school in Jackson, Mississippi (see Appendix 1, pp. 207–208).[23] Students were asked to check off school-clinic services ever used: About one-third had used the clinic for sports and health examinations, 26 percent for counseling in general, 28 percent for contraceptive counseling, 22 percent for contraceptive supplies, and 15 percent for immunizations. The researchers found few significant differences in pregnancy-prevention practices between clinic users and nonusers; however, they did find that 77 percent of the students who had ever used the school clinic to obtain contraceptives had used an effective method at last intercourse, compared with 48 percent of the students who had not used the clinic for this purpose. Between 1979 and 1990, more than 7,200 adolescents were served by the Jackson school-based programs. Among the 180 student mothers followed up, only 10 experienced a repeat pregnancy and the pregnancy-related dropout rate decreased from about 50 percent to zero.

Scattered results from preliminary studies around the country show small positive impacts. One question that is often raised is whether the mere presence of a clinic in a school influences the sexual activity rate. Research on the effect of clinics on the incidence of sexual activity among the students has yielded no evidence that the rates increase after the clinic opens.[23(pp9–10)] A two-year follow-up survey in Kansas City revealed almost no change in reported sexual behavior.[41] Following a three-year school-clinic demonstration project in Baltimore, Zabin et al. found a postponement of first intercourse that averaged seven months among program participants.[42]

A survey conducted by the Houston school-based clinic program showed that clinic users were more than twice as likely to use contraception every time they had sex as those who had not been to the clinic and they were less than half as likely never to use contraception.[43] Among students who were already sexually active, clinic patients in Kansas City showed higher rates of contraceptive use than nonpatients, and a striking increase in use of condoms among males. In Baltimore, younger female students and males in the experimental schools were much more likely to use birth control than those in the control schools, and in St. Paul, female contraceptive users had an extremely high rate of continuation: 91 percent were still using the method (mostly the pill) after a year and 78 percent after two years of use.[44] (Free-standing family planning clinics report a twelve-month program dropout rate of close to 50 percent.[45])

The Kansas City program reported a substantial drop in substance use during a two-year period.[41] This program places high priority on teaching healthy life-styles and reducing risk-taking behaviors through group and individual counseling. The Kansas City SBC also reported changes in mental-health outcomes: reductions in hopelessness, suicidal ideation, and low self-esteem. The Pinelands, New Jersey, program reported reductions in suspensions, dropouts, and births among students two years after the program started and the Hackensack, New Jersey, program showed a reduction in fights, which they attributed to conflict-resolution interventions.[46] Almost three-fourths of New York City students who used SBCs thought that the clinic had improved their health and more than a third stated that the clinic had improved their school attendance. Most (91 percent) stated that the clinic had improved their ability to get health care when they needed it and 88 percent stated that the clinic had improved their knowledge of and ability to take care of their bodies.[47]

At this point in time, the primary evidence that school-based programs are having an impact lies in utilization figures, with large proportions of student bodies enrolled and using services. One study found that the highest risk students (with multiple problem behaviors) were the heaviest users of the clinic.[48(p22)] Screening and assessments have resulted in extensive case findings—particularly heart murmurs, asthma and other respiratory diseases, need for immunization, sexual abuse, parasites, sexually transmitted diseases, and other problems that beset disadvantaged youth.

The school-based mental-health programs can document extensive hours of counseling and treatment. In New Brunswick, more than one-fourth of the student body has received intensive psychological care. These same students and their families did not use the local community mental health center for services because of costs and perceived inaccessibility. A clinic in Quincy, Florida, reported that about one student a week comes in saying that he or she is either contemplating or has attempted suicide.[49(p3)] Most of the cases found in school clinics require counseling and crisis intervention for depression, stress, and severe family problems, rather than long-term treatment for psychoses and conduct disorders.

No data are available about the outcomes of the provision of direct mental-health services to adolescents in schools, nor have new research findings been reported from current replications of the Comer process. We would expect that achievement and attendance rates would improve in communities that recognize the importance of mental-health interventions.

Categorical programs have been identified that can document improvement in categorical outcomes such as pregnancy prevention and lower substance use.[1] Comprehensive programs targeted to a specific population can produce some successes, such as teen parents programs that reduce repeat pregnancies and improve school completion.

Finally, parents, students, teachers, school administrators, and program staffs have extremely positive attitudes toward the concept of one-stop services located in schools. A Harris Poll found that 80 percent of parents and 81 percent of teachers believe that developing school programs to provide counseling and support services to children with emotional, mental, social, or family problems would "help a lot" to improve educational outcomes.[50] The public does not fear that attention to reproductive-health issues will increase the level of sexual activity among students. In fact, a survey of public attitudes toward provision of birth control information and contraceptives in schools showed an approval rating of 73 percent.[51] Approval was highest among African-American respondents (88 percent) and unmarried people (86 percent). Fully 80 percent approved of school clinic referrals to family-planning clinics.

The AIDS scare has begun to have an impact on policies regarding the distribution of condoms in schools. In recent months, New York City, Philadelphia, Los Angeles, San Francisco, and Baltimore authorities have revised policies to make condoms available to students. In New York City condoms are being distributed by teachers and other staff who volunteer to be trained for this mission. In Baltimore, the nine school-based clinics initiated a policy to distribute contraceptives after a parent survey showed wide approval.

In summary, school-based programs are developing at a rapid rate because they are providing services to a very needy population, junior and senior high school students who have little access to other sources of care. They bring into disadvantaged school systems committed and caring staff workers who can give all of their attention to the physical and psychosocial needs of the students. The development of these diverse programs is taking place all around the country despite trying conditions that include competition for scarce resources, acute shortages of nurse practitioners, and a constant struggle to maintain services.

LIMITATIONS OF
SCHOOL-BASED PROGRAMS

Two issues frequently arise in discussions about the merits of placing services in schools: the problem of negotiating governance between school systems and community agencies, and the lack of long-term funding.

Governance

Given the complex processes involved when one or more community agencies moves into a school system, it is surprising that these models are being replicated as rapidly as they are. Each party has its own board of directors, policies, funding, accounting procedures, personnel practices, and insurance. There are different union contracts and salary structures in schools and outside health and social service agencies. Working out the details for collaboration requires endless planning and negotiation.

From the point of view of the community agencies, school boards are often inflexible. Many initiatives have been delayed because of difficult policy decisions, for example, the use of school facilities, reproductive-health care, and personnel practices. Often, the host school is already overcrowded and finding adequate space for a clinic requires extensive remodeling. Clinic hours differ from those of the school, necessitating arrangements with the custodial staff. The school nurse may feel threatened by the new facility and raise objections to procedures that conflict with her turf.

One might think that policies regarding birth control create the most conflict. This has not generally been the case. Only one or two clinics have failed to open because of community dissension. So much has been made of this issue that it is typically dealt with early in the planning process. Few school systems allow distribution of contraceptives on site and almost all programs allow for parental consent. These policies have assuaged critics but they have also limited the effectiveness of school-based clinics in their work with sexually active teenagers in regard to compliance with contraceptive methods. As pointed out above, these policies are currently under review in light of the AIDS epidemic.

Operating a school-based clinic requires constant nurturing of the relationship between the clinic program and the school. The key player in these ongoing negotiations is the school principal. As the primary gatekeeper, the principal facilitates access to students, promotes good working relationships between the school staff and the program staff, and makes sure the building is safe and clean. If the principal does not cooperate, the program will not work.

School clinics open the door to many turf issues. One question that frequently arises when a program is placed in a school with existing support personnel such as a psychologist, a social worker, or even a guidance counselor, is who is in charge of mental health "cases." This becomes particularly sensitive in dealing with special education students. Ensuring confidentiality can be very difficult in situations in which school and clinic staff are both involved.

Similar questions have been raised about the "ownership" of health-promotion curricula. If the school-based clinic is providing extensive individual and group counseling, is it necessary to use school time for health-promotion curricula? If clinic personnel are willing to go into classrooms and take on the responsibility for sex-education, substance-abuse and suicide-prevention, and violence workshops, what is the role of school health educators? If the clinic assumes the health-promotion role, is it necessary to train teachers to do sex education and substance-abuse prevention?

Teachers in schools with clinics are sometimes reluctant to allow students to leave classes to make clinic visits. They may also be threatened by the confidential relationship between clinic counselors and students. In some cases, stress-related behavior derives from negative school experiences, and specific teachers have been implicated in lowering student's expectations and accused of failing to teach. Clinic practitioners may have negative views of school discipline policies that rely heavily on suspension and expulsion and practices such as tracking and grade retention that have been shown to undermine achievement.

Many school systems are driven by the desire to raise test scores and lower dropout rates. Teachers are frustrated because they believe that the students' behavioral problems and the social environments of the communities in which the schools are located stand in the way of achievement. School-restructuring efforts try to create a learning community equalizing outcomes for all students. In some instances, the school-based clinic programs have become involved with school restructuring because they see that they cannot successfully treat the students' psychosocial problems without massive changes in the way the students are treated in school.

Funding

School-based health and social service programs derive funds from diverse sources. More than half of the funding derives from Maternal and Child Health and other state health department grants.[18(p2)] Few programs are adequately funded and almost all of them rely on a mix of resources that require complicated and time-consuming accounting procedures. Each source of funds has its own regulations and eligibility. Foundation support is time-limited. The twenty-three Robert Wood Johnson grants have now reached their limit and those programs have to find other sources of funding, what the foundation calls "institutionalization."

One approach to long-term funding being appraised by RWJ-supported researchers and others is to increase the use of Medicaid funds for eligible students, particularly in light of new provisions to stimulate the use of Early Periodic Screening Treatment and Diagnosis programs. It has been estimated that about one-third of the students served in school-based clinics are eligible for Medicaid but only about 3 percent of the services are financed by such reimbursements. A recent survey found that the major barriers to the use of Medicaid or private insurance by school-based clinics were (1) students did not know whether their families were Medicaid or private insurance recipients; (2) time and costs of paperwork involved in billing were prohibitive; (3) state Medicaid or private insurance companies refused to pay for services; (4) Medicaid did not recognize schools as qualified medical providers; and (5) confidentiality issues.[52] Clinics administered by private community health agencies and hospitals or medical schools were the most likely to be using Medicaid. The tighter the link to a medical base, the more likely a program is to have access to third-party funds. Increasingly, clinics are placing Medicaid eligibility workers on school sites to help students with eligibility determinations. In some communities and states, the concept of declaring an entire school Medicaid-eligible is being explored. This would cut down on the bureaucratic hassle and ensure continuity of funding and confidentiality.

Another important source of support of school-based centers is a line item in the state budget, as in the New Jersey Department of Human Resources and the Kentucky Department of Education. The limitations of this approach are that only enough money may be included for demonstration projects, as in New Jersey, or that the grants may be very small, as in Kentucky. At one point, the state of Michigan developed a plan to fund 100 school-based clinics, but the appropriation so far covers only 20 such programs. The continuity of state funds depends on continuing legislative approval, not easily guaranteed during this period of fiscal constraints, and a change of governor can bring changes in priorities (although the school-based program has weathered changes in administration in most states). A further limitation is that state funds usually have restrictions, particularly prohibiting distribution of contraception and/or counseling regarding abortion.

In summary, many issues remain to be resolved in regard to the creation of one-stop centers in schools, issues that are similar despite the significant differences in the health, mental-health, and social services models. All programs suffer from shortages of funding and most operate in a crisis mode. The demand for services in schools is often overwhelming. Although most of the current school-based programs follow a medical model, starting with assessments, screening, and physical examinations, the most frequently cited unmet need is for mental-health counseling. The acute shortage of emergency psychiatric and day-treatment facilities for adolescents and the shortage of bilingual mental-health clinicians are widespread. As new staff and services are brought into centers, the utilization rates increase.

An observation of one inner-city project showed that:

> As soon as the doors of a new clinic site open, mobs of students pour in seeking minor items like bandaids, ice packs and sanitary napkins, producing a steady stream of work for the staff. At the same time, a small number of students are identified who have been battered, are severely depressed, have burdensome family problems, are taking drugs or require a complex mix of many different kinds of services. The new clinics are overwhelmed by the two extreme ends of the spectrum of needs and find little time to reach the vast majority of students in between. Reorganization of the work load, targeting high risk individuals and the development of specialized protocols have alleviated this problem somewhat, but the clinic staff perceive it as one which school based clinics can never overcome. As they say, "it goes with the territory."[29(p33)]

The absence of evaluation and the minimal published literature on the subject produce an impression of haphazard diffusion of an idea, implemented at widely disparate levels of effectiveness. With the exception of some of the state-supported programs, each program is packaged in a different way and there is no central system for monitoring quality. A common problem is the complexity of governance in a model that brings the services, staff, and funding from an outside community agency into a school.

OUTLOOK FOR ONE-STOP CENTERS IN SCHOOLS

In disadvantaged communities, schools cannot address the challenge of raising the quality of education and at the same time attend to the problems of young people and their families without a substantial mobilization of health and social services resources. Poverty rates among youth are growing, housing is deteriorating, and violence threatens everyone. These worsening conditions are accelerating the drive among concerned people to find new solutions that incorporate the linkage between educational achievement and adolescent health. While school-based services will not solve the underlying problems of poverty and discrimination, they are perceived by both health and educational practitioners as one potentially cost-effective approach to alleviating the symptoms. Young people can receive support to stay in school, manage their psychosocial problems, prepare for the work force, and experience positive relationships with caring adults. Thus, the idea of packaging services together and putting them in a central place like a school is very attractive.

Thus far, the school-based clinic model has been conceived as an intervention for "high-risk" communities. Many but not all of the clinics are located in metropolitan areas with the highest incidence of the "new morbidities"—teen pregnancy, sexually transmitted diseases, AIDS, drug abuse, violence, and depression—and the highest school failure and dropout rates. Although advocates of this model acknowledge that there are high-risk adolescents in affluent communities as well, there is no consensus on whether every school should have such a center or only those schools that serve disadvantaged populations. Suburban youth, who make up the majority of high school students, increasingly lack parental support and also need the attention of caring adults to help them get through their teen years. They also must learn to deal with a fragmented health, mental-health, and social service system. Suburban schools, because they have larger budgets than city schools, are more likely to employ support personnel including psychologists, speech therapists, school nurses, and guidance counselors. In order to ensure that all adolescents have access to the full range of services they need, suburban schools might take an intermediate step by assigning a staff member in every school to foster coordination with community agencies (as recommended in *Turning Points*[11]). This would entail schoolwide planning for individual counseling, crisis intervention, family involvement, and systematic referrals for services along with follow-up.

My own vision of the ideal community school is a center in a school that brings together those services most needed in that community. At the high school level, these might include health, mental-health, and career-training and job-placement services; after-school recreation and cultural events; parent education; and public-assistance and community police force programs. Most importantly, the center would facilitate arrangements for individual and family counseling. The employment of youth advocates who assist students with family and school problems would ensure that those most in need receive the services they require as soon as possible. Health-promotion activities such as pregnancy and substance-use prevention would become the responsibility of the center staff. The schoolhouse doors would be open most of the time, including evenings, weekends, and summers.

Community schools set up to serve elementary school populations would include preschool and after-school care, parent training, home visiting, educational programs for parents, and other health and social services. Experience to date suggests that once a school community enters the process of thinking about centralizing services in schools, almost any public or private community agency can be transported from its community base into the school facility. Edward Zigler of Yale University has long articulated the need for "Schools of the 21st Century" incorporating these services. His model is being replicated in more than 200 schools throughout the nation (particularly in Kentucky and Connecticut).[53]

The bottom line here, of course, is how to make this vision a reality. If the current crop of school-based clinics are having a hard time maintaining their bases of support, how can community schools be institutionalized on a large enough scale to have any impact? Schools, community agencies, foundations, states, and the federal government have various roles in meeting this challenge. The primary role for school systems is to encourage the development of these collaborative relationships, to make it known that they are willing to use their facilities to host an array of services. The role of the community agencies is to gear up to provide their services in new locations, much as hospitals and health departments organize satellite clinics. Community agencies have to be prepared to deal with the ambiguities and frustrations that arise in negotiations with school systems. Schools and community agencies together have to hammer out the governance arrangements that will assure efficient functioning of the center.

Articulate grass-roots support is an essential component in gaining the ear and pocketbook of both the citizenry and the decision-makers. Parents, students, and community leaders can make their voices heard at budget hearings and planning sessions.

Foundations have already played an important role in funding demonstration projects, but they must be prepared to do more. It is unlikely that evaluation will be conducted on a large enough scale without extensive foundation support. One of the advantages of foundations is that they can assist grantees to monitor programs and document processes.

Many states are already heavily involved in the extension of the school-based clinic model. These state programs, usually placed in state health or human resources departments, need to develop collaborative relationships with state education agencies. In some states, collaboration is legislatively mandated, while in others governors have created child- and youth-services "mini-cabinets" to foster integration of services. Together, state agencies need to be able to provide technical assistance to communities, monitor the quantity and quality of the services, and organize training and conferences. States can promote the development of school-based centers not only through funding, but also by waiving various regulations in regard to Medicaid and other state-controlled resources.

The federal government has played virtually no role in the advancement of these new kinds of service models. Yet the potential for moving from demonstration programs to institutionalization lies within the power of Congress, which in 1990 passed but did not fund the Young Americans Act. This legislation would create a central commission and council for generating a coordinated federal response to the multiple needs of children. Funds would be provided to states for planning and coordination. Congress could also create a new cabinet-level agency and integrate the hundreds of categorical youth-serving programs into a more rational delivery system.

The federal government could be instrumental in changing policies now to allow categorical funds to be used to design and implement community-school collaboratives. Possible sources of funds in addition to Medicaid include Drug Free Schools, Office of Substance Abuse Prevention, Juvenile Justice, Division of Adolescent and School

Health of the Centers for Disease Control, and other AIDS prevention monies. It is possible that the mission of Chapter 1 to aid economically disadvantaged children could be expanded to encompass their health and psychosocial needs as well as educational remediation. There are definitely signs in Washington that integration of youth and family services is the direction of the future, but almost all of the proposed school-based efforts are directed toward preschool or elementary school children, prior to the age of puberty.

All health and social indicators confirm that our society will have to move rapidly to enable disadvantaged adolescents to mature into responsible, literate, productive adults. The combined forces of the educational, health, and welfare systems working together are necessary to counteract the effects of the decaying social environment on this generation of youth. The traditional approaches to health and psychosocial problems are not working. New school-based centers of health and mental-health care are emerging but they will remain in the demonstration phase or disappear completely without significant support and attention.

APPENDIX 1
JACKSON-HINDS COMPREHENSIVE HEALTH CENTER'S SCHOOL-BASED CLINICS

The federally funded Comprehensive Health Center in Jackson, Mississippi, currently operates school-based health services in four high schools, three middle schools, and one elementary school. In 1979, when the program was first initiated at Lanier High School, the staff found many conditions that demonstrated the extensive unmet needs of the students, including urinary tract infections, anemia, heart murmurs, and psychosocial problems. In a student body of 960, they found more than 90 girls who were either pregnant or already had a child. Some 25 percent of the pregnancies had occurred while the youngsters were in junior high, leading the program to extend resources to an inner-city junior high school and a second high school the following year. The other clinics were added in the late 1980s.

Clinics are located in whatever rooms schools can make available. At Lanier High School, two small rooms near the principal's office are equipped as clinics. Group counseling and health-education classes are provided in a large classroom with private offices for individual counseling. The infant-care center is located in a mobile unit attached to the school. The staff at Lanier includes a physician, a nurse practitioner, a licensed practical nurse, two nurse assistants, and an educator/counselor, all part-time workers.

The school-based clinic protocol includes a medical history and routine lab tests of hematocrit, hemoglobin, and urinalysis. Each enrolled student completes a psychosocial assessment that reveals risk levels for substance abuse, violence, suicide, pregnancy, sexually transmitted diseases (STDs), accidents, and family conflict. Depending on indications from the health history and assessment tool, the student is scheduled for a visit with the physician and/or counselor. However, the clinic is always open, from 8:00 A.M. to 5:00 P.M., for walk-in visits for emergency care and crisis intervention.

Clinic staff conduct individual and group counseling sessions. If sexually active, students are given birth-control methods including condoms and followed up bi-monthly. Staff also dispense formal health instruction about specific issues such as compliance with medication protocols or treatment of acne, and informal "rap sessions" on parenting, the reproductive health system, birth-control methods, sexual values, STDs, and substance abuse. The counseling and clinic services are closely coordinated. Enrollees in the school clinic are referred to the primary community health center for routine dental screening, cleaning, and fluoride application. This facility is always open to students after school hours and on weekends and holidays.

Arrangements for early prenatal care are made through the obstetrical department of the health center. Teen mothers are carefully monitored throughout their pregnancies with special attention paid to keeping the young women in school as long as possible and getting them back within a month after delivery. Day care is provided at the school. Young mothers are counseled and instructed about child development and parenting skills. The Day Care Center is also used for teaching child psychology to high school students.[23,54,55]

APPENDIX 2
NEW JERSEY SCHOOL-BASED
YOUTH SERVICES PROGRAM

The School-Based Youth Services Program (SBYSP) has served as a model for other states. Following a competitive process, grants were made by the New Jersey Department of Human Services in 1987 to 29 communities for collaborative projects to be operated jointly by the school system and one or more local nonprofit or public health, mental health, or youth-serving agencies and to be located in or near the school. Based on the theme of "one-stop services," each project had to provide core services including mental health and family counseling, drug and alcohol counseling, educational remediation, recreation, and employment services at one site. Health services had to be available on site or by referral. In addition, child care, teen parenting, family planning examinations and referral for contraception, transportation, and hotlines could be provided with the grant (but not contraceptives or referral for abortion services). All centers had to be open after school, weekends, and during vacations.[56]

APPENDIX 3
SCHOOL-BASED YOUTH SERVICES PROGRAM, NEW BRUNSWICK (N.J.) PUBLIC SCHOOLS

This mental health program was initiated in New Brunswick High School in 1988, funded by the New Jersey School-Based Centers program. It is operated by the Community Mental Health Center, which is part of the University of Medicine and Dentistry of New Jersey. The program was stimulated by New Brunswick Tomorrow, a local business sponsored effort that is trying to revitalize New Brunswick. In 1991, New Brunswick School-Based Youth Services Program (SBYSP) was awarded new state funds to expand services into five local elementary schools.

The SBYSP is a centralized service delivery system that integrates existing school programs, creates new services within schools, and links a network of youth-service providers. Although its primary thrust is mental-health promotion and treatment, it "looks like" a comprehensive youth center in a school setting. Currently, the program has ten full-time core staff members, including eight clinicians (psychologists and social workers), one of whom serves as the director. The staff conduct individual, group, and family therapy and serve as consultants to school personnel and other agencies involved with adolescents. An activities/outreach worker plans and supervises recreational activities and outreach contacts at the high school. Specialized part-time staff include a pregnancy/parenting counselor, a substance abuse counselor, and consultants in suicide prevention, "social problems," and medical care. A number of student interns from Rutgers University Graduate Schools have field placements in this program and there are also some volunteers.

The facility at New Brunswick High School is located in the old band room, fixed up very attractively to resemble a game room in a settlement house, with television, pingpong, and other active games, comfortable furniture, and books and tapes for the students to borrow. Private offices where students can go for individual psychological counseling ring the main room. The center offers tutoring, mentoring, group activities, recreational outings, and educational trips. A number of "therapeutic" groups have been organized: social problem solving, substance abuse, Children of Alcoholics, and coping skills for gifted and talented. Students are referred to the local neighborhood health center for health services and treatment. Children of teen parents are offered transportation to child-care centers.

Of the 650 students in the New Brunswick High School, 91 percent are enrolled in the program and have parental consent statements on file. During the past two years, one in four of the enrolled students has been involved in active mental-health counseling with one of the clinicians. Many of the students, especially the girls, appear to be clinically depressed. According to Gail Reynolds, the director, the demand for services is overwhelming. Many of the problems require immediate and time-consuming interventions with the family, school, and social agencies. After a student has made three visits, parents must come in for counseling sessions. Staff make home visits in order to involve parents.

In the process of setting up the program within the school, the superintendent was a key player and supportive from the start. The first summer was spent overcoming the resistance of the people in the school, preparing the school staff, and working out referral procedures with the school's four guidance counselors and the teachers. Reynolds meets with the counselors once a month and with the principal and vice-principal weekly. Relationships with school staff are complex and vitally important to the functioning of the center. One problem that had to be overcome was convincing the maintenance staff to allow the premises to stay open after 3:00 P.M. The center is open all day and into the evening, and all summer.[57,58]

Notes

1. Dryfoos JG. *Adolescents-at-Risk: Prevalence and Prevention.* New York, NY: Oxford University Press; 1990.

2. Tyack D. Health and social services in public schools: historical perspectives. In: *The Future of Children: School-Linked Services,* vol 2. Los Altos,

Calif: Center for the Future of Children, David and Lucile Packard Foundation; 1992:19–31.

3. Cronin GE, Young WM. *400 Navels: The Future of School Health in America.* Bloomington, Ind: Phi Delta Kappa; 1979.

4. Heller HC. The need for a core, interdisciplinary life sciences curriculum in the middle grades. *Teachers Coll Rec.* 1993;94:645–652.

5. Ambach GM. Linking health and education in the middle grades. *Teachers Coll Rec.* 1993;94:653–654.

6. Meier D. Transforming schools into powerful communities. *Teachers Coll Rec.* 1993;94:654–658.

7. Comer JP. The potential effects of community organization on the future of our youth. *Teachers Coll Rec.* 1993;94:658–661.

8. Lavin AT, Shapiro GR, Weill KS. Creating an agenda for school-based health promotion: a review of selected reports. *J Sch Health.* 1992;62: 212–228.

9. National Commission on the Role of the School and the Community in Improving Adolescent Health. *Code Blue: Uniting for Healthier Youth.* Washington, DC: American Medical Association, National Association of State Boards of Education; 1990.

10. US Congress, Office of Technology Assessment. *Adolescent Health; vol 1: Summary and Policy Options.* Washington, DC: US GPO; 1991.

11. Task Force on Education of Young Adolescents. *Turning Points: Preparing American Youth for the 21st Century.* Washington, DC: Carnegie Council on Adolescent Development; 1989.

12. This discussion focuses on actual health services. However, schools are involved in other health-related activities, such as providing health education, paying attention to nutrition, and maintaining a healthy and safe school environment. An unknown number of school systems employ health educators, school psychologists, and other special-education experts.

13. Lear JG, Gleicher HB, St Germaine A, Porter PJ. Reorganizing health care for adolescents: the experience of the school-based adolescent health care program. *J Adolesc Health.* 1991;12:450–458.

14. Nader P. School health services. In: Wallace HM, Ryan G, Oglesby AC, eds. *Maternal and Child Health Practices.* 3rd ed. Oakland, Calif: Third Party Publishing; 1988.

15. National Center for Education Statistics. *National Education Longitudinal Study of 1988: User's Manual.* Washington, DC: US Department of Education; 1990.

16. An earlier school-based clinic started in 1965 provided comprehensive health services primarily to young children in Cambridge, Mass. Porter P. School Health is a place, not a discipline. *J Sch Health.* 1987;57:417–418.

17. Edwards LE, Steinman ME, Arnold KA, Hakanson EY. Adolescent pregnancy prevention services in high school clinics. *Fam Plann Perspect.* 1980;12:6–14.

18. Center for Population Options. School-based and school-linked clinics [fact sheet]. Washington, DC: Center for Population Options; 1991.

19. Dryfoos JG. School and community-based prevention programs. In: Coupey S, Klerman L, eds. *Adolescent Sexuality: Preventing Unhealthy Consequences.* Philadelphia. Pa: Hanley and Belfus; 1991.

20. Robert Wood Johnson Foundation. *Making Connections.* Princeton, NJ: Robert Wood Johnson Foundation; undated.

21. Waszak CS, Neidell S. *School-Based and School-Linked Clinics: Update 1991.* Washington, DC: Center for Population Options; 1992.

22. Center for Population Options, *School-Based Clinics: Update 1990.* Washington, DC: Center for Population Options; 1991.

23. Kirby D, Waszak CS, Ziegler J. *An Assessment of Six School-Based Clinics: Services, Impact, and Potential.* Washington, DC: Center for Population Options; 1989.

24. Brindis CD et al. *Utilization Patterns Among California's School-Based Health Centers: A Comparison of the School Year 1989–1990 with the Baseline Year of 1988–1989.* San Francisco, Calif: Center for Reproductive Health Policy Research; 1991.

25. *San Jose School Health Centers 1990–91 Annual Report.* San Jose, Calif: San Jose Medical Center; 1991.

26. Adelman HS, Taylor L. Mental health facets of the school-based center movement: need and opportunity for research and development. *J Ment Health Adm.* 1991;18:272–283.

27. *Mental Health Network News,* various issues.

28. *Mental Health Network News.* 1991;2:1–2.

29. Dryfoos JG. Bringing health and social services into inner-city junior high schools. *Report to the Center for Population and Family Health*, Columbia University School of Public Health, New York; 1991.

30. Comer JP. Improving American educational roles for parents. In: *Hearing Before the Select Committee on Children, Youth, and Families, June 7, 1984.* Washington, DC: US GPO; 1984:55–60.

31. Melaville A, Blank M. *What It Takes: Structuring Interagency Partnerships to Connect Children and Families with Comprehensive Services.* Washington, DC: Education and Human Services Consortium; 1991.

32. Weiss H. *Family Support and Education, Programs, and the Public Schools.* Cambridge, Mass: Harvard Family Research Project; 1988.

33. Nickel P, Delany H. *Working with Teen Parents: A Survey of Promising Approaches.* Chicago, Ill: Family Resource Coalition; 1985.

34. Center for the Study of Social Policy. *New Futures in Pittsburgh: A Mid-Point Assessment.* Washington, DC: Center for the Study of Social Policy; 1991.

35. Wehlage G, Smith G, Lipman P. Restructuring urban schools: the new futures experience. *Am Educ Res J.* 1992;29:51–93.

36. National Institute of Alcohol Abuse and Alcoholism. *Prevention Plus: Involving Schools, Parents, and the Community in Alcohol and Drug Education.* Washington, DC: US Department of Health and Human Services; 1984.

37. Inwood House. *Community Outreach Program: Teen Choice—A Model Program Addressing the Problem of Teenage Pregnancy.* New York, NY: Inwood House; 1987.

38. Allen JP, Philliber S, Hoggson N. School-based prevention of teenage pregnancy and school dropout: process evaluation of the national replication of the Teen Outreach Program. *Am J Community Psychol.* 1990;18:505–524.

39. Siegel L, Kriebel T. Evaluation of school-based high school health services. *J Sch Health.* 1987;57:323–327.

40. Kaplan DW. *School Health Care-Online! School-Based Clinic Management Information System.* Denver, Colo: Children's Hospital; 1992.

41. Kitzi G. Presentation at the third annual conference of the Support Center for School-Based Clinics, Denver, Colo.; 1986.

42. Zabin LS, Hirsch MB, Smith EA, Streett R, Hardy JB. Evaluation of a pregnancy prevention program for urban teenagers. *Fam Plann Perspect.* 1986;18:119–126.

43. Galavotti C, Lovick S. The effect of school-based clinic use on adolescent contraceptive effectiveness. Presented at: National Conference on School-Based Clinics; November 1987; Kansas City, Mo.

44. Edwards L, Arnold-Sheeran K. Presented at: meeting of the American Public Health Association; November 1985.

45. Shea J, Herceg-Baron R, Furstenberg F. Clinic continuation rates according to age, method of contraception, and agency. Presented at: annual meeting of the National Family Planning and Reproductive Health Association; March 1982.

46. Kean T. Presented at: Carnegie Council on Adolescent Development; April 14, 1992; Washington, DC.

47. Welfare Research Inc. *Health Services for High School Students: Short-Term Assessment of New York City High School-Based Clinics.* Report to New York City Board of Education; June 3, 1987.

48. Stout J. *School-Based Health Clinics: Are They Addressing the Needs of the Students?* [master's thesis]. Seattle, Wash: University of Washington; 1991.

49. Center for Population Options. *Clinic News,* April 1986:3.

50. Metropolitan Life, Louis Harris and Associates. *The American Teacher, 1988.* New York, NY: Metropolitan Life; 1989.

51. Planned Parenthood Federation of America, Louis Harris and Associates. *Public Attitudes Toward Teenage Pregnancy, Sex Education, and Birth Control.* New York. NY: Planned Parenthood Federation of America; 1988.

52. Palfrey JS, McGaughey MJ, Cooperman PJ, Fenton T, McManus MA. Financing health services in school-based clinics. *J Adolesc Health.* 1991;3:233–239.

53. Yale Bush Center in Child Development and Social Policy; 1992.

54. *A Community-Based Education and Intervention System.* Jackson, Miss: Jackson-Hinds School-Based Adolescent Health Program; undated.

55. Information provided by Dr. Aaron Shirley, director of the Jackson-Hinds Community Health Center.

56. Levy J, Shepardson W. A look at current school-linked service efforts. In: *The Future of Children: School-Linked Services.* Los Altos, Calif: Center for the Future of Children, David and Lucile Packard Foundation; 1992:141–142.

57. New Brunswick Public Schools. *School-Based Youth Services Programs.* New Brunswick, NJ: New Brunswick Public Schools; undated.

58. Discussions with Gail Reynolds, director, New Brunswick Public Schools.

CHAPTER 11

Addressing Barriers to Learning

Beyond School-Linked Services and Full-Service Schools

Howard S. Adelman, Linda Taylor, 1997

School-linked services, integrated services, school-based clinics, one-stop shopping, wraparound services, seamless service delivery, comprehensive school health, co-location of services, restructuring—such terms are associated with a host of system reforms. Ample support for pursuing these reforms is found in the considerable agreement about deficiencies in outcome efficacy and cost-efficiency and in a growing consensus about directions for change.[1–10] The call is for moving from fragmentation to coordinated/integrated intervention and from narrowly focused, problem-specific, and specialist-oriented services to comprehensive general approaches.

In pursuing these trends, it is essential to attend to issues they engender. Of particular importance is the continuing confusion about such matters as (1) What systems are systemic reformers talking

---

about? (2) Coordinated or integrated services? (3) How comprehensive is comprehensive? This article will address each of these questions in turn, in an effort to clarify key issues and discuss implications for moving ahead with system reforms that can address a full range of barriers to student learning.

WHAT SYSTEMS ARE REFORMERS TALKING ABOUT?

System changes that play a role in addressing barriers to learning are found in two reform movements. One set of initiatives aims at restructuring community health and human services; the other movement encompasses efforts to reform education. Each domain has implications for the other and encompasses a host of issues that require exploration.

Community Health and Human Services

Concern about the fragmented way in which community health and human services are planned and implemented has renewed the 1960s human-service integration movement.[11–13] The hope is to better meet the needs of those served and use existing resources to serve greater numbers. To these ends, there is considerable interest in connecting with school sites.

SCHOOL-LINKED SERVICES—CONCEPT AND CONCERNS. Initiatives to restructure community health and human services have fostered the concept of school-linked services, and contribute to the burgeoning of school-based and school-linked health clinics.[3,14] At the outset, a distinction should be made between school-*linked* and school-*based.* In practice, the terms encompass two separate dimensions (1) where programs/services are located, and (2) who owns them. Literally, school-based indicates activity carried out on a campus, and school-linked refers to off-campus activity with formal connections to a school site. In either case, services may be owned by schools or a community-based organization; in some cases, they are co-owned. As commonly used, the term school-linked refers to community owned on- and off-campus services and is strongly associated with the notion of coordinated services.

The movement toward school-linked services aims at enhancing access to services, reducing redundancy, improving case management, coordinating resources, and increasing efficacy. In pursuing these desirable goals, however, the tendency is to think mainly in terms of coordinating community services—and putting some on school sites. This emphasis downplays the need to weave community resources together with the resources that schools already own and operate. As a result, initiatives for school-linked services have led some policy makers to the mistaken impression that such an approach can effectively meet the needs of schools in addressing barriers to learning.

The movement also colludes with the misguided tendency of some legislators to view school-linked services as a way to free up the funds underwriting school-owned services. In pursuing school-linked services, care must be taken that the dwindling pool of school and community-owned resources is not diminished further. The reality is that even when one adds together community and school assets, the total set of services in economically impoverished locales is woefully inadequate.[5]

SERVICES/PROGRAMS. As the concept of school-linked services spreads, the terms "services" and "programs" increasingly are used interchangeably. This leads to some confusion, especially since addressing a full range of barriers to learning requires going beyond a focus on services. Services themselves should be differentiated to distinguish between narrow-band, clinical services and broad-band public health and social services.[16] Furthermore, although services can be provided as part of a program, not all are. For example, counseling to ameliorate a mental health problem can be offered on an ad-hoc basis or as one element of a multifaceted program. Pervasive and severe psychosocial problems, such as substance abuse, teen pregnancy, physical and sexual abuse, gang violence, and delinquency, require multifaceted, programmatic interventions. Besides providing services to correct existing problems, such interventions encompass primary prevention (e.g., public-health programs that target groups seen as "at risk") and a broad range of open-enrollment didactic, enrichment, and recreation programs. Differentiating services and programs helps mediate against tendencies to limit the range of interventions for addressing barriers to learning. The distinction also underscores the breadth of activity that requires coordination and integration.

ONE-STOP SHOPPING AND WRAPAROUND SERVICES. A set of accessible programs is essential for addressing barriers to learning. The term "wraparound services" reflects the desire to develop a sufficient range of interventions to meet the needs of those served, a point that will be underscored in the discussion of comprehensive approaches, below.

In enhancing access, location is a fundamental consideration. Increasingly, schools are seen as a logical access point, and this has accelerated advocacy for school-community collaborations. Various forms of such collaboration are being tested around the country. For instance, many projects are trying to demonstrate "one-stop shopping"—a family service or resource center, established at or near a school, with an array of medical, mental health, and social services.[3,7,17–20] State-wide initiatives in California, Florida, Kentucky, New Jersey, and Oregon, among others, are exploring the possibility of developing strong relationships between schools and public and private community agencies.[21,22]

STATE OF THE ART. In analyzing emerging school-linked service initiatives, Franklin and Streeter[23] categorized five alternative approaches—informal, coordinated, partnerships, collaborations, and integrated services. These were conceptualized as differing in terms of the degree of system change required. As would be anticipated, most initial efforts focus on developing informal relationships and beginning to coordinate services.

A review by Knapp[24] underscored the extent to which contemporary literature on school-linked services is heavy on advocacy and prescription and light on findings. Each day brings additional reports from projects such as New Jersey's School-Based Youth Services Program, the Healthy Start Initiative in California, the Beacons Schools in New York, Cities-in-Schools, and the New Futures Initiative. Not surprisingly, findings primarily reflect how hard it is to institutionalize such collaborations. New Futures represents one of the most ambitious efforts. Thus, reports from the initiative's on-site evaluators[25] are particularly instructive. They have detailed the project's limited success and cautioned that its deficiencies arose from defining collaboration mainly in institutional terms and failing to involve community members in problem solving. This produced "a top-down strategy that was too disabled to see the day-by-day effects of policy." The evaluators concluded:

> Collaboration should not be seen primarily as a problem of getting professionals and human service agencies to work together more efficiently and effectively. This goal, though laudable, does not respond to the core problems. . . . Instead, the major issue is how to get whole communities, the haves and the have-nots, to engage in the difficult task of community development.[25(pp36–37)]

Keeping the difficulties in mind, a reasonable inference from available data is that school-community collaborations can be successful and cost-effective over the long run. Stationing community agency staff at schools allows easier access for students and families—especially in areas with underserved and hard-to-reach populations. Such efforts not only provide services, they seem to encourage schools to open their doors in ways that enhance family involvement. Analyses suggest that better outcomes are associated with empowering children and families and having the capability to address diverse constituencies and contexts.[24] Families using school-based centers have been described as becoming interested in contributing to school and community by providing social-support networks for new students and families, teaching each other coping skills, participating in school governance, and helping create a psychological sense of community.[25]

At the same time, it is clear that initiatives for school-linked services produce tension between school district pupil-services personnel and their counterparts in community-based organizations. When "outside" professionals are brought in, school specialist staff often view the move as discounting their skills and threatening their jobs. These concerns are aggravated whenever policy makers appear to overestimate the promise of school-linked services with regard to addressing the full range of barriers to learning. And, ironically, by downplaying school-owned resources, the school-linked services movement has allowed educators to ignore the need for restructuring the various education support programs and services that schools own and operate.

Restructuring Education

The literature on school restructuring is filled with statements affirming that factors interfering with student learning must be addressed if the educational mission is to succeed.[26–31] Moreover, the need for services that enable students to benefit from instruction is clearly acknowledged by the educational bureaucracy at state and national levels (e.g., by bodies such as departments of education, the Council of Chief State School Officers, and associations of school boards).

Despite widespread recognition of need, the school-reform movement continues to pay scant attention to education support programs and services. Leaders of comprehensive educational reform seem content to call for "coordinated" and "school-linked" services and concomitantly ignore fundamental considerations related to restructuring school-owned and operated psychosocial and health programs. Thus, it is not surprising that relatively little has been done at any administrative level to establish the leadership and infrastructure required for essential reform of this facet of school activity.

The necessity for restructuring education support programs is evident from observing school operations. Factors such as categorical funding and the lack of effective mechanisms for coordination and integration lead to piecemeal design of delivery systems and disjointed implementation of programs and services. In some schools, for example, a student identified as at risk for dropout, suicide, and substance abuse may be involved in three counseling programs operating independently of each other. Functionally, much of the activity focuses on individuals and small groups and is carried out in a "clinical" fashion.[16] Organizationally, practitioners at a school site operate in relative isolation and usually are not included in new governance bodies as schools move toward school-based management and shared decision making. Further, time for on-the-job professional education remains exceedingly limited,[32] and little or no attention is paid to cross-disciplinary training.[9,33] In addition, aides and volunteers working in this area still receive little or no formal training before or after they are assigned duties.

All of this contributes to maintaining an enterprise that is narrowly focused, fragmented, and oriented to discrete problems and specialized services—and one that is not a prominent part of a school's organizational structure and daily functions. Based on their status in the administrative structure, it seems reasonable to conclude that the prevailing view of pupil services, in policy and practice, is that they are desirable but not essential. Because of their devalued status in the educational hierarchy, such "auxiliary" or "support" services too often are among those deemed dispensable as budgets tighten. Indeed, many districts have cut back a significant portion of their pupil services' staff in recent years, thereby further limiting the ability of schools to address barriers to learning and enhance healthy development.

As districts move to decentralize authority and empower all stakeholders, realignment is likely with respect to how pupil personnel professionals are governed and how they are involved in school governance and collective bargaining.[34,35] Ultimately, of course, this will determine how many are employed. Unfortunately, if restructuring education support programs and services continues not to be a high priority, emerging realignments probably will not translate into important reforms and may even exacerbate current deficiencies.

COORDINATED OR INTEGRATED?

Use of the term "integrated" permeates the literature on school-linked services. Its frequent occurrence conveys a long-term aim, and one that will not be easy to attain. The difficulties associated with integrating community health and human services are well established. Comparable difficulties exist for any effort to integrate school-owned programs and services. And the complications undoubtedly will be multiplied exponentially when efforts are made to integrate community and school-owned interventions.

True integration involves blending of resources and shared governance. At this stage of system reform focused on school-community collaboration, the emphasis is mainly on increasing communication, cooperation, and coordination—sometimes with a focus on enhancing case management, sometimes to enhance use of resources.

As an aid in discussing integrated interventions, it is helpful to differentiate key dimensions relevant to school-community collaborative arrangements, such as (1) focus of collaborative efforts (specific programs and services or major systemic reform), (2) scope of collaboration (number of programs and services involved; horizontal collaboration within and among schools/agencies; vertical collaboration within a catchment area and among different levels of jurisdictions), (3) ownership (programs and services owned by school, community, public-private, shared ownership), (4) location (programs and services are school-linked or school-based), and (5) degree of cohesiveness among multiple interventions serving the same student/family (unconnected, communicating, cooperating, coordinated, integrated). Brief consideration of the focus and scope of such arrangements and the problem of ownership may help to clarify some basic concerns.

Focus and Scope: Integration for What?

A major emphasis in restructuring health and human services is to ensure coordination of service delivery through enhancing case management. In doing so, redundancies should be detected and outcome efficacy and cost-effectiveness improved. Case management usually focuses on enhancing coordination, rather than on the more complicated considerations involved in integrating interventions.

When the aim is to enhance productivity of resources, reforms tend to focus on systemic factors producing redundancy and interfering with programs, services, and staff working together. The ultimate vision is one of total integration. However, there are many institutionalized factors that mediate against establishing this vision in the short run (e.g., categorical funding for programs, conflicts between education law and health law related to matters such as confidentiality and consent, turf protection, guild and union prerogatives, narrow specialist training). Because of the problem's scope, current system reform focuses mainly on (1) creating horizontal cooperative arrangements to enhance resource coordination at the school and community level and (2) exploring vertical cooperative arrangements at various jurisdictional levels. For the vision of integrating school and community resources to become a reality, entities at federal, state, and local levels must redefine policy and their focus and scope of operation.[10,36–38] Essential policy and bureaucratic redefinitions are more apt to occur if simultaneous efforts are made at all levels (top-down, bottom-up, and sideways).

The Problem of Ownership

At the most fundamental level, the intent to integrate programs and services must deal effectively with the problems of ownership and distribution of power. Funds and resources must be blended and power redistributed. For entities throughout a community (e.g., schools, health, social service, safety, and recreational agencies) to be integrated, new models for governance at various jurisdictional levels will be required. Such new models will reflect how power has been redistributed, and the new governance bodies will have responsibility for guiding the use of blended resources.

Given the range of stakeholders with vested interests, it seems inevitable that consensus-building regarding redistribution of property and other resources will require a shared commitment to the process of system change and a lengthy period of transition. And none of this is likely without potent and focused leadership and a sound infrastructure to support change.

HOW COMPREHENSIVE IS COMPREHENSIVE?

In responding to the troubling and the troubled, schools tend to rely overly on narrowly focused and time-intensive interventions. Given sparse resources, this means serving a small proportion of the many students who require assistance and doing so in a noncomprehensive way. The deficiencies of such an approach have led to calls for increased comprehensiveness—both to better address the needs of those served and to serve greater numbers.

A Team with Wide Appeal

Comprehensiveness is becoming a buzzword. Health providers pursue comprehensive systems of care; states establish initiatives for comprehensive school-linked services; school health professionals talk about comprehensive school health; school-based clinics aspire to be comprehensive health centers. Increasing use of the term masks the fact that comprehensiveness, like integration, is a vision for the future—not a reality of the day.

Comprehensiveness requires holistic and developmental perspectives that are translated into an extensive continuum of programs focused on individuals, families, and environment. Such a continuum ranges from primary prevention and early-age intervention, through approaches for treating problems soon after onset, to treatment for severe and chronic problems. Included are programs designed to promote and maintain safety at home and at school, programs to promote and maintain physical and mental health, preschool programs, early school-adjustment programs, programs to improve and augment ongoing social and academic supports, programs to intervene prior to referral for intensive treatments, and programs providing intensive treatment.[39] This scope of activity underscores the need to develop formal mechanisms for long-lasting interprogram collaboration.[40]

Comprehensiveness also requires balancing problem-specific and specialist-oriented services with less categorical, cross-disciplinary programs. The specialized approaches that currently dominate school and community interventions are shaped primarily by two factors. One involves funding agency regulations and guidelines; for example, those related to legislatively mandated compensatory and special-education programs and to categorical programs for addressing social problems such as substance abuse, gang and on-campus violence, and teen pregnancy. The other shaping force is the prevailing intervention models taught by various fields of specialization, such as counseling, school and clinical psychology, and social work. There is growing consensus that specialist-oriented activity must be balanced with a generalist perspective in order to develop a comprehensive, integrated approach.[41]

School-Focused Examples

School settings are the focus for several initiatives that aspire to comprehensiveness. Three prime examples are: (1) comprehensive school-based health centers, (2) the comprehensive school health model, and (3) full-service schools.

COMPREHENSIVE SCHOOL-BASED HEALTH CENTERS. Many of the now more than 900 school-based or school-linked health clinics are described as comprehensive centers.[3,42–44] This reflects the fact that the problems students bring to such clinics require much more than medical intervention.

The school-based clinic movement was created in response to concerns about teen pregnancy and a desire to enhance access to physical health care for underserved youth. Soon after opening, most clinics find it essential to address mental health and psychosocial concerns. The need to do so reflects two basic realities. First, since some students' physical complaints are psychogenic, treatment of various medical problems is aided by psychological intervention. Second, in a large number of cases, students come to clinics primarily for help with nonmedical problems, such as personal adjustment and peer and family relationship problems, emotional distress, problems related to physical and sexual abuse, and concerns stemming from use of alcohol and other drugs. Indeed, up to 50% of clinic visits are for nonmedical concerns.[45–47] Thus, as these clinics evolve, so does the provision of counseling, psychological, and social services in the schools. At the same time, given the limited number of staff at such clinics, it is not surprising that the demand for psychosocial interventions quickly outstrips the resources available. Because school-based and school-linked health clinics can provide only a restricted range of interventions to a limited number of students, the desire of such clinics to be comprehensive centers in the full sense of the term remains thwarted.

COMPREHENSIVE SCHOOL HEALTH. Up until the 1980s, school health programs were seen as encompassing health education, health services, and health environments. Over the last decade, school health advocates[48,49] have championed a model encompassing the following eight components: health education; health services; biophysical and psychosocial environments; counseling, psychological, and social services; integrated efforts of schools and communities to improve health; food service; physical education and activity; and health programs for faculty and staff.

To foster development of each state's capacity to move toward comprehensive school health programming, the Centers for Disease Control and Prevention (CDC) set in motion an initiative to support an enhanced administrative infrastructure designed to increase interagency coordination.[50] In addition, the Educational Development Center, funded under a cooperative agreement with CDC's Division of Adolescent and School Health, has initiated a large-scale project to clarify how national organizations and state and local education and health agencies can advance school health programs.[51]

The focus on comprehensive school health is admirable. However, in restricting its emphasis to health, it tends to engender resistance from school policy makers who do not understand how they can afford a comprehensive focus on health and still accomplish their primary mission of educating students. Reform-minded policy makers may be more open to proposals encompassing a broad range of programs to enhance healthy development if such programs are part of a comprehensive approach for addressing barriers to learning.

FULL-SERVICE SCHOOLS. Dryfoos[3,17] encompassed the trend to develop school-based primary health clinics, youth service programs, community schools, and similar activity under the rubric of "full-service schools," crediting the term to Florida's comprehensive school-based legislation. As she noted:

> Much of the rhetoric in support of the full service schools concept has been presented in the language of systems change, calling for radical reform of the way educational, health, and welfare agencies provide services. Consensus has formed around the goals of one-stop, seamless service provision, whether in a school- or community-based agency, along with empowerment of the target population.... Most of the programs have moved services from one place to another; for example, a medical unit from a hospital or health department relocates into a school through a contractual agreement, or staff of a community mental health center is reassigned to a school, or a grant to a school creates a coordinator in a center. As the program expands, the center staff work with the school to draw in additional services, fostering more contracts between the schools and community agencies. But few of the school systems or the agencies have changed their governance. The outside agency is not involved in school restructuring or school policy, nor is the school system involved in the governance of the provider agency. The result is not yet a new organizational entity,

but the school is an improved institution and on the path to becoming a different kind of institution that is significantly responsive to the needs of the community.[3(p169)]

Although full-service schools reflect the desire for comprehensiveness, the reality remains much less than the vision. As long as such efforts are shaped primarily by a school-linked services model (i.e., initiatives to restructure to community health and human services), resources will remain too limited to allow for a comprehensive continuum of programs.

In sum, with respect to addressing barriers to learning, comprehensiveness requires more than outreach to link with community resources, more than coordination of school-owned services, and more than coordination of school and community services. Moving toward comprehensiveness encompasses restructuring and enhancing (1) school-owned programs and services and (2) community resources; in the process, it is essential to (3) weave school and community resources together. The result is not simply a reallocation or relocation of resources; it is a total transformation of the nature and scope of intervention activity.

IMPLICATIONS FOR MOVING AHEAD

Policy makers and reform leaders have yet to come to grips with the realities of addressing barriers to learning. A few preliminary steps have been taken. For example, to facilitate reform by countering what has been described as a "hardening of the categories," there are trends toward granting (1) flexibility in the use of categorical funds and (2) temporary waivers from regulatory restrictions. There also is renewed interest in cross-disciplinary training—with several universities already testing interprofessional collaboration programs.[35,52]

One reason for the limited progress is the lack of a unifying concept around which advocates and decision makers can rally. A related problem is the dearth of models clarifying the nature and scope of essential programs, services, and infrastructure mechanisms. The following brief sections are intended to illuminate each of these matters.

A Unifying Concept

Despite the argument that schools should not be expected to operate nonacademic programs, it is commonplace to find educators citing the need for health and social services as ways to enable students to learn and perform. Also, increasing numbers of schools are reaching out to expand services that can support and enrich the educational process. Thus, there is little doubt that educators are aware of the value of health (mental and physical) and psychosocial interventions. In spite of this, efforts to create a comprehensive approach still are not assigned a high priority.

The problem is that the primary nature of relevant activity has not been effectively thrust before policy makers and education reformers. Some demonstrations are attracting attention, but they do not convey the message that interventions addressing barriers to teaching and learning are *essential* to successful school reform.

The next step in moving toward a comprehensive approach is to see to it that policy makers at all levels are aware that, if school reform is to produce desired student outcomes, school and community reformers must expand their vision beyond the restructuring of instructional and management functions; they must recognize that there is a third primary (i.e., *necessary*) set of functions involved in enabling teaching and learning. This essential third facet of school and community restructuring has been called the Enabling Component.[16,39,53] Such a component stresses integration of enabling programs and services with instructional and management components. Emergence of a cohesive enabling component requires (1) weaving together what is available at a school; (2) expanding it by integrating school and community resources; and (3) enhancing access to community programs and services by linking as many as feasible to programs at the school.

The concept of an enabling component provides a unifying focus around which to formulate policy. Adoption of an inclusive unifying concept is seen as pivotal in convincing policy makers to recognize enabling activity as essential if schools are to attain their goals. The value of rallying around a broad unifying concept has been demonstrated in California, where in 1995 the type of policy shift outlined here was drafted into a proposed (although not enacted) urban education bill (AB784). In addition, the concept has been adopted by one of the original nine national "break the mold" models supported by the New American Schools Development Corporation.[54]

A Programmatic Focus

Operationalizing an enabling component requires formulating a carefully delimited framework of basic programmatic areas and creating an infrastructure to support enabling activity. Based on analyses of extant school and community activity, enabling activity can be clustered into six basic programmatic areas that address barriers to learning and enhance healthy development. These encompass interventions to (1) enhance classroom-based efforts to enable learning, (2) provide prescribed student and family assistance, (3) respond to and prevent crises, (4) support transitions, (5) increase home involvement in schooling, and (6) develop greater community involvement and support—including recruitment of volunteers. These six areas have been described in detail elsewhere;[53] a brief overview follows.

CLASSROOM-FOCUSED ENABLING. The intent here is to enhance classroom-based efforts to enable learning and productive classroom functioning by increasing teacher effectiveness in preventing and handling problems. This is accomplished by providing personalized professional development and enhanced resources to expand a teacher's array of strategies for working with a wider range of individual differences. For example, teachers learn to use peer tutoring and volunteers (as well as home involvement) to enhance social and academic support; they learn to increase their range of accommodative strategies and their ability to teach students compensatory strategies; and, as appropriate, they are provided support in the classroom by resource and itinerant teachers and counselors. Only when clearly necessary is temporary out-of-class help provided. In addition, programs are directed at developing the capabilities of aides, volunteers, and any others who help in classrooms or work with teachers to enable learning. With a view to further preventing learning, behavior, emotional, and health problems, there is also an effort to enhance those facets of classroom curricula designed to foster socioemotional and physical development.

STUDENT AND FAMILY ASSISTANCE. Some problems cannot be handled without special interventions; thus the need for student and family assistance. The emphasis is on providing special services in a personalized way to assist with a broad range of needs. To begin with, available social, physical and mental health programs in the school and community are used. As community outreach brings in other resources, they are linked to existing activity in an integrated manner. Special attention is paid to enhancing systems for pre-referral intervention, triage, case and resource management, direct services to meet immediate needs, and referral for special services and special-education resources and placements. Ongoing efforts are made to expand and enhance resources.

CRISIS ASSISTANCE AND PREVENTION. The intent here is to respond to, minimize the impact of, and prevent crises. Work in this area requires systems and programs for emergency/crisis response at a site, throughout a school complex, and community-wide (including a program to ensure follow-up care); it also encompasses prevention programs for school and community to address school safety and violence reduction, suicide prevention, child-abuse prevention, and so forth. Crisis assistance includes ensuring that immediate emergency and follow-up care is provided so that students are able to resume learning without undue delay. Prevention activity creates a safe and productive environment and develops the type of attitudes and capacities that students and their families need to deal with violence and other threats to safety.

SUPPORT FOR TRANSITIONS. This area involves planning, developing, and maintaining a comprehensive focus on the many transition concerns confronting students and their families. Such efforts aim at reducing alienation and increasing positive attitudes and involvement related to school and various learning activities. Examples of interventions include (1) programs to establish a welcoming and socially supportive school community, especially for new arrivals; (2) counseling and articulation programs to support grade-to-grade and school-to-school transitions, moving to and from special education, going to college, moving to post-school living and work; and (3) programs for before- and after-school and intersession to enrich learning and provide recreation in a safe environment.

HOME INVOLVEMENT IN SCHOOLING. Efforts to enhance home involvement must range from programs to address specific learning and support needs of adults in the home to approaches that empower legitimate parent representatives to become full partners in school governance. Examples include programs designed to (1) address specific learning and support needs of adults in the home, such as English-as-a-Second-Language classes and mutual-support groups; (2) help those in the home meet their basic obligations to the student, such as instruction in parenting and in helping with schoolwork; (3) improve communication about matters essential to the student and family; (4) enhance the home-school connection and sense of community, (5) enhance participation in making decisions that are essential to the student; (6) enhance home support related to the student's basic learning and development; (7) mobilize those at home to engage in problem-solving related to student needs; and (8) elicit help (support, collaborations, and partnerships) from those at home with respect to meeting classroom, school, and community needs. The context for some of this activity may be a parent center (which may be part of a family service center facility if one has been established at the site).

COMMUNITY OUTREACH. Outreach to the community is used to build linkages and collaborations, develop greater involvement in schooling, and enhance support for efforts to enable learning. Outreach is made to (1) public and private community agencies, universities, colleges, organizations, and facilities; (2) businesses and professional organizations and groups; and (3) volunteer service programs, organizations, and clubs. Activities include (1) programs to recruit community involvement and support (e.g., linkages and integration with community health and social services; cadres of volunteers, mentors, and individuals with special expertise and resources; local businesses encouraged to adopt a school and provide resources, awards, incentives, and jobs; formal partnership arrangements), (2) systems and programs specifically designed to train, screen, and maintain volunteers (e.g., parents, college students, senior citizens, peer and cross-age tutors and counselors, and professionals-in-training to provide direct help for staff and students—especially targeted students); (3) outreach programs for hard-to-involve students and families (e.g., children who don't come to school regularly—including truants and dropouts); and (4) programs to enhance community-school connections and sense of community (e.g., orientations, open houses, performances and cultural and sports events, festivals and celebrations, workshops and fairs).

Ultimately, a comprehensive set of programs to address barriers and enhance healthy development must be woven into the fabric of every school. In addition, neighboring schools need to link together to maximize use of limited school and community resources. Over time, by working toward developing a comprehensive, integrated approach, every school can be seen, once more, as a key element of its community. When schools are viewed as a valued and integrated part of every community, talk of school and community as separate entities can cease; talk of education as if it were the sole function of schools will end; and the major role schools can play in enhancing healthy development will be understood and appreciated.

Building an Infrastructure

An infrastructure of mechanisms must be created for restructuring resources in ways that enhance the efficacy of each programmatic area and facilitate coordination among enabling activities. It must also establish mechanisms for enhancing resources by developing direct linkages between school and community programs; for facilitating integration of school and community resources; and for integrating the instructional, enabling, and management components.[53]

Once policy makers recognize the essential nature of a component for addressing barriers to learning, it should be easier to weave together all enabling activity (including special and compensatory education), and elevate the status of programs to enhance healthy development. It also should be less difficult to gain acceptance of the need for fundamental policy shifts to reshape programs of pre- and in-service education.

A policy shift and programmatic focus are necessary but not sufficient. For significant systemic change to occur, policy and program commitments must be demonstrated through allocation/redeployment of resources (e.g., finances, personnel, time, space, equipment) that can adequately operationalize policy and promising practices. In particular, there must be sufficient resources to develop an effective structural foundation for system change. Existing infrastructure mechanisms must be modified in ways that guarantee new policy directions are translated into appropriate daily practices. Well-designed infrastructure mechanisms ensure that there is local ownership, a critical mass of committed stakeholders, processes that can overcome barriers to stakeholders working together effectively, and strategies that can mobilize and maintain proactive effort so that changes are implemented and renewed over time.

Institutionalizing a comprehensive, integrated approach requires redesigning mechanisms with respect to at least five basic infrastructure concerns: (1) governance, (2) planning and implementation associated with specific organizational and program objectives, (3) coordination/integration for cohesion, (4) daily leadership; and (5) communication and information management. In reforming mechanisms, new collaborative arrangements must be established, and authority must be redistributed—all of which is easy to propose and extremely hard to accomplish. Reform obviously requires providing adequate support (time, space, materials, equipment)—not just initially, but over time—

to those who operate the mechanisms. And there must be appropriate incentives and safeguards for those undertaking the tasks.

In terms of task focus, infrastructure changes must attend to (1) interweaving school and community resources for addressing barriers to learning (a component to enable learning), direct facilitation of learning (instruction), and system management; (2) reframing in-service programs—including an emphasis on cross-training; and (3) establishing appropriate forms of quality improvement, accountability, and self-renewal. Clearly, all this requires greater involvement of professionals providing health and human services, and other programs addressing barriers to learning—and this means involvement in every facet of the system, especially governance.

CONCLUSIONS

As the Carnegie Council on Adolescent Development succinctly concluded: "School systems are not responsible for meeting every need of their students. But when the need directly affects learning, the school must meet the challenge."[27(p7)] School-community collaboratives represent a promising direction for efforts to generate essential interventions. However, steps must be taken to counter the piecemeal and fragmented approach that characterizes most school and community efforts.

As emphasized throughout this article, effectively meeting the challenges of addressing persistent barriers to learning and enhancing healthy development requires melding resources of home, school, and community to create a comprehensive, integrated approach. (This requirement is not met simply by participation in a multidisciplinary team that discusses cases or coordinates resources.) Its realization involves a policy shift in which development of such an approach is placed on a par with current reforms related to instruction and school management. Creation of the approach proposed here also involves new roles for professionals who work in schools and communities, and requires shifting priorities and redeploying time for program coordination, development, and leadership.[55]

Clearly, staff currently providing health and human services can contribute a great deal to the creation of a comprehensive, integrated approach. Equally evident is the fact that they cannot do so as long as they are completely consumed by their daily caseloads. Their role must be a multifaceted one—providing services as well as vision and leadership that transforms the ways in which schools address barriers to learning and enhance healthy development.

Notes

1. Adler L, Gardner S, eds. *The Politics of Linking Schools and Social Services.* Washington, DC: Falmer Press; 1994.

2. Cahill M. *Schools and Communities: A Continuum of Relationships.* New York, NY: Youth Development Institute, Fund for the City of New York; 1994.

3. Dryfoos JG. *Full-Service Schools: A Revolution in Health and Social Services for Children, Youth, and Families.* San Francisco, Calif: Jossey-Bass; 1994.

4. Hooper-Briar K, Lawson H. *Serving Children, Youth, and Family Through Interprofessional Collaboration and Service Integration: A Framework for Action.* Oxford, Ohio: Danforth Foundation, Institute for Educational Renewal at Miami University; 1994.

5. Koppich JE, Kirst MW, eds. Integrating services for children: prospects and pitfalls. *Educ Urban Soc.* 1993;25(2) [special issue].

6. Kusserow RP. *Services Integration for Families and Children in Crisis.* Washington, DC: US Department of Health and Human Services; 1993.

7. Melaville A, Blank M. *What It Takes: Structuring Interagency Partnerships to Connect Children and Families with Comprehensive Services.* Washington, DC: Education and Human Services Consortium; 1991.

8. Sheridan SM. Fostering school/community relationships. In Thomas A, Grimes J, eds. *Best Practices in School Psychology,* vol 3. Washington, DC: National Association for School Psychologists; 1995:203–212.

9. US Department of Education, Office of Educational Research and Improvement, American Educational Research Association, American Association of Colleges for Teacher Education, Association of Teacher Education, National Center on Education in the Inner Cities. *School-Linked Comprehensive Services for Children and Families: What We Know and What We Need to Know.* Washington, DC: US Department of Education; 1995.

10. US General Accounting Office. *School-Linked Services: A Comprehensive Strategy for Aiding Students at Risk for School Failure.* Washington, DC: US General Accounting Office; 1993.

11. Agranoff R. Human service integration: past and present challenges in public administration. *Public Admin Rev.* 1991;51:533–542.

12. Tyack DB. Health and social services in public schools: historical perspectives. *Future Child.* 1992;2:19–31.

13. Weiss CH. Nothing as practical as good theory: exploring theory-based evaluation for comprehensive community initiatives for children and families. In: Connell JB, Kubish AC, Schorr L, Weiss CH, eds. *New Approaches to Evaluating Community Initiatives: Concepts, Methods, and Contexts.* Washington, DC: Aspen Institute; 1995:65–92.

14. Center for the Future of Children Staff. Analysis. *Future Child.* 1992;2:6–188.

15. Koyanagi C, Gaines S. *All Systems Fail.* Washington, DC: National Mental Health Association; 1993.

16. Adelman HS. Clinical psychology: beyond psychopathology and clinical interventions. *Clin Psych: Sci Prac.* 1995;2:28–44.

17. Dryfoos JG. Full-service schools: revolution or fad? *J Res Adolesc.* 1995;5: 147–172.

18. Holtzman WH. Community renewal, family preservation, and child development through the School of the Future. In: Holtzman WH, ed. *School of the Future.* Austin, Tex: American Psychological Association, Hogg Foundation for Mental Health; 1992:3–18.

19. Kagan SL, Rivera AM, Parker FL. *Collaboration in Action: Reshaping Services for Young Children and Their Families.* New Haven, Conn: Bush Center on Child Development and Social Policy, Yale University; 1990.

20. Kirst MW. Improving children's services: overcoming barriers, creating new opportunities. *Phi Delta Kappan.* 1991;72:615–618.

21. First PF, Curcio JL, Young DL. State full-service school initiatives: new notions of policy development. In: Adler L, Gardner S, eds. *The Politics of Linking Schools and School Services.* Washington, DC: Falmer Press; 1994:63–74.

22. Palaich RM, Whitney TN, Paolino AR. *Changing Delivery Systems: Addressing the Fragmentation in Children and Youth Services.* Denver, Colo: Education Commission of the States; 1991.

23, Franklin C, Streeter CL. School reform: linking public schools with human services. *Soc Work.* 1995;40:773–782.

24. Knapp MS. How shall we study comprehensive collaborative services for children and families? *Educ Res.* 1995;24:5–16.

25. White JA, Wehlage G. Community collaboration: if it is such a good idea, why is it so hard to do? *Educ Eval Policy Anal.* 1995;17:23–38.

26. Barth RS. *Improving Schools From Within: Teachers, Parents, and Principles Can Make a Difference.* San Francisco, Calif: Jossey-Bass; 1990.

27. Carnegie Council on Adolescent Development, Task Force on Education of Young Adolescents. *Turning Points: Preparing American Youth for the 21st Century.* Washington, DC: Carnegie Council on Adolescent Development; 1989.

28. Elmore RF, Associates. *Restructuring Schools: The Next Generation of Educational Reform.* San Francisco, Calif: Jossey-Bass; 1990.

29. Lieberman A, Miller L. Restructuring schools: what matters and what works. *Phi Delta Kappan.* 1990;71:759–764.

30. Newmann FM. Beyond common sense in educational restructuring: the issues of content and linkage. *Educ Rev.* 1993;22:4–13, 22.

31. Wang MC, Haertel GD, Walberg HJ. The effectiveness of collaborative school-linked services. In: Flaxman E, Passow AH, eds. *Changing Populations, Changing Schools.* 94th yearbook of the National Society for the Study of Education, pt 2. Chicago, Ill: University of Chicago Press; 1995:253–270.

32. National Education Commission on Time and Learning. *Prisoners of Time.* Washington, DC: US GPO; 1994.

33. Lawson H, Hooper-Briar K. *Expanding Partnerships: Involving Colleges and Universities in Interprofessional Collaboration and Service Integration.* Oxford, Ohio: Danforth Foundation, Institute for Educational Renewal at Miami University; 1994.

34. Hill P, Bonan J. *Decentralization and Accountability in Public Education.* Santa Monica, Calif: RAND Corporation; 1991.

35. Streeter CL, Franklin C. Site-based management in public education: opportunities and challenges for school social workers. *Soc Work Educ.* 1993;15:71–81.

36. Bruner C. *Thinking Collaboratively: Ten Questions and Answers to Help Policy Makers Improve Children's Services.* Washington, DC: Educational and Human Services Consortium; 1991.

37. Kahn A, Kamerman S. *Integrating Service Integration: An Overview of Initiatives, Issues, and Possibilities.* New York, NY: National Center for Children in Poverty; 1992.

38. Stoner CR. School/community collaboration: comparing three initiatives. *Phi Delta Kappan.* 1995;76:794–800.

39. Adelman HS, Taylor L. *On Understanding Intervention in Psychology and Education.* Westport, Conn: Praeger; 1994.

40. Adelman HS. School-linked mental health interventions: toward mechanisms for service coordination and integration. *J Community Psychol.* 1993;21:309–319.

41. Henggeler SW. A consensus: conclusions of the APA Task Force report on innovative models of mental health services for children, adolescents, and their families. *J Clin Psychol.* 1995;23:3–6.

42. Advocates for Youth. *School-Based and School-Linked Health Centers: The Facts.* Washington, DC: Advocates for Youth; 1994.

43. Robert Wood Johnson Foundation. *Making the Grade: State and Local Partnerships to Establish School-Based Health Centers.* Princeton, NJ: Robert Wood Johnson Foundation; 1993.

44. Schlitt JJ, Rickett KD, Montgomery LL, Lear JG. *State Initiatives to Support School-Based Health Centers: A National Survey.* Washington, DC: Robert Wood Johnson Foundation; 1994.

45. Adelman HS, Barker LA, Nelson P. A study of a school-based clinic: who uses it and who doesn't? *J Clin Child Psychol.* 1993;22:52–59.

46. Center for Reproductive Health Policy Research. *Annual Report: Evaluation of California's Comprehensive School-Based Health Centers.* San Francisco, Calif: Center for Reproductive Health Policy Research; 1989.

47. Robert Wood Johnson Foundation. *Annual Report.* Princeton, NJ: Robert Wood Johnson Foundation; 1989.

48. Allensworth DD, Kolbe LJ. The comprehensive school health program: exploring an expanded concept. *J Sch Health.* 1987;57:409–473.

49. Kolbe LJ. Increasing the impact of school health programs: emerging research perspectives. *Health Educ.* 1986;17:47–52.

50. Kolbe LJ. An essential strategy to improve the health and education of Americans. *Prev Med.* 1993;22:544–560.

51. Marx E, Wooley SF, with Northrup D, eds. *Health Is Academic: A Guide to Coordinated School Health Programs.* New York, NY: Teachers College Press; 1998.

52. Knapp MS, Barnard K, Brandon RN., Gehrke NJ, Smith AJ, Teuther EL. University-based preparation for collaborative interprofessional practice. In: Adler L, Gardner S, eds. *The Politics of Linking Schools and School Services.* Washington, DC: Falmer Press; 1994:137–152.

53. Adelman HS. *Restructuring Support Services: Toward a Comprehensive Approach.* Kent, Ohio: American School Health Association; 1996.

54. Los Angeles Educational Partnership. *Learning Center Model: A Design for a New Learning Community.* Los Angeles, Calif: Los Angeles Educational Partnership; 1995.

55. Taylor L, Adelman HS. Mental health in the schools: promising directions for practice. *Adolesc Med.* 1996;7:303–317.

—∿— Grant Report Summaries from the Robert Wood Johnson Foundation

ENGAGING HIGHER EDUCATION IN REGIONAL HEALTH PROBLEMS

(last updated January 2003)

The National Commission on Partnerships for Children's Health held a conference of southeastern state officials and higher education representatives on ways to form regional child health collaborations in October 2000. The commission aims to engage higher education in working with state and local agencies on the health and welfare of children and families. The Robert Wood Johnson Foundation provided a $49,050 grant to the Harvard School of Public Health in support of the conference.

STUDY OF SCHOOLS' ROLES IN RESOLVING HEALTH AND SOCIAL ISSUES CONFRONTING YOUTH

(last updated February 2000)

This grant to the National Association of State Boards of Education (NASBE) provided partial support for a study of the roles and responsibilities of public schools in addressing health and related social problems confronting today's children and youth. Many educators believe that they are compelled to intervene in the health and social environment affecting students, their families, and the community, even as a strong "back to basics" reform movement denies any role for schools outside of academics.

Under this grant, NASBE—which represents state boards of education nationwide—formed a 16-member study group (including 15 members of state boards of education) to conduct the study, which included three formal meetings and the preparation and dissemination of a project report. During its first meeting in January 1999, the group discussed the impact of family, community, and social dynamics on child and adolescent development and educational achievement. At its second meeting in March 1999, the group explored the budgetary implications of schools' attempts to address these health and social issues and to develop strategies for building partnerships needed to form a common understanding and vision for the schools. At its third meeting in June 1999, the group drafted recommendations on the role of state boards of education in promoting school attention to health and other social issues affecting students. At each meeting, the group heard presentations from a number of educators, practitioners, and researchers.

In its final report, titled *The Future Is Now: Addressing Social Issues in Schools of the 21st Century,* the study group reached the following conclusions:

> *Schools have an important role to play in addressing the needs of students by helping them succeed academically and by supporting the growth that will enable them to lead successful, productive adult lives.* The question is not whether schools should address nonacademic barriers to learning but rather what schools can do both alone and with others to support learning.

The group recommended that state boards of education do the following:

> *Set standards for creating positive school environments that foster academic achievement and support the development of children and youth.* Examples include setting high academic standards for all students, providing academic support services for students at risk of failure, and reducing class and school size.

> *Take a leadership role in creating a shared vision and sense of responsibility with others for helping children and youth to succeed academically in school and to become productive members of society.* To this end, they should foster collaboration with other state policymakers and agencies and initiate a dialogue with schools, families, and communities to develop a local understanding of what is needed to support student learning and a successful transition to adulthood.

Work collaboratively with other policymakers in the development and implementation of early childhood and pre-kindergarten programs. Children with a strong and healthy developmental foundation are more likely to come to school ready to learn.

Work with schools and others to combine and coordinate resources across agencies and in the public and private sectors in support of children's success. They can help schools maximize funding in support of students by reviewing and streamlining regulations and policies; targeting funds to schools serving populations more in need; providing technical assistance to help local schools to identify, access, and best utilize additional resources; and providing guidelines for pooling resources with other entities.

School-Based Health Centers

Reprints of Key Reports and Articles

CHAPTER 12

Back to School

A Health Care Strategy for Youth

James A. Morone, Elizabeth H. Kilbreth,
Kathryn M. Langwell, 2001

E leven million children have no health insurance. Ambitious efforts to reach them—such as the State Children's Health Insurance Program (SCHIP)—have gotten bogged down in the states, which enroll fewer than half of the eligible kids.[1,2] For teenagers, access to health care is especially tricky. Teens face problems—substance abuse, reproductive health needs, and depression, among others—that are difficult to face and can land them in serious trouble. However, ignoring the problems of adolescents can lead to even bigger troubles: one million unintended pregnancies a year, three million sexually transmitted diseases, more than four thousand suicides, and flashes of school violence. The adolescent and young adult death rate in the United States is high—1.5 deaths per thousand young males. (In contrast, the rate is 0.7 in England, 0.6 in Sweden, and 0.9 in Germany.) In the United States, one of every three youth deaths comes from

---

This chapter originally appeared as Morone JA, Kilbreth EH, Langwell KM. Back to school: a health care strategy for youth. *Health Aff.* 2001;20(1): 122–136. Copyright © 2001. Reprinted with permission from Copyright Clearance Center, Inc.

Table 12.1   Number and Regional Distribution of School-Based
Health Centers, 1996 and 1998.

Region	1996	1998
Mid-Atlantic and New England	379	422
Southwest and Rocky Mountain	155	233
Southeast and South-Central	180	212
Midwest	109	173
Pacific Coast	77	114
Total	**900**	**1,154**

homicide, suicide, or acquired immunodeficiency syndrome (AIDS).[3,4]

One response, now stirring across the nation, springs from a simple intuition: Put the health care where the kids are. Communities are opening health centers in the schools, especially in poor neighborhoods. Local hospitals, community health centers, or public health departments often run school-based health centers (SBHCs).

The idea sounds simple, but the centers have raised all kinds of objections. They do not fit the logic of managed care. They look like a throwback to the community health center model last touted in the 1960s. And they enrage some social conservatives; critics worry about encouraging promiscuity, turning schools into social service centers, and undermining parental authority. SBHCs kindle anxieties about difficult matters: How should a community deal with adolescents who drink, use illegal drugs, or have high-risk sex?

Despite the hurdles, SBHCs have spread rapidly—from roughly 150 centers (covering an estimated 137,000 children) in 1990 to more than 1,300 centers (covering 1.1 million) today.[5–8] Ten years ago SBHCs were concentrated in the Northeast; now they operate in forty-five states and the District of Columbia (see Table 12.1).[9] The centers offer a simple, relatively inexpensive way to whittle away at the problems of children's health care. While most policy analyses focus on the big-ticket items, such as SCHIP and Medicaid, SBHCs are tackling the same problems, one school at a time.

Will the school centers grow into an important feature of the American health care landscape? Will they effectively address young people's health needs? It is too soon to tell. But despite all the red flags they send up, SBHCs may prove to be an important innovation that fits the political temper of our time.

A SNAPSHOT OF CHILDREN'S HEALTH

During the past two years we have visited SBHCs across the country.[10] The first thing to strike us was the sheer level of need. Kids, and their schools, face extraordinary pressures. They have to cope with all of the tensions of American society. The data are familiar. Child poverty rates may be falling, but almost one of every five children (18.7 percent) lives below the poverty line. The economy grows stronger, but homelessness continues to rise—perhaps as much as 50 percent in the past decade; some seven million persons, mostly families with children, are at high risk of homelessness. We are experiencing the second-largest immigration wave in American history; almost one of every ten persons in the United States was born abroad. Even schools in small cities face students speaking many different languages (in the case of Woonsocket, Rhode Island, thirty-five).[11,12] But the statistics failed to prepare us for what we saw and heard, traveling from school to school.

In an Oregon elementary school, a student's mother stormed into the classroom and began to scream at her child. The mother, it turned out, had just been released from prison. Her three children had been living in a garage with their grandmother, sleeping in sleeping bags. Their only meals were the free breakfast and lunch provided at the school. In Colorado a Mexican American child came into the clinic complaining of a sore throat. When approached by the clinician, the child recoiled in fear. He had never seen a tongue depressor before.

One New England school board sternly forbade any birth-control services in the local SBHC. School officials accepted the decision without protest. They understood that there were deeply held views on all sides of the issue. Still, teachers in the high school we visited faced a stubborn reality: forty pregnant girls. In Louisiana a rural, largely African American parish is home to 9,000 children and three physicians. None of the doctors are pediatricians, two are over age sixty-five, and only one accepts Medicaid. For most children in the parish, the SBHC is their first and only source of regular care.

Across the country we saw clinic providers overwhelmed by the mental health needs of their students. The staffs see depression, anxiety, phobias, eating disorders, self-mutilation, substance abuse, uncontrolled anger, and the sheer stress from broken homes and life below the poverty line. Clinic staff routinely deal with multiple suicide attempts during each academic year. In that same Louisiana parish, for example, five high school students attempted suicide on the same day. The teens did not seem to know one another, and no one ever figured out the cause.

We heard these kinds of stories everywhere we went. They reminded us that behind the data and the policy debates lies a sharp reality: American youth face enormous health care needs. We found ourselves sobered by the scope of the problem. Anyone interested in questions about our children and their health care ought to plant those hard images front and center.

A NEW MODEL FOR AGE-OLD PROBLEMS

Today's SBHCs are a far cry from yesterday's school nurse. The health centers are designed to deliver comprehensive primary, preventive, and acute care. Most are staffed by nurse practitioners, nurses, mental health care providers, and aides. Many include part-time physicians on a regular schedule; some are training sites for medical students. SBHCs often have lab facilities for routine blood tests, and some even offer dental care.

Students either make appointments or walk in. The centers conduct comprehensive physical exams, treat chronic conditions (such as asthma), diagnose injuries, treat sexually transmitted diseases, monitor mental health problems, and—we heard this all the time—offer a trained adult ear when children (or their parents) need to talk. The clinicians educate parents, consult with teachers, and teach students about anger management, nutrition, and sex.

Most important, providers in the SBHCs are experts in adolescent and child health care. When the clinics work well, staff members win a reputation among students for compassionate, confidential, and nonjudgmental treatment. Students actually use the services. They have a safe place to take their aches and anxieties.

History of SBHCs

The SBHC idea goes back to the late 1960s and early 1970s. It flowed from two very different public health impulses. First, pediatricians organized school clinics in cities such as Dallas, Minneapolis–St. Paul, and Cambridge, Massachusetts. These early efforts shaped the model. A small circle of policy entrepreneurs began championing the school clinics. The Robert Wood Johnson Foundation (RWJF) jump-started broader interest through funding initiatives starting in 1978.[13] In the 1980s a handful of state and local policymakers picked up the idea. Gov. Lowell Weicker Jr. of Connecticut, for example, imagined a SBHC in every school (although he left office, in 1995, fewer than fifty schools into the campaign). More recently, the federal government dipped a funding toe into the field with a grant program titled Healthy Schools, Healthy Communities, launched in 1994.[14,15]

The second impulse proved more controversial. In the mid-1980s organizations such as the Children's Defense Fund began to publicize the teen pregnancy crisis. Between 1970 and 1989 the teen pregnancy rate among young white teens (ages fifteen to seventeen) rose 250 percent. Sexually transmitted disease rates also rose sharply. (Despite all of the "underclass" hype, the pregnancy rate for young black women, while much higher, declined 13 percent during the same period.)[16(p1099)] Public health advocates and politicians scrambled for solutions. Joy Dryfoos, who is often considered the "mother" of the SBHC movement, wrote a series of influential articles promoting family planning through SBHCs.[17–20]

In the early 1990s family planning in SBHCs got a more flamboyant advocate. In her autobiography, former U.S. surgeon general Joycelyn Elders gleefully describes her first press conference as director of the Arkansas Department of Health. Reporters were sleepily going through the motions until she promised to reduce teen pregnancy. "How?" they asked, stirring to life. Elders responded:

> "We're going to have . . . school-based clinics," [I said]. Now they were all wide awake. Somebody said, "School-based health clinics? Does that mean you're going to distribute condoms in schools?" I said, "Yes it does. We aren't going to put them on their lunch trays. But yes, we intend to distribute condoms."[21(p242)]

Gov. Bill Clinton, concluded Elders, looked like he was "trying hard to swallow something." The image of condoms on the cafeteria trays would haunt school clinics and their advocates. But that politically combustible image was just the hottest in a series of challenges to come.

BARRIERS TO THE SPREAD OF SCHOOL-BASED CENTERS

SBHCs have a lot going for them. They offer access to services for kids who are not getting health care. They reach teens who might be afraid or embarrassed to confide in their parents. They can be invaluable for working parents who cannot take time from their jobs to deal with sick calls from school—an especially urgent issue now that welfare reform has pushed many poor people into low-wage, often precarious jobs. They are bargains compared with the large insurance programs that states normally wrestle over—"decimal dust" in the budget process, one program manager told us.[22] All of these advantages did not get the SBHCs very far until they solved three basic challenges: negotiating the culture wars, getting funded, and managing partisan politics.

The Culture Wars

Opening an SBHC often means confronting the image of condoms on the cafeteria trays. Teen health care raises all of the thorny issues surrounding sexuality and reproductive health. As a result, the centers face instant enemies almost everywhere. In the Northeast, Roman Catholic bishops are chary of birth control. In the South and West, conservative Christians see a danger to family values. On the airwaves, Laura Schlessinger ("Dr. Laura") skewers the health centers for snatching moral guidance from parents and placing it in the hands of secular school officials.

These are not easy issues. Some parents are comfortable with school programs that promote safer sex. Many would want their children treated for sexually transmitted diseases as swiftly and efficiently as possible. Other parents are horrified at the implicit message—such services condone promiscuity, they say. The issue is further complicated by the question of parental notification. Many providers are reluctant to violate students' requests for confidentiality. But shouldn't parents know? Of course, clinic staff can urge children to inform their parents. But should they be required to do so?

For all the political passion, most SBHC supporters have learned to defuse the critics. Some former skeptics—many Catholic bishops, for example—have become forceful allies. How? The most important strategy is the most obvious: compromise. Everywhere, clinic staff repeat the same mantra: You do what the community will accept. Naturally, the local norms vary enormously. New York legislation requires SBHCs to provide reproductive health services, either on site or by "active referral." Louisiana's authorizing legislation, on the other hand, explicitly prohibits dispensing contraceptives or counseling for abortions on school grounds; some Louisiana communities do not permit testing for sexually transmitted diseases and explicitly forbid pelvic exams for adolescent girls.[23]

Since school politics normally plays out on the local level, the pattern can vary within a single state. Take Maryland, for example, where local taxes fund education and local school boards make the rules. In Baltimore, SBHCs offer a full range of reproductive services. In Maryland's affluent District of Columbia suburbs, program sponsors scrupulously sidestep the issue. School board meetings are televised. As one official told us, "Those people have to get elected—they aren't going to talk dirty on television." Instead, reforming energy gets concentrated onto the safer ground of elementary schools. Some communities in rural Maryland have worked out an unofficial compromise. SBHCs do not treat any reproductive health problem except sexually transmitted diseases. But parents and school board members live comfortably with the unstated but broadly recognized policy (reported to us by a board member) that center staff refer students to community-based services—and even accompany them if they need transportation or emotional support.

The sticking point often comes with parental consent and notification. The issues sometime trip up even savvy political advocates. In California, SBHC legislation that left parental notification up to the local centers stirred a rally of 10,000 parents and a governor's veto.[24] Even the simpler matter of permission has to be negotiated. Most places simply ask parents to fill out blanket consent forms, a necessary ticket for access to the health centers. The forms allow parents with strong objections to take their kids out of the system. Different school systems have sampled all kinds of approaches: Some ask for a single form when the child enters school; others require an annual form; and—in one short-lived maneuver—a skeptical state committee proposed requiring parental consent for every possible clinical service on a form that went on for pages.

Quiet Victories

And yet the school clinics thrive, even in culturally conservative states where arguments against social services might have found a sympathetic audience. In South Carolina, for example, the number of centers jumped from three to twenty-two in the past four years. In Louisiana an all-out campaign by the Christian Coalition failed to dislodge the health centers; by the time the battle was over, the legislature had used its tobacco settlement funds to lock in a long-term SBHC funding stream.

The health centers have defused fears of creeping socialism with another classic bit of political wisdom: Build a constituency for your service. Some communities introduce the clinics in the lower schools, where sex, violence, and substance abuse are not major issues. As the children move up the grades, parents push to keep their health services, which means extending them to older youth. Once parents turn into stakeholders defending "their" social entitlements, the ideologues face an uphill battle. Ultimately, children and parents telling personal health care stories are the most effective way to quell the culture wars.

Supporters often dig up dramatic cases. For example, an African American high school student electrified a legislative task force on youth violence in Louisiana. He calmly described how his plan to shoot his abusive stepfather was diverted by mental health counselors in a school-based anger management class. "This spring," he summed up softly, "I'm graduating high school instead of doing time." Any adult in the packed hearing room who had ever had an abusive relationship or an angry divorce could understand the young man's anguish.

But Where's the Money?

A decade ago, advocates imagined school health centers playing an important role in that long-awaited Shangri-La, national health insurance. Ironically, the Clinton administration proposal, with its emphasis on managed competition, spurred an industry surge toward market competition and managed care. SBHCs were not ready for that.

Most public clinics (community health centers, hospital clinics, and SBHCs) had been operating worlds apart from managed care. They generally served low-income persons who were irrelevant to the commercial managed care industry. Most SBHCs had never billed for services. Staff did not know the children's insurance status. Neither did the children. The centers were not wired for sophisticated record keeping and did not have the staff (much less the funding) to track down coverage data or bill the payers. On the contrary, many staff members worked up a warm contempt for the insurance industry and its "insurance-ese."

The great shift in Medicaid policy changed all that. By the mid-1990s every state had turned to managed care for its Medicaid populations. The school centers and their medical sponsors spent the end of the decade scrambling to catch up. They never succeeded.

Many managed care organizations rely on a "gatekeeper" to control costs. Enrollees get a primary care provider who authorizes most services. SBHCs normally cannot operate as the gatekeeper since they do not provide coverage twenty-four hours a day, seven days a week.[25] As a result, school clinics have to negotiate a marriage with an outside primary care organization. The predictable difficulties always spring up: Who is responsible for what? What may the SBHC do without prior authorization? And, most important, what about payment?

The basic problem is both simple and intractable: Limited funds have to be stretched across two facilities. Medicaid capitation rates for school-age children generally range from $6 to $10 a month. Medicaid providers and health plans are reluctant to split such meager payment with the schools. And children are likely to use the school health services far more often than the models predicted when rates were set—precisely the point of the SBHC exercise.

Some SBHCs, backed up by a community health center or a local hospital, do serve as the primary care provider. But the clinics are in the schools to improve access to health care services, not to guard the gates. Children walk in without appointments. Clinics respond to kids in crisis by calling in mental health professionals without waiting for authorization. Payers rightly distrust the SBHCs—their mission makes them terrible gatekeepers.

These organizational tensions defeat even good-faith efforts by managed care organizations and SBHCs to forge working relationships. When they negotiate an agreement—no easy job—the school clinics still find their billings routinely denied. SBHCs have sunk enormous energy into gearing up for managed care. Many now have far better record-keeping systems than they did a decade ago, and they routinely report utilization information to their state health departments. The effort may have made the centers more credible among state health policymakers. But SBHCs do not bring in much cash. The most recent survey of twenty-six states indicates that no SBHC receives more than 10 percent of its revenue from third-party billings to managed care contractors. (J.G. Lear, personal communication, October 14, 2000).[26]

To make matters worse, the SBHC clientele reflects the usual crazy-quilt of insurance coverage. Students are covered by many different carriers. The SBHC's poor and working-class populations are likely to be uninsured. Even eligible children have often failed to enroll in public programs such as Medicaid or SCHIP. These coverage problems are compounded by the welfare reform law of 1996. The reform split income assistance from Medicaid; persons who are not receiving cash benefits are now far less likely to sign up for Medicaid. In some places, lawsuits charge state officials with actively driving away persons who qualify for Medicaid.[2]

So where will SBHCs get their funding? Across all states' programs, about 61 percent of SBHC funding comes from state appropriations,

Table 12.2   **Aggregate National Funding Sources for School-Based Health Centers (1999).**

Source	Dollars	% of Total Revenues
State general funds	29,000,000	60.8
Maternal and child health block grant	9,270,000	19.4
Medicaid fee-for-service reimbursement	8,200,000	17.2
Medicaid managed care reimbursement	700,000	1.5
Private insurance reimbursement	500,000	1.0
Total	**47,670,000**	

Note: Total does not reflect miscellaneous additional sources of revenue, such as founation grants, dollar and in-kind contributions from sponsoring organizations such as hospitals, or local school or health department funds.

and another 19 percent from state allocation of maternal and child health block grant funds (Table 12.2).[9] Medicaid fee-for-service payments account for 17.2 percent of total revenues (most of this in New York). Payments from billings to managed care companies—for both Medicaid and commercial insurance enrollees—amount to less than 2 percent of SBHC monies. Of course, winning a dedicated budget line raises still another challenge: To survive and flourish, the school clinics have to negotiate state politics.

Partisan Politics

The 1990s did not appear to be an auspicious period for social welfare innovations on the state level. The 1994 election—marked by Newt Gingrich's celebrated "Contract with America"—was one of the greatest electoral routs in U.S. history. The Republican Party won both houses of Congress. Republicans also captured control of both houses of the legislature in eleven new states (in 1994) and took fifteen new governors' offices (between 1993 and 1996). Political scientists are still puzzling out the implications for governance. The last political sea change of this size occurred in the trough of the Great Depression, between 1930 and 1932.

A shift of such magnitude rattles the policy establishment. Changes in administration normally signal a change in priorities. In some states liberal administrations had embraced SBHCs. Weicker (a liberal independent in Connecticut) and Mario Cuomo (a liberal Democrat in New York) had been perhaps the most active proponents of the school clinics. Their administrations were replaced by conservative Republican John Rowland in Connecticut and moderate Republican George Pataki in New York. Neither would be expected to make the same kind of commitment to what were, after all, the signature programs of their political rivals. The same diffidence could be expected of the rising conservative politicians around the nation.

Sure enough, there seemed to be a major backlash brewing. In North Carolina the new Republican House majority explicitly forbade any of the state's SCHIP money from going to SBHCs. In Louisiana, where a Republican governor loosely affiliated with the Christian Coalition had bolted from out of nowhere to win, conservatives set out to abolish the school centers. However, once the smoke from that first partisan volley had cleared, it became obvious that school centers would be perfectly compatible with the new Republican era. In the second half of the 1990s the number of SBHCs around the nation more than tripled. North Carolina repealed the bar on funds; as we saw above, Louisiana turned positively generous toward its school centers.

In large measure, success was due to classic interest-group politics. Respectable locals—parents, teachers, and health care providers—went to their legislators and told heartwarming stories about their kids and their SBHCs. This is the kind of language that all legislators understand, regardless of party label. Legislators are always primed to deliver concrete benefits to "responsible" community members. SBHCs make the perfect constituent service. They combine education and health care. They will not bust the budget. They are simple to understand. They are local. They offer fine photo opportunities. They can be doled out slowly, one school at a time.

In brief, expanding the number of SBHCs fits neatly into the dynamics of American state politics: responsive, low cost, and local. And the clinics offer political relief from all the complex, health policy brain-busters that torment state legislators. Connecticut may have elected a conservative Republican governor, but when we visited the state, the legislature had seven different bills before it, each authorizing another new school health clinic.

STATE GOVERNMENTS IN ACTION

SBHCs involve two unusual political twists: activists in the bureaucracy (which sounds like an oxymoron), and links across three normally unconnected policy areas.

Bureaucratic Activists

From a distance, SBHCs glint with a kind of Jeffersonian haze: Local activists build clinics, round up local providers, mollify opponents and uneasy parents, and then march to the state capital for funding. The reality is different.

In every case we studied, the innovating spark flew not up from the grassroots but down from state government. Sometimes governors championed the reform; when governors were hostile or indifferent, the push often came from health administrators. State officials organized the centers, dug up seed money, compiled data on health care needs, and formed steering committees to draw in the major stakeholders (medical societies, child advocacy groups, and government agencies). State officials even organized local supporters, who eventually ended up lobbying the legislature for more support. And they guided school officials into the health care thickets.

For example, one local school built its clinic with no thought to privacy or antiseptic conditions. These health care novices constructed examining rooms with half-walls (so that anyone could hear everything) and wall-to-wall carpet. A state health official quickly provided "technical assistance," gently explaining that the carpet would be difficult to keep sterile and had to go.

The political pattern seems to turn conventional wisdom upside down. Aren't state agencies just repositories of fossilized bureaucrats? One provider even proposed a motto for her state department of health: "Don't just do something—stand there!" Activists, in the usual view, rise up from the grassroots and struggle against these unfeeling, red-tape recalcitrants. In contrast to our romantic memories of the 1960s, we found social activists operating in offices throughout the state health bureaucracies. Many are seriously committed to more and better health care. They helped to organize the local activists who then rose up to champion children's health care.

The role played by bureaucratic innovators introduces a classic political theme: the interplay between government action and grassroots mobilization. Some social movements rise up against unfriendly or unresponsive governments—for example, the first wave of AIDS activists (in the early 1980s) or the antiwar movement (in the 1960s). In other cases, government decisions open the door for activists; the U.S. Supreme Court's ruling in *Brown* v. *Board of Education* helped to transform civil rights agitation into a mass movement in the 1950s, and ambiguous New Deal legislation unleashed the great labor movements in the 1930s.[27]

The bureaucratic activists we observed did not quite fit either of these models. They operated without the sanction of federal policy and, in some instances, independent of state political leadership. Rather than acting within the organizational framework of their state agencies, they reached into the communities to create support for programs, often support that had not existed or had lain dormant. Here is a new twist on health politics: mavericks within the state bureaucracies organizing the grassroots.

Health, Education, and Crime

The school clinics stand at the intersection of three very different policy domains: health, education, and criminal justice. Each system operates on different principles. Each has its own assumptions, rules, actors, forms of funding, policy debates, and patterns of power. They even seem to speak different languages—to someone in education, for example, "primary care" goes to the kids in grade school. A successful SBHC program requires "multilingual" leaders.

Obviously, the school clinics bridge the gap between health and education. That means negotiating two radically different authority structures. Health care programs run on federal and state funds guided by federal and state rules. The chain of command invariably runs through the state capital. Education inverts all that. Local taxes (sometimes mixed with state money) fund the schools; local boards make the important decisions. In health care, the state Medicaid agency is a major player; in education, there is rarely a state agency with comparable muscle (or money).

SBHCs are also in the criminal justice business. Mental health issues shade into violence prevention. Substance abuse straddles the blurry line between health problems and criminal matters. Moreover, the school centers find themselves thrust into a major debate on juvenile justice policy. Crime policy specialists face off between tough-minded advocates of "zero tolerance" on the one hand and those who emphasize education, treatment, and rehabilitation on the other. In recent years the proponents of "getting tough" have enjoyed the stronger hand; states have legislated mandatory sentences, pushed young people into adult courts, and introduced a host of zero-tolerance policies in the schools. But critics have now begun to challenge these harsh moves.[28]

Skeptics of zero tolerance find allies in the school-based health centers. The clinics offer a different way to address youth violence and substance abuse. The partnership between reformers in juvenile justice and health care—still in its infancy—hints at a new, health-based approach to reaching troubled kids. The clinics offer a vehicle through which the juvenile justice "doves" can shift the balance from harsh sanctions to the education and treatment regimes more familiar to public health advocates.

TOWARD A YOUTH-FRIENDLY HEALTH CARE SYSTEM

SBHCs are no substitute for Medicaid or private health insurance. As the only option for school-age children, the small clinics would quickly be overwhelmed by demand. What they do offer is a potentially important—perhaps crucial—addition to a youth-friendly health care system.

In a sense, the clinics complement the managed care ideal. In theory, managed care offers a professionally monitored gateway into integrated and comprehensive health services, organized in a way that breaks both providers and consumers of their presumed addiction to overtreatment. In practice, managed care organizations ration care with relatively blunt instruments that do not always identify essential care, especially for treating mental illness and substance abuse. It takes persistence and skill to get around the barriers.

SBHCs offer almost the reverse. They do not offer a comprehensive, much less an integrated, care model. And they are organized on the reverse assumption: that adolescents underuse health care services. SBHC culture encourages repeat visits, active outreach, and leisurely paced visits, where children are encouraged to open up about anxieties or high-risk behavior that may underlie their health complaints. The centers fill the gaps in health education, counseling and mental health care. They are well placed to reach the many kids who fall through the cracks of the health care system.

Terrible events, such as the shootings at Colorado's Columbine High School, might have provoked a national conversation about our children and their needs. Instead, they provoked thin debates between congressional conservatives touting the Ten Commandments and liberals answering with gun control. Meanwhile, in the trenches, schools face pressing needs with limited resources. SBHCs offer a small response with the potential to do a lot of good. They are a simple, inexpensive way to get care to underserved children and reluctant teenagers. They help working parents—especially low-wage workers—who cannot take time off for sick children. They pose an alternative to the harsh zero-tolerance policies that throw young people—minorities first—out of the education system at the first sign of trouble. They offer state legislators a health care solution that works across party lines.

It is too early to know how far school clinics can take children's health care. But this reform is moving steadily across the states, spreading far beyond the familiar health policy innovators. For all the barriers they face, the school clinics might just fit the political temper of the times. They are certainly worth keeping an eye on. They are also, we believe, a reform well worth encouraging.

Notes

1. Ho D. Eligible children not being signed up for health insurance. *Boston Globe.* August 10, 2000:A3.

2. Thompson F. Federalism and health care policy. In: Hackey R, Rochefort D, eds. *State Health Policy.* Lawrence, Kans: University Press of Kansas; 2001.

3. World Health Organization. *World Health Statistics Annual, 1996.* Geneva, Switzerland: World Health Organization; 1998.

4. US Department of Education, US Department of Justice. *Annual Report on School Safety,* 1999. Washington, DC: US GPO; 2000.

5. Robert Wood Johnson Foundation. Making the Grade [Web site]. Available at: http://www.gwu.edu/~mtg/index.htm.

6. National Assembly on School-Based Health Care [Web site]. Available at: http://www.nasbhc.org.

7. J. G. Lear, Making the Grade National Program Office, Washington, DC.

8. Advocates for Youth, Center for Population Options, Washington, DC.

9. Making the Grade National Program Office. *School-Based Health Centers: National Survey, 1997–1998 Report.* January 1999. Available at: http://www.gwu.edu/~mtg/sbhcs/papers/98natlreport.htm. Accessed November 6, 2000.

10. In 1998 and 1999 we visited schools at multiple sites (ranging from Brooklyn, New York, to rural Oregon) across nine states as part of an evaluation of the Robert Wood Johnson Foundation's Making the Grade initiative. The program is designed to encourage state development of SBHCs. The nine states were Colorado, Connecticut, Louisiana, Maryland, New York, North

Carolina, Oregon, Rhode Island, and Vermont. We especially focused on the policy questions raised by the school centers. What are the advantages and the pitfalls of SBHCs? Are they financially sustainable? With what sources of funding? And what about the politics? Do communities need clinics if most children can be enrolled in an insurance program? We talked with a broad range of people, including legislators, state officials, school principals, students, parents, advocates, skeptics, and health care providers.

11. Terry D. US child poverty rate fell as economy grew, but is above 1979 level. *New York Times.* August 11, 2000:A10.

12. Tichenor T. *Controlling the Community.* Princeton, NJ: Princeton University Press; 2001:chap. 10.

13. The RWJF first underwrote school health services in four states in 1978. Between 1981 and 1989 the foundation promoted community health centers in eight cities. Five of these cities established primary care centers in schools as a part of this program. Then, in 1986, the RWJF launched the School-Based Adolescent Health Care Program and awarded nineteen six-year grants to public and private institutions to set up health centers in twenty-four high schools in fourteen cities. Finally, the Making the Grade initiative, launched in 1993, awarded grants to states to create state sponsorship, sustainable funding strategies, and regulatory oversight of SBHCs. Through these various initiatives the RWJF has, at one time or another, supported the development of school-based health care in twenty-one states. Twenty-four other states, plus the District of Columbia, have adopted the strategy.

14. The program funds thirty-three organizations to establish new school-based health centers in twenty-three states.

15. Health Resources and Services Administration. Healthy Schools, Healthy Communities program [fact sheet]. Rockville, Md: US Department of Health and Human Services; 2000. Available at: http://bphc.hrsa.gov/hshc/hshcfact.htm. Accessed July 28, 2000.

16. US Congress. House Committee on Ways and Means. *1992 Green Book Overview of Entitlement Programs.* Washington, DC: US GPO; 1992.

17. Dryfoos JG. The incidence and outcome of adolescent pregnancy in the United States. *J Biosoc Sci.* 1978;5(suppl):85–99.

18. Dryfoos JG, Heisler T. Contraceptive services for adolescents: an overview. *Fam Plann Perspect.* 1978;10:223–225, 229–233.

19. Dryfoos JG. What President Bush can do about family planning [editorial]. *Am J Public Health.* 1989;79:689–690.

20. Dryfoos JG. School-based health clinics: three years of experience. *Fam Plann Perspect.* 1988;20:193–200.

21. Elders J, Chanoff D. *Joycelyn Elders, M.D.: From Sharecropper's Daughter to Surgeon General of the United States of America.* New York, NY: Morrow; 1996.

22. SBHCs offer efficiencies through their use of mid-level practitioners. However, the lower salary costs of the staff may be offset by the longer visit time taken with each student. Obviously, the major reason that SBHCs are low cost is because they are, so far, small programs. Costs will increase as the programs expand to reach more children. However, one thing making SBHCs politically attractive is that they can be carefully targeted and incrementally funded.

23. Act 1055, House Bill 169L, signed by Louisiana Governor Charles E. "Buddy" Roemer II, 1991.

24. Holgate K. Angry parents storm state capitol to protest school health bill. October 1, 1999. Available at: http://www.karenholgate.com/ar991001.shtml.

25. Managed care organizations require that their primary care gatekeepers provide access twenty-four hours a day, seven days a week for their patients so that persons with acute or emergency conditions can get medical advice or authorization for emergency care at any time. This means that even physicians in solo practices have to have arrangements with colleagues to cover for each other twenty-four hours a day. Most SBHCs operate only during school hours and are closed for the summer and are thus not positioned to share on-call requirements with full-time medical practices.

26. Koppelman J, Lear JG. *From the Margins to the Mainstream: Institutionalizing School-Based Health Centers.* Washington, DC: Making the Grade National Program Office; 2000.

27. Morone JA. *The Democratic Wish: Popular Participation and the Limits of American Government.* 2nd ed. New Haven, Conn: Yale University Press; 1998.

28. Rethinking zero tolerance [editorial]. *Boston Globe.* August 17, 2000:A19.

CHAPTER 13

Creating Access to Care for Children and Youth

School-Based Health Center Census, 1998–1999

National Assembly on School-Based Health Care: report by
John J. Schlitt, John S. Santelli, Linda Juszczak, Claire D. Brindis,
Robert Nystrom, Jonathan D. Klein, David W. Kaplan, Michelle D.
Seibou, 2000

In the early 1970s, poor access to health care, troubling statistics on risk-taking behaviors, and teen pregnancy motivated public school and community health care leaders from Dallas, Texas, St. Paul, Minnesota, and Cambridge, Massachusetts to create the first primary health care programs in schools. These early pioneers demonstrated that health care could be delivered in a setting most familiar and accessible to young people: their school. The services were organized around students' unique physical and emotional development needs in an easily accessible environment that was cul-

---

This chapter was originally issued as a report for the National Assembly on School-Based Health Care, by Schlitt JJ, Santelli JS, Juszczak L, Brindis CD, Nystrom R, Klein JD, Kaplan DW, Seibou MD. *Creating access to care for children and youth: School-Based Health Center Census 1998–1999*. Washington, DC: National Assembly on School-Based Health Care; June 2000. Reprinted with permission from the National Assembly on School-Based Health Care.

turally sensitive, comfortable, and safe. Wide acceptance by students, their families, and the schools provided compelling evidence that a success story was in the making.[1-3]

The school-based health center prototype inspired education and health care policy makers around the country who sought creative strategies for addressing health problems that affect learning. With the investment of resources and political will from federal, local and state governments, national and community foundations, health care organizations, and schools, hundreds of communities have followed suit in the three decades since the first center doors opened.[4-7] In 1998, school-based health centers numbered nearly 1,200—a ten-fold increase from 120 in 1988. No longer primarily in urban high schools, health centers now operate in diverse areas in 45 states, serving students in every grade. The expansion of these centers into America's rural and suburban schools is a powerful reminder that access to health care is not only a problem for inner-city teenagers. It also illustrates the way that school-based health centers have been embraced by communities and individuals from divergent political perspectives.[8]

The thirty-year anniversary of school-based health centers affords an opportunity to reflect on the exponential growth of school-based health centers, the political and social forces that have shaped the field, and the emerging trends that will both challenge and sustain it tomorrow. Many of the compelling reasons that sparked this successful innovation in the early 1970s still exist today. Schools continue to be burdened by students who cannot take full advantage of their educational experience because of poor physical and emotional health. The health indicators associated with high-risk behaviors that have plagued our nation in recent decades remain, and new challenges have emerged. Gun violence in our schools and the emergence of HIV/AIDS have prompted public calls for more effective prevention and early intervention services targeted at school-aged youth. Each of these issues has strengthened the resolve of the education and health care sectors to seek collaborative solutions to health problems that are preventable.

An important fundamental public policy shift within the past ten years is also having a dramatic impact on school-based health care. As federal and state health care reforms and insurance expansions unfold, the initial rationale for serving uninsured children and adolescents in school-based health centers is being reconsidered. Managed care is transforming the business of primary care in many communities, prompting school-based health care providers to examine the roles they can and should play in health care markets with increasing cost and utilization controls, and new quality assurance requirements. Health care reforms have had a profound effect in how centers view themselves, their relationships with students and families, and their role within the larger health care system.[9–13]

In spite of rapid changes within our nation's health care systems, there are clear indications that challenges to meeting the health care needs of some school-age children and youth remain. Many are not eligible for expanded health care coverage or do not receive coverage due to inadequate educational outreach; in 1999 more than 2 million children ages 13–18 were not enrolled in public insurance despite being eligible. Inadequate coverage for important preventive and mental health care and cost-sharing requirements create additional barriers for insured children and teens seeking services. Recent reports have found that one in seven adolescents was uninsured and that 20% had gone without heath care they thought they needed.[14,15] When they do utilize health care services, many young people report that their needs for critical guidance and education to support sound decision-making are not being met.[16] For many school-aged children and adolescents, location, convenience, confidentiality, and trust matter a great deal. These challenges to our nation's health care systems are likely to keep school-based health centers well positioned to serve as an attractive child- and adolescent-focused health care access strategy.

ABOUT THE NATIONAL ASSEMBLY

The National Assembly on School-Based Health Care is a multidisciplinary membership association dedicated to promoting access to health care for children and adolescents through school-based settings. Created in 1995, the National Assembly serves as the collegial home for the multiple disciplines involved in school-based health care. The National Assembly conducted the 1998–99 Census of School Health Centers (Census 1998–99) to:

- Collect specific information on the current status of SBHCs, including services, clinic policies, staffing and utilization, and populations served.

- Create a database of SBHCs for future National Assembly efforts in advocacy, policy making, and research. This database will also form the basis of a national directory of school health centers.

- Assess the information, resource, and technical assistance needs of SBHCs and National Assembly staff.
- Assess the current prevention activities provided by SBHCs both in health centers and in classrooms.
- Assess quality assurance mechanisms and relationships between SBHCs and managed care organizations, including both professional and financial relationships.
- Provide a better understanding of the role of SBHCs in meeting the health needs of uninsured school-aged children.
- Promote widespread dissemination of the survey findings to policy makers, practitioners, researchers, and advocates.

The 1998–99 census builds on the longstanding work of Advocates for Youth and its Support Center for School-Based and School-Linked Health Centers. Since 1986, the Support Center has tracked and reported the movement's growth and programmatic trends. Its "School-Based Health Care Update" series has served as one of the field's early chronicles. With the creation of the National Assembly, Advocates for Youth leaders agreed that it was time to transfer the survey of school-based health centers to the new membership organization.

Creating Access to Care documents findings from the largest data collection and analysis of its kind, and illustrates emerging themes that will assist in program planning, development, and evaluation of school-based health centers. The report highlights:

- A broad and comprehensive range of primary and mental health care services;
- Acceptance of the health center by students and their parents as demonstrated by the centers' enrollment;
- An expansion into rural and suburban communities, and middle and elementary grades;
- An interdisciplinary health care team model;
- An expansive emphasis on prevention through classroom and health center education and health promotion activities; and
- Operations built upon health professional quality standards, including computerized encounter tracking and third-party billing systems, continuous quality improvement mechanisms, and national accreditation.

METHODS

Information for the 1998–99 Census of School Health Centers was collected through a questionnaire that was mailed to health centers in December 1998. A total of 806 school-based health centers (centers located in a school or on a school campus) responded, representing a 70% response rate. A nonresponders questionnaire was conducted for centers that had not returned a completed survey. The characteristics of responding and nonresponding health centers were similar. An expanded description of the methodology can be found in Appendix A (pp. 287–290).

SCHOOL-BASED HEALTH CENTER CHARACTERISTICS

Table 13.1 depicts the distribution of 1,135 school-based health centers throughout 45 states. The geographic location of schools served by health centers was described as urban (56%), rural (30%), and suburban (14%). The types of school settings were characterized as elementary (30%), combined elementary-middle (7%), middle (12%), combined middle-high (5%), high (41%), and combined K–12 (5%). Half of the health centers (399, or 51%) were located in schools that included but were not limited to high school grades. More than one-third served elementary grades (331, or 42%). Twenty-nine percent (228) served in schools that included middle grades seven and eight.

The average school size was 1,004 for all schools, with a majority of schools (61%) serving between 500 and 1,500 students. Average enrollment by school type included 698 students in elementary schools, 811 in middle schools, and 1,316 in high schools.

Health centers were asked to report on the number of students in the school, health center enrollees (students who have registered with the clinic and had a consent form on file), and health center users each year. Information was collected separately for the school in which the health center was located ("health center school") and for each additional school it served ("linked schools"). Of the 806 centers that completed the questionnaire, 252 (31%) reported serving one or more linked schools. Of those reporting one or more linked schools, 36% served one additional school and 22% reported two additional schools. The total number of linked schools was 848 and the average number was 3.4.

The average center was located in a school of 1,004 students; 642 (64%) students enrolled, and 537 students used the center at least once.

An estimated 1.1 million students (2% of the nation's school enrollment) attended schools with a school-based health center in

1998–99.[17] An additional 310,000 to 750,000 students attended schools that were linked to a school with a health center.[18]

Among students who had access to school-based health centers, nearly two-thirds were minorities. The tradition of establishing school-based health centers in communities with unmet health needs and inadequate health care resources is reflected in the substantial number of schools located in low-income communities in which racial/ethnic minorities often live. Thus, African American (29%), Hispanic (26%), Asian (4%), and Native American children and adolescents (3%) were among those served by school-based health centers.

SCHOOL-BASED HEALTH CENTERS ARE WIDELY ACCEPTED, WIDELY USED. School-based health center enrollment and utilization data illustrate the health centers' success in attracting students. The average student body enrollment rate of 64% represents acceptance by the majority of students and the parents and guardians who provide consent for their children's use of the services. Health center utilization by 83% of enrollees also provides important validation of the health centers' ability to meet diverse student needs. Descriptions of health center users from various studies have shown that the demographic makeup of users reflects the population of the school.[4,19,20] Health center users have also been reported to be those with the greatest physical and mental health needs.[21,22]

School-Based Health Center Sponsors

School-based health centers represent a partnership between schools (or school districts) and health care organizations. The health partner is critical to the development of the health center facility, as well as its operations and staffing, supervision of clinicians, and provision of medical back-up for complicated cases and after-hours care when the center is not open. Hospitals, local health departments, and community health centers represent 73% of school-based health center sponsors. Also serving as health care sponsors were university medical centers (5%) and nonprofit health care agencies (9%). Although less common, some health centers are administered by the school or school district (10%) employing direct service providers to staff the centers.

Age of Health Centers

The median age of the health centers was four years and the average was six years. Six percent of health centers opened within the last year, 17% within the past two years. Nearly 60% of health centers have been in

Table 13.1   Distribution of School-Based Health Centers by State, Community Type, Grades Served, and Age of Center.

	All	Resp	Resp Rate	Community Type			Grades Served			Age of Center (in yrs)			
				Rural	Sub	Urban	Elem	Midd	High	< 2	2–4	5–9	10+
AK	1	0	0%	n/a	n/a	n/a	n/a	n/a	n/a	n/a	n/a	n/a	n/ac
AL	4	4	100%	0	1	3	0	1	3	0	0	2	2
AR	21	17	81%	15	0	2	10	8	10	2	3	6	3
AZ	79	45	57%	14	11	21	32	10	8	8	31	4	0
CA	63	53	84%	9	12	37	23	10	23	7	25	12	7
CO	30	26	87%	4	3	20	7	9	14	2	11	2	1
CT	51	25	49%	2	3	20	10	9	8	5	14	4	2
DC	1	1	100%	0	0	1	0	0	1	0	1	0	0
DE	26	19	73%	8	6	5	0	2	19	5	8	2	4
FL	50	31	62%	12	8	11	9	6	21	3	9	13	3
GA	6	2	33%	2	0	0	0	1	1	0	0	0	2
HI	3	1	33%	0	1	0	0	0	1	0	1	0	0
IA	15	9	60%	6	2	2	2	3	8	3	4	2	0
IL	31	25	81%	2	2	22	12	9	12	2	7	1	3
IN	14	13	93%	4	0	9	3	4	7	0	8	3	2
KS	1	0	0%	n/a	n/a	n/a	n/a	n/a	n/a	n/a	n/a	n/a	n/ac
KY	34	30	88%	21	5	4	9	13	16	0	7	17	4
LA	31	23	74%	11	1	11	8	11	9	4	11	4	4
MA	39	37	95%	2	2	34	6	9	26	1	17	10	8
MD	42	34	81%	4	16	15	21	4	8	11	14	1	6
ME	15	8	53%	6	0	2	0	1	8	2	4	1	1
MI	33	19	58%	2	3	23	8	7	9	6	9	0	4
MN	22	21	95%	1	0	20	2	7	19	1	5	1	14

Table 13.1 Distribution of School-Based Health Centers by State, Community Type, Grades Served, and Age of Center (*Continued*).

	All	Resp	Resp Rate	Community Type			Grades Served			Age of Center (in yrs)			
				Rural	Sub	Urban	Elem	Midd	High	< 2	2–4	5–9	10+
MO	9	9	100%	0	1	8	5	1	5	5	4	0	0
MS	4	2	50%	1	0	1	2	1	0	0	2	0	0
MT	1	0	0%	n/a	n/a	n/a	n/a	n/a	n/a	n/a	n/a	n/a	n/ac
NC	40	27	68%	20	2	11	5	9	14	7	10	7	3
NH	3	3	100%	0	3	0	2	0	1	0	0	3	0
NJ	18	13	72%	5	1	8	2	3	11	0	1	2	10
NM	31	27	87%	19	2	10	8	8	20	1	10	7	8
NY	154	97	63%	17	4	76	56	40	36	12	22	17	39
OH	13	11	85%	8	2	5	8	1	2	8	3	0	0
OK	10	8	80%	1	0	7	5	3	1	1	7	0	0
OR	39	32	82%	10	17	5	6	6	22	7	5	6	12
PA	28	20	71%	2	1	18	8	7	7	2	3	12	2
RI	3	2	67%	0	0	2	0	2	1	0	1	0	1
SC	3	2	67%	1	1	0	0	0	2	0	1	1	0
TN	13	9	69%	6	0	3	3	3	5	2	4	2	1
TX	69	47	68%	9	12	29	33	5	14	10	27	6	1
UT	2	0	0%	n/a	n/a	n/a	n/a	n/a	n/a	n/a	n/a	n/a	n/ac
VA	13	11	85%	6	0	6	5	3	5	0	8	2	1
WA	7	5	71%	0	0	5	5	0	5	0	2	3	0
WI	30	12	40%	0	0	12	10	1	1	10	1	1	0
WV	34	26	76%	24	0	2	11	11	16	3	21	1	1
	1135	806	71%	254	122	470	331	227	398	130	321	155	149

operation four years or less. In all, 20% had been operating for ten years or more; only 1% have been in operation for twenty years or more.

SCHOOL-BASED HEALTH CENTER STAFF

School-based health centers were asked to list the members of their health care team and the hours on-site each week.

Ninety-two percent of the health centers employed a combination of physicians, physician assistants, or nurse practitioners to provide physical health services. Physical health services staff collectively averaged 27 hours per week on-site. Physicians were part of the team in 50% of reporting programs, providing services and supervision on-site for an average of six hours a week. The sole medical provider in 7% of health centers, the physician was more likely to work in collaboration with other health care providers with diagnostic and prescriptive authority, including nurse practitioners and, less frequently, physician assistants. Nurse practitioners spent an average of 25 hours per week in 76% of SBHCs. Physician assistants practiced in 12% of school-based health centers for an average of 20 hours per week.

Mental health professionals were part of the clinical team in 57% of the health centers for an average of 33 hours a week. Clinical social workers and mental health counselors were the professionals most frequently on-site, followed by psychologists, substance abuse counselors and psychiatrists.

Most health centers (>90%) employed support staff to maximize the efficiency of the clinical practitioners and to support daily operations. Clinical support was most often provided by registered or practical nursing staff, found in 55% of health centers for an average of 32 hours per week. Other types of support came from health aides (39% of centers) and administrative assistants (52% of centers). Additional administrative oversight was provided by a director in 24% of health centers for an average of 22 hours per week.

A smaller number of school-based health centers augmented this core team with additional staff, including health educators (in 19% of health centers), social service workers (19%) and nutritionists (14%). Centers listed dental care professionals the least frequently of all staff members.

SCHOOL-BASED HEALTH CENTERS EMBRACE AN INTERDISCIPLINARY APPROACH. The interdisciplinary team approach to school-based health care is one of the model's greatest strengths. As evidenced by the census data, most health centers respond to the complex health care needs of high-risk children and adolescents with staff from multiple disciplines who bring diverse experience and expertise: the primary care practitioner with diagnostic and treatment ability, the mental health professional to explore emotional and psychosocial dimensions that sometimes underlie somatic concerns, and the educator to impart knowledge and social skills. Once considered unattainable because of limited resources, the interdisciplinary team is now a recognized standard. Credit is owed to funders, including state health departments, the Robert Wood Johnson Foundation, and the federal grant program, Healthy Schools, Healthy Communities, whose staffing standards have influenced the model's implementation nationwide. An Advocates for Youth update from school year 1991–92 reported that fewer than 30% of health centers employed mental health professionals. In the subsequent seven years, that figure reached nearly 60 percent.[23-25]

SCHOOL-BASED HEALTH CENTER OPERATIONS/AFTER-HOURS CARE

Health centers were asked to report on their operating hours and policies for health care access when they are closed. Most health centers (69%) were open more than 30 hours a week, or six hours or more a day, five days a week. An additional 17% were open between eight and 30 hours a week; 14% were open less than eight hours a week. Half of all school-based health centers operated during the summer months (48%), with summer hours similar to general operation hours during the school year.

Seventy percent of health centers provided some source of pre-arranged emergency and after-hours care when centers were closed. Half the health centers provided, at a minimum, telephone information for local emergency services. The most frequently cited source of care was provided on-call by the health centers' sponsoring agency (59%). A small percentage (17%) offered on-call services through another external health care agency.

SBHC AS KEY ACCESS POINT. The business of school-based health care is, for most health centers, a full-time job. After-school hours, school vacations, and summer months create unique challenges to the health centers. Because the health centers often become the primary provider by default for uninsured and underinsured students, being available to students when needed is an important access standard. Most health centers appear to fulfill many aspects of the role of the primary care provider, serving as first contact, providing continuous care, and ensuring coordination through referrals and linkages to other sources of care.[26,27]

SCOPE OF SERVICES

School-based health centers were asked to identify four categories of services provided on-site: physical health care, reproductive health care, mental health care, and health education, and risk reduction services.

Physical Health Services

The vast majority of health centers (89%) provided the basic tools of primary preventive care; the most common components in the school-based health care scope of service were comprehensive health assessments, anticipatory guidance, vision and hearing screenings, immunizations, treatment of acute illness, laboratory services, and prescription services. The most frequently cited immunizations provided were hepatitis B, measles-mumps-rubella (MMR), diphtheria and tetanus toxoids (DTT), and oral poliovirus. More than half of the health centers provided preventive oral health services in the form of dental screenings. A much smaller proportion of programs made available comprehensive dental care and sealants.

SCHOOL-BASED HEALTH CENTERS AS PRIMARY CARE SITES. The spectrum of physical health services delivered in school-based health centers closely resembles the services provided in other primary care practice settings. The one-stop shopping model allows students to be assessed, diagnosed, treated on-site and, if appropriate, returned to the classroom. On-site laboratory tests and prescriptions reduce the need for off-site referrals, which often are ignored or not followed through by students because of inadequate transportation or resources. National and local program evaluations have confirmed that students who access school-based health centers make greater number of visits to a health care provider when compared to national adolescent utilization rates.[28,29] The most common types of visits for physical health services reported in the literature include well-child exams and health supervision, acute illness, respiratory and ear, nose and throat problems, and injuries.[30,31]

Reproductive Health Services

Survey respondents were asked to identify whether reproductive health services were available on-site, referred to an off-site provider, or not provided at all. On-site reproductive services, including related counseling, education, and testing, were, of course, more commonly a part of health care practices in middle and high schools than in elementary schools. Thus, for this section, only data from health centers serving middle and high school health centers are analyzed.

Middle and high school health centers were more likely to provide on-site treatment for sexually transmitted diseases (73%), HIV/AIDS counseling (77%), and diagnostic services such as pregnancy testing (85%) than contraceptive services. Family planning services most often encompassed birth control counseling (72%) and follow up (61%). A minority of health centers neither provided on-site nor referred to an off-site provider for any sexual health services.

Three of four school-based health centers serving middle and high school grades reported that contraception was not dispensed on-site. The majority of health centers, however, arranged for services off-site by referral. Among health centers not dispensing, 4% adopted the policy voluntarily; the majority of health centers do not dispense at the direction of the school (29%), the school district (73%), or state (12%). Half or more of school-based health centers were not prohibited from dispensing contraceptives in Missouri (88%), Minnesota (57%), California (53%), and Texas (50%).

SCHOOL-BASED HEALTH CENTERS ARE RESPONSIVE TO THE COMMUNITY. Although it affords unprecedented access opportunities to school-aged youth, the school as health care setting is unique in that the content of care is at times a matter of public discourse and decision-making.[22] The inclusion of reproductive health care, which is potentially a source of controversy, is typically based on input from the community, school, families, and students. While some communities have fully embraced family planning in school-based health care as a strategy to prevent pregnancy and STD, many more have limited the range of on-site reproductive health services out of deference to community concerns and fear of community opposition. Utilization studies suggest that, in practice, reproductive health care—when available—accounts for 10–17% of clinical visits.[47,33,34]

Mental Health Services

Mental health and counseling services provided by health centers included crisis intervention (79%), case management (70%), comprehensive evaluation and treatment (69%), substance abuse (57%), and the assessment and treatment of learning problems (39%). Group counseling was used by health centers to offer peer support (59%), grief counseling (53%), classroom behavior modification (49%), substance use prevention and treatment (41%), and gang intervention (26%).

SCHOOL-BASED HEALTH CENTERS REDUCE BARRIERS TO MENTAL HEALTH CARE. In studies of school-based health center service utilization, mental health counseling is repeatedly identified as the leading reason for visits by students. Placing counseling in the context of school-based primary health care normalizes it and makes seeking help acceptable. Particularly for students at risk of health compromising behaviors, the health center provides a safe place to explore developmental and emotional adjustment issues, and serves to engage students in building positive social skills that minimize their health risks and strengthen protective factors. Several studies have shown that the barriers experienced in traditional mental health settings—stigma, non-compliance, inadequate access—are overcome in school-based settings.[28,35–37] One study in particular found that, compared to traditional providers, school-based health centers substantially increase access to and utilization of mental health and substance abuse care.[38]

Prevention and Health Promotion Services

Health centers were asked to list the prevention and health promotion services they provided on six topics: tobacco, alcohol, HIV, pregnancy, injury, and violence. Respondents specified the setting for these activities as health center–based, classroom-based, or other (for example, health fair). More than 60% of health centers conducted some level of prevention services in the clinical setting, with little differences across the six topics. Many health centers extended prevention activities into the classrooms as well. Half of the centers offered classroom educational sessions on tobacco, alcohol, and HIV prevention. Slightly fewer of the health centers covered violence, pregnancy, and injury prevention topics. Tobacco and alcohol prevention were also the topic most likely to be addressed in other school-wide health promotion activities such as health fairs, education campaigns, and general assemblies.

SCHOOL-BASED HEALTH CENTERS TARGET HEALTH THREATS. Because of their unique setting, public health orientation, and proximity to children and youth at risk, school-based health centers can play an important role in influencing the small number of risk behaviors that present the greatest threats to health. Interpersonal connections in the clinical setting and small group support enable providers to ask the questions young people rarely hear, assess their risks for health threats, and assist in the development of social skills and competencies for avoiding these risks. Augmenting these services with the classroom and school-wide activities reported here reinforces the community values and norms that support student wellness beyond the clinic walls.

SCHOOL-BASED HEALTH CARE POLICIES

As providers of health care to school-age children, school-based health care professionals have an obligation of accountability to both the students and their families who benefit from their services, as well as to public and other funders responsible for their financial support. School-based health centers were asked to describe their policies and procedures for obtaining parental consent, tracking patient care visits, billing third parties, assuring quality of care, and training professionals. The activity described here suggests that efforts to deliver the highest standard of care in accordance with health care industry practice are commonplace across most health centers.

Parental Consent

Health centers were asked to identify their parental permission policies regarding enrollment and use of any and all services offered by the centers. Parental consent to enroll in the health center was a requirement for 94% of responding health centers. Twelve percent indicated that students needed parental consent for each visit to the center. Nearly two-thirds (64%) of the health centers allowed parents to restrict access to a specific service (for example through an enrollment form that includes a list of services from which the parents can choose to exclude their child).

Health centers were asked to identify services offered on-site that, in accordance with state law, a student could receive without parental consent. The most frequently cited service of this type was emergency care, identified by 47% of health centers, followed by STD treatment (41%), drug and alcohol counseling (35%), family planning (33%), mental health counseling (29%), and prenatal care (23%).

PARENTAL EXCLUSIONS. When parents have the opportunity to select services to exclude from the health provider's scope of care for their child, a great majority do not exercise this option. Anecdotal evidence suggests anywhere from 1%–5% of signed consent forms include certain exclusions, typically for birth control and mental health services.[34]

Encounter Tracking System

Health centers were asked to describe their mechanisms for documenting and tracking patient visits. Computer-based patient tracking systems were used by 88% of health centers. Of these, 43% used School HealthCare ONLINE! (a system developed specifically for school-based health centers), and 41% used their sponsoring agency's medical tracking system. Paper record forms were used in combination with computer systems in 75% of health centers. Ten percent used paper record forms only. Nearly three of four health centers (73%) bill Medicaid and/or other third-party insurers for student-patient encounters.

PATIENT CARE REVENUE IN SCHOOL-BASED HEALTH CENTERS. Billing third party payers for health care services provided to insured students has become increasingly commonplace in school-based health centers. Studies of school-based health care revenues from Medicaid and other third party payers, however, have consistently found that insurance remains an elusive and complicated means of financial support. Although the experience differs from community to community, a high volume of uninsured and underinsured students, the difficulty in securing insurance information, confidentiality, Medicaid managed care, and the provision of non-reimbursable services have contributed to limited revenue recovery—on average 5–10 percent of the health centers' operating budgets.[10,13,40]

Standards of Care

Health centers identified the use of standards and quality assurance mechanisms to guide and assess health center program operations. The survey included four areas: the use of professional standards of clinical care, the use of standards for quality assurance measures, components of quality assurance, and sources of health center accreditation or certification.

PROFESSIONAL STANDARDS. Health centers identified which of five nationally recognized clinical health care standards they use. Ninety-two percent indicated the use of at least one standard, 69% indicated two or more. Centers used Medicaid's Early, Periodic Screening, Diagnosis and Treatment (EPSDT) standard most frequently (73%). The American Medical Association's Guidelines for Adolescent Preventive Services (GAPS) standard was used more often in older populations; the American Academy of Pediatrics' clinical standards and the federal Maternal and Child Health Bureau's Bright Futures, were used more frequently in elementary grades.

QUALITY ASSURANCE MEASURES. Quality assurance benchmarks in health care are used as performance assessment tools. Two prominent industry standards are the Health Plan Employer Data and Information Set (HEDIS), developed by the National Committee on Quality Assurance (identified by 8% of health centers), and the Joint Commission on Accreditation of Healthcare Organizations' assessment guide (identified by 35%). Several state health departments have also created performance review tools specific to school-based health care, with 31% of health centers reporting use of these tools. A majority of health centers (65%) reported using quality assurance benchmarks established by themselves or their sponsoring agency.

COMPONENTS OF QUALITY ASSURANCE SYSTEMS. Health centers identified which of seven common components of a quality assurance system they used to measure quality of care. Among the 97% that responded to at least one category, staff credentialing and chart audits were identified most often; assessment of patient knowledge was less common.

ACCREDITATION. Thirty-one percent of health centers reported having successfully participated in their sponsoring institution's accrediting process through the Joint Commission on Accreditation of Healthcare Organizations (JCAHO). One-third of health centers (34%) reported being certified by a state government entity.

TRAINING IN THE HEALTH CENTER. Three of four health centers (75%) reported that they serve as training sites for health care professionals, including physicians, nurses, physician assistants and social workers. The setting provides unique preservice experience in an interdisciplinary practice with unprecedented opportunities to work with school-age youth in their natural environment.

HEALTH CENTER CHARACTERISTICS BY GRADE, GEOGRAPHY, AGE, SPONSOR, AND STATE

Do school-based health centers share common characteristics, regardless of geographic location, school setting, or longevity? For example, does a school-based health center in a rural high school resemble its counterpart in an inner city, or an elementary-based center? Do sponsoring agencies approach the organization of services in a similar fashion? Do programs evolve as they mature? The following section examines the effects of location, setting, age, sponsorship, and state boundaries on the school-based health center's scope of services, staffing, and operation policies (see Tables 13.2 to 13.5).

BY GRADES SERVED. With few exceptions, the organization of school-based health care in elementary, middle and high school grades varied little across most operations and services. Some differences did emerge that appear to be related to school size as well as to the developmental needs of the target population. For example, health centers in schools with grades 10, 11, or 12 were more likely to operate for 30 hours or more per week and to have more hours of primary and mental health care staff on-site than schools with grades 6, 7, or 8. Middle grade schools, in turn, reported more operational hours than those in schools serving grades 5 or below. The likelihood of offering counseling and prevention services also increased as the age of the students increased. While health centers serving elementary grades were more likely to require parental permission for every visit, they also reported greater rates of enrollment and utilization than centers serving middle and high school grades.

BY COMMUNITY TYPE AND GEOGRAPHY. Centers in urban communities more frequently reported a broader scope of services and more on-site primary care and mental health staff hours than their suburban and rural counterparts. Urban centers were also more likely to provide operating hours when schools are closed. Services were strikingly different between urban and rural centers for prescriptions, psychosocial assessment, dispensing of medications, and STD diagnoses and treatment. Rural health centers were more likely to be involved in classroom health promotion and prevention education. Although a greater proportion of suburban centers required parental consent for every visit, suburban programs also were more likely to allow adolescents to consent to family planning. Although suburban centers reported higher student enrollment rates, utilization was greater by students in rural and urban centers.

Table 13.3 outlines key operations, services and policies by state. Data were aggregated for those states with ten or more health centers included in the response.

BY SPONSOR TYPE. The effects of health center sponsorship did not appear to follow consistent patterns. Health centers sponsored by public health departments and schools had fewer on-site primary care hours, and were less likely to offer comprehensive services, such as prescriptions, or to provide after-hours care. School sponsorship was associated with greater on-site mental health presence, and greater frequency of counseling services. In contrast to medical providers (who traditionally have quality assurance required by accreditation or funding sources), health centers with school sponsors were least likely to engage in quality assurance activities, such as patient satisfaction surveys and medical record reviews. School sponsored programs were also least likely to bill for third-party revenue. Public health departments, community health centers, and non-profit agencies were most likely to allow students to consent to family planning and more frequently offered on-site reproductive health services.

BY AGE OF CENTER. In examining health centers by longevity, we observed patterns across the four age groups. The older the health center, the more likely it was to operate 30 hours or more a week. The oldest programs (10 years or more) were also more likely to have parity between mental health and primary care, averaging 30 hours a week for both types of providers. The availability of reproductive health services among centers was also strongly linked to the center's age. The older the health center, the greater likelihood that reproductive health services, including family planning, were offered on-site and that adolescents were able to consent for these services. That the oldest health centers reported higher enrollment than their younger programs is not surprising, as developing a solid base of registrants takes considerable outreach, education and time. We are unsure, however, why the proportion of students at a school using the health center somewhat decreases among older programs.

Table 13.2 Select Operations, Services and Policies by Grades Served, Geographic Location, Sponsorship and Age of Center.

	Grades Served			Community Type			Age of SBHC (years)				Sponsor Type					
	Elem	Middle	High	Urban	Suburb	Rural	<2	2–4	5–9	10+	HD	CHC	Schl	Hosp	Univ	NPO
Primary care	20	24	28	30	24	16	24	24	24	30	20	29	19	28	24	26
Mental health	12	19	23	22	19	13	17	14	18	30	14	18	23	16	24	20
Operation Hours	%	%	%	%	%	%	%	%	%	%	%	%	%	%	%	%
>30 hrs/week	57	72	78	71	72	65	58	62	72	88	71	72	76	65	73	64
Summer operations	47	48	49	55	50	33	42	49	45	55	48	41	41	56	54	35
Services On-Site	%	%	%	%	%	%	%	%	%	%	%	%	%	%	%	%
Prescriptions	91	87	90	96	89	79	94	92	84	89	77	97	77	95	98	94
Medications dispensed	55	56	65	74	51	44	65	58	58	72	52	59	37	70	71	81
STD diagnosis and treatment	30	55	77	63	51	46	42	52	57	75	61	63	34	51	48	74
Birth control	—	22	28	32	25	14	21	19	21	41	29	22	13	25	15	32
Psychological development assessment	72	75	73	81	74	59	70	72	73	72	68	71	58	79	93	73
Individual substance abuse counseling	42	57	70	55	52	64	55	53	60	70	56	53	67	53	51	73
Tobacco prevention in classroom	45	59	57	46	52	62	54	51	54	52	57	41	56	51	62	54

Table 13.2   Select Operations, Services and Policies by Grades Served, Geographic Location, Sponsorship and Age of Center. (*Continued*).

	Grades Served			Community Type			Age of SBHC (years)				Sponsor Type					
	Elem	Middle	High	Urban	Suburb	Rural	<2	2–4	5–9	10+	HD	CHC	Schl	Hosp	Univ	NPO
Policies	%	%	%	%	%	%	%	%	%	%	%	%	%	%	%	%
Parental consent for every visit	18	10	8	11	21	9	13	16	10	4	9	9	17	12	24	12
Bill third party	75	78	71	77	71	66	76	69	75	71	82	85	51	64	76	79
Chart audits	84	89	88	88	91	82	82	83	93	91	90	89	71	87	88	94
Patient survey	66	73	76	74	82	63	64	73	72	77	70	80	59	70	68	86
Acceptance of SBHC	%	%	%	%	%	%	%	%	%	%	%	%	%	%	%	%
Students enrolled	70	68	60	62	69	67	52	66	64	66	66	68	55	64	66	59
Students visited at least once	63	58	50	51	44	65	62	55	53	48	64	50	60	46	90	48

Table 13.3   Percent of SBHCs Providing Selected Primary Care and Reproductive Health Services by State for States with 10 or More SBHCs.

State	After Hours Care	Anticipatory Immunizations	Guidance	Comp Assessment	Lab	Prescription	Dental Sealant	Condoms On-Site	Condoms Refer	STD On-Site	STD Refer	Gynecological Exams On-Site	Gynecological Exams Refer	Pregnancy Test On-Site	Pregnancy Test Refer
AR	13	87	53	93	44	13	0	23	38	21	43	23	39	43	21
AZ	64	67	91	91	82	84	22	7	36	16	59	9	55	20	52
CA	70	100	94	96	81	92	26	55	31	63	24	60	25	63	24
CO	96	100	100	92	100	100	5	19	81	85	15	81	19	92	8
CT	96	100	100	100	96	100	8	12	72	72	12	76	8	68	16
DE	74	100	100	95	100	81	0	0	95	84	16	74	26	89	11
FL	29	65	90	87	55	81	3	17	66	30	53	33	50	77	10
IL	92	100	100	100	100	96	14	36	60	52	44	52	44	52	44
IN	46	69	100	100	100	100	44	0	85	86	0	85	0	85	0
KY	28	100	100	93	90	37	14	7	67	26	57	11	67	83	10
LA	100	100	100	100	100	91	9	0	50	61	39	74	26	100	0
MA	97	100	100	100	97	100	5	38	57	81	14	73	22	81	14
MD	62	97	100	100	85	100	21	28	22	44	16	44	16	41	9
MI	68	95	95	95	95	89	31	0	74	63	32	63	32	68	26
MN	71	100	100	100	100	100	6	52	48	95	5	95	5	100	0
NC	74	96	88	100	100	100	4	4	77	67	15	63	19	67	15
NJ	92	62	77	77	62	62	0	0	92	54	38	58	33	62	31
NM	62	52	92	85	70	85	8	27	62	59	30	63	26	74	15
NY	94	99	97	99	97	99	25	31	54	63	29	50	43	69	23
OH	18	100	100	100	100	91	0	0	18	9	82	81	82	9	82
OR	55	100	100	91	91	91	6	47	34	81	9	55	9	84	6
PA	75	90	100	100	100	100	15	10	50	55	15	55	25	75	0
TX	68	98	98	96	94	100	18	24	41	55	21	54	24	59	17
VA	9	45	91	91	100	100	0	9	73	27	73	27	73	36	55
WI	17	67	67	92	58	100	0	0	83	17	67	25	50	33	50
WV	100	100	96	100	96	100	4	0	85	46	42	31	58	62	27

Table 13.4   Selected Counseling and Prevention Services by State for States with 10 or More SBHCs.

State	Comp Individual Evaluation & Treatment (%)	Individual Substance Abuse Counseling (%)	Classroom Education on Tobacco (%)	Classroom Education on Violence (%)
AR	47	33	44	50
AZ	22	38	24	24
CA	74	61	43	34
CO	96	85	46	38
CT	96	92	44	52
DE	89	100	68	58
FL	90	76	65	71
IL	75	25	80	68
IN	92	50	54	77
KY	55	48	70	50
LA	96	83	83	87
MA	81	65	57	38
MD	70	52	38	53
MI	74	63	74	74
MN	86	62	95	67
NC	62	77	63	48
NJ	85	67	62	46
NM	68	81	74	70
NY	84	48	30	26
OH	18	73	100	91
OR	66	81	53	13
PA	45	30	50	25
TX	51	23	34	26
VA	36	9	9	9
WI	25	25	42	50
WV	64	68	85	62

Health centers that have been existence for ten years or greater were much more likely to provide family planning services on site than younger centers (41% versus 20% for birth control). Does this reflect an evolution in programming, that as health centers become more established within the school and community, and more familiar with the specific needs of students, they are in a more favorable policy environment to increase access to other services such as reproductive health? Or were programs established ten years ago or earlier more likely to have included special services such as on-site contraception from the start? Data collected from centers in 1988 by Advocates for Youth show that the average rate of health centers dispensing birth control was 20%, less than the 1998–99 rate of 26%, supporting the argument that service scope does evolve over time.

Table 13.5 Percentage of SBHCs using Selected Tools and Policies by State for States with 10 or More SBHCs.

State	Any Computer-Based Encounter System	Medicaid Billing	Any Use of Professional Standards	Any Use of QA Measures	Any Use of QA Tools	Accreditation			Serves Training Site
						JCAHO	State	Other	
AR	79	73	94	96	100	0	10	10	23
AZ	88	20	89	78	98	23	81	22	64
CA	82	88	89	83	91	27	54	13	78
CO	88	77	96	88	100	13	13	13	74
CT	100	96	100	100	100	36	48	18	90
DE	100	5	95	100	100	72	11	0	94
FL	86	43	77	81	97	36	11	4	50
IL	96	88	96	92	100	57	29	42	56
IN	100	46	85	77	100	31	31	0	100
KY	86	100	97	90	100	5	55	9	82
LA	100	100	100	100	100	36	68	26	100
MA	100	97	97	97	100	52	82	18	91
MD	100	100	97	79	97	0	39	11	90
MI	100	53	84	89	100	0	50	0	82
MN	95	70	71	71	100	19	5	52	67
NC	96	67	74	93	100	15	0	16	58
NJ	90	15	38	77	85	64	18	0	78
NM	96	63	74	89	100	35	22	19	65
NY	80	94	88	93	98	43	55	6	89
OH	18	82	91	100	100	73	0	0	91
OR	97	56	94	84	100	3	3	7	66
PA	95	35	85	60	100	33	0	0	83
TX	73	91	98	89	91	43	19	0	73
VA	90	27	73	73	91	50	0	9	36
WI	92	75	100	50	83	0	0	0	75
WV	94	100	96	92	100	17	0	24	87

SCHOOL-BASED, SCHOOL-LINKED, AND MOBILE HEALTH CENTERS

School-based health centers represent one of several models for linking health care services with school-aged children and adolescents. The confluence of community resources, political will, and, most certainly, student need, will dictate whether, how often, and what types of health care can be made accessible through school sites. Health centers that do not operate on school property but in close proximity to the school are often called school-linked health centers. Located across the street, or within a short distance that can be traveled by foot, bus, or automobile, school-linked centers are less affected by school policies, and generally provide more comprehensive services. The "link" implies ties to the school through the participation of health center staff in classroom activity and through referrals to the center by school staff to ensure access.

On-site delivery of health services by a traveling health care team in temporary or portable space is called a mobile health center. Staff of mobile centers rotates from school to school, typically in a set pattern for a prescribed period of time in each school. This strategy is likely motivated by a desire to maximize community resources so that a health program could serve a greater number of students across multiple schools.

Both of these models are less commonly found than school-based health centers: the 846 centers that responded to the survey included only 28 school-linked and twelve mobile health centers. Data on school-linked and mobile health centers are included here to compare and contrast services, staffing, and operations across the three models (see Table 13.6).

School-linked health centers had a greater presence in the suburbs than school-based and mobile programs. School-linked programs in our sample were also older: 40% were ten years of age or older (compared to 20% of school-based centers) and only 8% opened in the last two years. Because they are freestanding, community-based health centers, the school-linked programs were more heavily staffed, with 50 hours each week of primary care—twice the amount of time provided in school-based programs. With the exception of reproductive health services, there were no differences in the scope of practice among school-based and school-linked centers. The linked programs were more likely to offer a comprehensive range of reproductive health and least likely to be prohibited from dispensing birth control. Unlike

Table 13.6   Health Center Demographics by Location.

	Link (n = 25–28)	Mobile (n = 8–12)	SBHC (n = 747–806)
Geography	%	%	%
Rural	36	17	30
Suburban	25	8	14
Urban	39	75	56
Grades Served			
Elementary	24	75	42
Middle	36	8	29
High	56	33	51
Age of Center			
< 2 Years	8	60	17
10 years +	40	0	20
Operations			
less than 8 hours/week	18	40	14
30+ hours/week	71	50	69
Summer hours	93	42	48
After hours	82	50	70
Services			
Comprehensive health assessment	96	67	95
Gynecological exams	82	25	53
STD treatment	82	25	56
Immunizations	96	67	91
Condoms	75	8	25
Counseling (any)	96	42	58
Group (any)	54	25	65
Tobacco (health center)	50	25	64
Tobacco (classroom)	46	25	52
Policies			
Parental consent for each visit	28	18	12
Prohibited from dispensing birth control	15	75	77
Perform chart audits	89	67	87
Bill Medicaid	82	58	73
Computer System	74	45	88
Staff	**Average Hours Per Week**		
Primary care	50	19	25
Mental health	25	3	19

school-based centers, school-linked programs reported a higher rate of requiring parental permission at each visit (28% versus 12%).

Mobile clinics that responded to the census were younger programs found largely in urban elementary schools. Compared to school-based and linked centers, mobile clinics were less likely to operate full-time, reported fewer hours of primary care, and offered significantly fewer hours of mental health care per week. Mobile centers were also less likely to deliver primary care or reproductive health services. Because of their limited time at each site, mobile clinics were less able to provide services that require a greater staff presence, including counseling and preventive health promotion and education within the classroom setting.

THE WIDENING DOMAIN OF SCHOOL-BASED HEALTH CENTERS

With more than half of all school-based health centers no older than four years, the 1998–99 census data demonstrate that despite a thirty-year history, the school-based health center movement is still growing and thriving. Illustrative of this growth are health centers in Arizona, Missouri, Mississippi, Ohio, Oklahoma, Wisconsin, and West Virginia, where many communities have only recently established school-based health centers. Nine in ten health centers in these states were opened within the last four years. Seventy percent of new health centers were located in elementary and middle schools, and one in two was administered by a community hospital, reflecting the growing interest of hospitals as sponsors of school-based programs.

The adoption of school-based health centers by communities and schools not associated with the model's early history suggests an expansion of school-based health care's domain. Comparisons of older health centers with those opened more recently demonstrate the trends of health centers over the past decade. Health centers ten years of age and older were more likely to be in urban schools and serve adolescents. Newer programs were more frequently found in rural schools where school-aged youth experienced similar health care barriers to those of their urban counterparts. With the prospect of reducing acute and minor illnesses and introducing preventive health services at earlier ages, the elementary school has also become a more popular setting for school-based health centers.

Perhaps one of the most important advances is that of health centers into suburban communities. When he pledged that any high school in Delaware that wanted a health center would have one, Governor Thomas Carper reframed the perception that the need for a youth-focused health care safety net has no socio-economic or geographic boundaries.

These expanded domains—rural and suburban communities, elementary and middle grades—signify the increasing universal appeal of school-based health care as access programs for children and youth regardless of their age, location or income.

TO THE FUTURE

The school-based health center model, as embodied in this report's data, remains highly variable, although these data bring the field closer to identifying a core set of services and access standards. The number of centers has expanded and now includes a larger percentage of centers in elementary and middle school grades, and in suburban and rural as well as urban communities. In addition to providing traditional primary care services, the centers are increasingly offering mental health and health education services targeting some of the most challenging health behaviors of children and adolescents. Additionally, many centers report having in place systems to evaluate operations and monitor the quality of care.

Questions that need to be considered regarding the operations and services provided by the model include: When is the full implementation of the model most appropriate? Are there efficiencies to be gained—and what effects or impact are compromised—with a model scaled back to minimal staffing and limited on-site operating hours? What is driving the growth in elementary schools and how is the model different from centers in high schools? The data also raise several concerns, including the lack of consistent after-hours care, the need for more dental and mental health services, the limitations on reproductive health services, and the need for a stronger prevention orientation. The latter is particularly important as health centers have an opportunity due to their strategic location within the school to implement broad-based community/school outreach and prevention activities. More than half the centers do not participate in classroom-based health education or health promotion and risk reduction activities. While these shortcomings would no doubt be resolved with additional resources and expanded staffing patterns, many of these school-based health centers face an uncertain financial future.

After thirty years of innovation, and fueled by a combination of federal, state, and local health care investments, the recent and rapid growth of school-based health centers suggests that the era of demonstration is over. While far from full-scale efforts, this health services model is continuing to gain momentum. The ability to sustain the growth of school-based health centers will depend on continued efforts to demonstrate their value in health care and education environments, both of which are experiencing their own accountability pressures. School-based health centers can make an increasingly important contribution to access to and utilization of health care for children and adolescents, but critical questions need to be addressed: Are school-based health centers substitutive or complementary care providers for children and adolescents? Will our nation's health care system support multiple points of entry for children and adolescents? How can school-based health centers play a measurable role in health promotion and disease prevention?

The National Assembly on School-Based Health Care stands committed to providing leadership and support to the burgeoning field so that we may clarify and respond to these critical questions. This fourth decade of school-based health care will see the articulation, promotion and adoption of national standards for the field, as well as the development of guidelines, tools and technical assistance for assuring high quality health care in school-based settings. We will promote the continued growth and integration of school-based health centers as an acceptable, comprehensive, accessible, and accountable source of health care—a view substantiated by the data in this report. At a time when so many factors are impeding the ability of this nation to provide high-quality education and health care to its children, school-based health centers are likely to play an increasingly important role in the solutions.

APPENDIX A

Methods

To guide the conduct of this Census, the National Assembly established a technical advisory committee (TAC) of school-based health center evaluators to provide advice on questionnaire preparation, sampling design, data analysis, report writing, and dissemination of results.

IDENTIFYING SCHOOL-BASED HEALTH CENTERS. We used a variety of sources to identify school-based health centers. We obtained lists of school-based health centers from the National Assembly membership database, Advocates for Youth, Making the Grade, the federal Healthy Schools, Healthy Communities program, and the National Association of Community Health Centers. We also contacted school and adolescent health coordinators in state health and education departments, state school-based health center associations, and individual members of the National Assembly in 1998 to identify health centers. After purging duplicate records, we identified 1,415 school-based and school-linked health centers. Because it was difficult to verify the continued existence of certain health centers or the correct classification of each program (e.g., school-based versus school-linked, primary care versus school nursing), the TAC decided to correct this number after reviewing survey responses and conducting a nonresponders survey (see Table 13.7).

QUESTIONNAIRE DEVELOPMENT. To ensure a good response rate, the TAC created an instrument that could be completed in less than 30 minutes by the person(s) most knowledgeable about the clinical care in the health center, such as the nurse practitioner or clinic director. The instrument was pre-tested at nine health centers. The final questionnaire was twelve pages long with a minimum of 225 questions, the majority of which could be answered by "yes" or "no." (More questions were possible if a health center served more than one school.) The questionnaire allowed open-ended responses (i.e., "Other") to 18 questions. The questionnaire included six content areas: school-based health center characteristics, student demographics, staffing and operations, services, health center policies, and technical assistance needs.

SURVEY ADMINISTRATION AND EFFORTS TO IMPROVE THE RESPONSE RATE. We mailed the questionnaire to health centers in December 1998. Nonresponders received a postcard in February 1999 and a second mailing of the questionnaire in April 1999. Incentives to complete were a copy of the report and either *A Guidebook for Evaluating School-Based Health Centers* by Brindis, Kaplan, and Phibbs, (University of Colorado and University of California, San Francisco, 1999) or a coupon worth $25 toward registration for the 1999 National Assembly conference in Washington, DC.

Table 13.7   **School-Based Health Center (SBHC) Survey Responders and Nonresponders by Geography, School Type, Grades and Age.**

	Responders %	Nonresponders %
Geography	(*n* = 806)	(*n* = 328)
Urban	56	64
Rural	30	26
Suburban	14	10
School	(*n* = 790)	(*n* = 326)
Elementary	30	30
Elementary-Middle	7	9
Middle	12	16
Middle-High	5	7
High	41	31
K–12	5	7
Duplicated Grades	(*n* = 790)	(*n* = 326)
Elementary	42	47
Middle	29	39
High	51	44
Age of SBHC	(*n* = 755)	(*n* = 244)
< 2 years	17	24
2–4 years	42	33
5–9 years	21	21
10 years +	20	22

SURVEY CONTENT, DATA CLEANING, AND DATA RECODING. National Assembly staff prior to data entry visually inspected all questionnaires; double entry procedures were used. Staff checked the data electronically for inconsistencies and "failure to follow skip" patterns. They imputed missing data where possible, based on other information in the question (e.g., a school-based health center in New York City with missing information on geographic location was recoded to "urban"). The TAC recoded all open-ended responses to existing categories, where possible, after review. For example, "mostly rural but partly suburban" was recoded to "rural." Where new categories were suggested, these were added to the dataset. Generally, the TAC used a minimum of 15 similar responses as a criterion for adding a new response category. A complete description of the variables and recoding decisions is available from the National Assembly.

A total of 846 completed questionnaires were received. Responders included 806 health centers operating in schools or on school property, 28 school-linked health centers, and 12 mobile programs. No response was obtained from 567 programs. A seven-question nonresponders questionnaire was mailed or conducted via telephone for centers that had not responded after repeated attempts. We also obtained data directly by having the state coordinators, National Assembly members living in the state, or National Assembly staff call the school or health center. The nonresponse survey allowed us to calculate nonresponse by program type and to eliminate from the database health centers that were no longer open or that were not providing primary care.

Of the 567 nonresponding programs, 97 (17%) had closed, 77 (13%) were not school-based health centers (these were primarily school nursing, non-primary care programs), 329 (63%) were school-based health centers, 19 (3%) were school-linked health centers, 21 (4%) were mobile programs, and 24 (4%) were of unknown type after repeated attempts to collect data. Adding responders and nonresponders, we estimated 1,135 school-based health centers (in schools or on school property), 47 school-linked health centers, and 32 mobile programs. The response rate was 70% for school-based health centers, 60% for school-linked health centers, and 36% for mobile programs. Responders and nonresponders showed small differences by location, grades served, and length of time open (see Table 13.7).

RESPONSE RATE/NONRESPONDERS SURVEY. Estimates for school-linked health centers and mobile programs are undercounts, as many of these programs were not collected in our identification process. As such, most of the analyses presented in this report are limited to school-based health centers (either in school or on the school campus).

ETHICAL REVIEW. The study was reviewed at the Centers for Disease Control and Prevention for human subjects protection.

Notes

1. Edwards LE, Steinman ME, Hakanson EY. An experimental comprehensive high school clinic. *Am J Public Health.* 1977;67:765–766.
2. Dryfoos JG. School-based health clinics: a new approach to preventing adolescent pregnancy? *Fam Plann Perspect.* 1985;17:70–75.

3. Kirby D. Comprehensive school-based health clinics: a growing movement to improve adolescent health and reduce teen-age pregnancy. *J Sch Health.* 1986;60(4):164–169.

4. Lear JG, Gleicher HB, St Germaine A, Porter PJ. Reorganizing health care for adolescents: the experience of the school-based adolescent health care program. *J Adolesc Health.* 1991;12:450–458.

5. Lovick SR, Wesson W. School-based clinics: update 1986. Houston, Tex: Support Center for School-Based Clinics, Center for Population Options; 1986.

6. Peak G, Hauser D. School-based health centers: update 1993. Washington, DC: Center for Population Options; 1994.

7. Fothergill K. *Update 1997: School-Based Health Centers.* Washington, DC: Advocates for Youth; 1998.

8. American Medical Association Council on Scientific Affairs. Providing medical services through school-based health programs. *JAMA.* 1990;261:1939–1942.

9. Brellochs C, Zimmerman D, Zink T, English A. School-based primary care in a managed care environment: options and issues. *Adolesc Med.* 1996;7:197–207.

10. Lear JG, Montgomery LL, Schlitt JJ, Rickett KD. Key issues affecting school-based health centers and Medicaid. *J Sch Health.* 1996;66(3):83–88.

11. Brindis CD, Sanghvi RV. School-based health clinics: remaining viable in a changing health care delivery system. *Ann Rev Public Health.* 1997;18: 567–587.

12. Zimmerman D, Santelli JS. School and adolescent health and managed care. *Am J Prev Med.* 1998;14(3S):60–66.

13. Schlitt JJ. *Critical Issues in Financing School-Based Health Centers.* Washington, DC: National Assembly on School-Based Health Care; 1999.

14. Newacheck PW, Brindis CD, Cart CU, Marchi K, Irwin CE. Adolescent health insurance coverage: recent changes and access to care. *Pediatrics.* 1999;104 (2 pt 1):195–202.

15. Ford C, Bearman P, Moody J. Foregone health care among adolescents. *JAMA.* 1999;282:2227–2234.

16. Children Now. *Adolescents and Managed Care: Partners in Transition.* Oakland, Calif, Children Now; 2000.

17. Overall, 91% (*n* = 731) of health centers were able to report school enrollment information. Based on an average school population of 1,004, this yielded a total of 733,924 students in schools served by a SBHC. This estimate rises to 797,600 students if one includes an estimated school enrollment for nonreporting schools, adjusting for the size of school by community type (urban, rural, suburban) and by grades served. If one considers the

329 health centers that did not respond to the initial survey but for which data were obtained from the nonresponder survey (and again adjust for community type and grades served), this estimate rises to 1,123,171 students.

18. Only 60% of 252 health centers reporting one or more linked schools also were able to report information on the school population at these linked schools. The 148 health centers reporting school population reported 3.4 linked schools per health center, 628 students per linked school, and therefore a combined school population of 2,114 students per health center. In the 148 schools that directly reported school population, a total of 312,856 students have access to school health centers through the school-health center linkage. Assuming that the 104 health centers not reporting school population served similar schools, this estimate rises to 532,700. Assuming that health centers that did not respond to the initial questionnaire but for which data were obtained from the nonresponders survey ($n = 329$), this estimate rises to 750,142 students.

19. Balassone ML, Bell M, Peterfreund N. A comparison of users and non-users of a school-based health and mental health clinic. *J Adolesc Health.* 1991;12:240–246.

20. Kisker EE, Hill J. Healthy caring: an outcome evaluation of the Robert Wood Johnson Foundation's school-based adolescent health care program. Princeton, NJ: Mathematica Policy Research; 1993.

21. Wolk LI, Kaplan DW. Frequent school-based clinic utilization: a comparative profile of problems and service needs. *J Adolesc Health.* 1993;14:458–463.

22. Pastore DR, Juszczak L, Fisher MM, Friedman MB. School-based clinic utilization: a survey of users and non-users. *Arch Dis Child Adolesc.* 1998;152:763–767.

23. Brellochs C, Fothergill K. Special report: defining school-based health center services. Atlanta, Ga: Centers for Disease Control and Prevention Division of Adolescent and School Health; 1994.

24. Schlitt JJ, Rickett KD, Montgomery LL, Lear JG. *State Initiatives to Support School-Based Health Centers: A National Survey.* Washington, DC: Robert Wood Johnson Foundation; 1994.

25. Waszak CS, Neidell S. *School-Based and School-Linked Clinics: Update 1991.* Washington, DC: Center for Population Options; 1992.

26. Brindis CD, Kapphahn C, McCarter V, Wolfe AL. The impact of health insurance status on adolescents' utilization of school-based clinic services: implications for health care reform. *J Adolesc Health.* 1995;16:18–25.

27. Santelli JS, Morreale M, Wigton A, Grason H. School health centers and primary care for adolescents: a review of the literature. *J Adolesc Health.* 1996;18:357–367.

28. Anglin TM, Naylor KE, Kaplan DW. Comprehensive school-based health care: high school students' use of medical, mental health, and substance abuse services. *Pediatrics.* 1996;97:318–330.

29. Kisker EE, Brown RS. Do school-based health centers improve adolescents' access to health care, health status, and risk-taking behavior? *J Adolesc Health.* 1996;18:335–343.

30. Kaplan DW. School-based health centers: primary care in high school. *Pediatr Ann.* 1995;24:192–200.

31. Borenstein PE, Harvilchuck JD, Rosenthal BH, Santelli JS. Patterns of ICD-9 diagnoses among adolescents using school-based clinics: diagnostic categories by school level and gender. *J Adolesc Health.* 1996;18:203–210.

32. Rienzo BA, Button, JW. The politics of school-based clinics: a community-level analysis. *J Sch Health.* 1993;63(6):266–272.

33. Fisher MM, Juszczak L, Friedman SB, Schneider M, Chapar G. School-based adolescent health care: review of a clinical service. *Am J Dis Child.* 1992;146:615–621.

34. Juszczak L, Fisher M. Dispensing contraceptives in school-based health centers. *J Pediatr Adolesc Gynecol.* 1997;10:45–48.

35. Walter HJ, Vaughan RD, Armstrong B, Krakoff RY, Tiezzi L, McCarthy JF. School-based health care for urban minority junior high school students. *Arch Pediatr Adolesc Med.* 1995;149:1221–1225.

36. Weist MD, Paskewitz DA, Warner BS, Flaherty LT. Treatment outcome of school-based mental health services for urban teenagers. *Community Ment Health J.* 1996;32:149–157.

37. US Department of Health and Human Services. *Mental Health: A Report of the Surgeon General.* Rockport, Md: US Department of Health and Human Services; 1999.

38. Kaplan DW, Calonge BN, Guernsey BP, Hanrahan MB. Managed care and school-based health centers: use of health services. *Arch of Pediatr Adolesc Med* 1998;152:25–33. (See Chapter Fifteen.)

39. Santelli JS, Alexander M, Farmer M, et al. Bringing parents into school clinics: parent attitudes toward school clinics and contraception. *J Adolesc Health.* 1992;13:269–274.

40. Grant R, Maggio L. The impact of Medicaid managed care on school-based clinics. *Res Sociol Health Care.* 1997;14:289–303.

CHAPTER 14

School-Based Health Centers

A Blueprint for Healthy Learners— Data from the 2001–2002 School-Based Health Center Census

National Assembly on School-Based Health Care: report by Linda Juszczak, John Schlitt, Michelle Odum, Caroline Barangan, and Deidre Washington, 2003

S chool-based health centers (SBHCs) provide on-site medical and mental health services that promote the health and educational success of school-aged children and adolescents.

Services are provided by a community health organization, in partnership with the school, and through a collaborative planning process that includes families and students, communities, school districts, and individual and agency health care providers.

Services typically offered in SBHCs are age-appropriate and address the most important health needs of children and youth.

The chapter was originally issued as a report by the National Assembly on School-Based Health Care. *School-based health centers: a blueprint for healthy learners. Data from the 2001–2002 School-Based Health Center Census.* Washington, DC: National Assembly on School-Based Health Care; 2003. Reprinted with permission from the National Assembly on School-Based Health Care.

There are approximately 1,500 SBHCs across the country supported by local, state, and federal public health and primary care grants, community foundations, and reimbursement from public and private health insurance.

The following data, drawn from a national survey of more than 1,100 SBHCs, illustrate their operations, staffing and services.

Reception

SBHCs are typically open 29 hours per week.

39% of SBHCs keep their doors open during summer months.

61% of SBHCs have pre-arranged sources of care when the SBHC is closed.

Of the 66% of SBHCs that are located in schools with a school nurse, more than half are co-located together.

67% of SBHCs bill Medicaid; 45% bill private insurance.

Waiting Room

62% of SBHCs serve students in the urban communities; 25% serve students from rural communties.

51% of students in schools with health centers are African American or Hispanic.

46% of SBHCs serve high school students; 50% serve middle school students; 45% serve elementary school students.

An estimate of 39% of students served by SBHCs have no other medical home.

65% of SBHCs also serve other populations such as family members of students, school faculty, and students from other schools.

Exam Room

Primary care is provided by physicians, physician assistants, and nurse practitioners. Most frequent medical services include:

- Treatment of acute illness (94%)
- Screening such as vision, hearing, scoliosis (91%)
- Asthma treatment (90%)
- Comprehensive physicals (89%)
- Sports physicals (87%)
- Immunizations (85%)

Lab and Pharmacy

> 82% of SBHCs offer laboratory testing on site.
>
> 90% of SBHCs prescribe medications.
>
> 57% of SBHCs dispense medications on site.
>
> 80% administer medications in the health center.

Prevention Central

Nurses, health educators, nutritionists and social workers provide critical education and skills building. Health topics are addressed in individual counseling, small group, classroom, and schoolwide settings. Health topics most frequently addressed by SBHCs include:

- Tobacco (87%)
- Alcohol and drug abuse (82%)
- Violence prevention & conflict resolution (82%)
- HIV/STD prevention (76%)

Counselor

Mental health professionals are present in 56% of SBHCs. Most frequent mental health services include:

- Assessment (74%)
- Crisis intervention (72%)
- Screening (71%)
- Grief and loss therapy (62%)
- Brief therapy (62%)

Conference Room

> Most frequent sponsors of SBHCs include hospitals (32%), health departments (17%), federal community health centers (17%), school districts (14%), and nonprofit agencies (12%).
>
> Most frequent community partners (non-sponsors) that provide staff and services include the school (60%), health department (41%), local hospital (29%) and mental health agency (26%).
>
> Many SBHCs provide training for health professionals, including nurse practitioners (55%), physicians (38%), and mental health providers (25%).
>
> SBHCs use a variety of evaluation tools to measure their quality of care and outcomes, including chart audits (88%), student health

assessments by paper and pencil (57%), parent surveys (44%), teacher surveys (40%), and computer surveys of student health (19%).

NATIONAL CENSUS SCHOOL YEAR 2001–2002

The National Assembly on School-Based Health Care conducted the 2001–2002 census of school-based health centers to:

- Collect specific information on the current status of SBHCs, including services, clinic policies, staffing and utilization, and populations served.

- Assess the current prevention activities provided by SBHCs both in health centers and in health centers and in classrooms.

- Assess quality assurance mechanisms.

- Provide a better understanding of the role of SBHCs in meeting the health needs of uninsured school-aged children and adolescents.

At the start of the census in November 2001, the number of SBHCs had grown to 1,385. Through the year-long census process, we found an additional 238 centers and removed 245 that had closed or were not health centers, for a final total of 1,378. A total of 1,165 centers responded (1,081 to a long survey; 84 to an abbreviated survey), representing an 85% response rate.

Schools

Settings for school-based health centers (SBHCs) are as varied as the types of schools in the United States. Traditional elementary, middle and high schools are the dominant setting, but a number of consolidated or combined schools also have health centers (see Figure 14.1).

School size also varies, with the majority of health centers (60%) in schools with 500–1,500 students. Twenty percent are in schools with less than 500 students, another 20% with more than 1,500 students.

Community

SBHCs are located in geographically diverse communities, with the majority (62%) in urban communities. One in four health centers

Figure 14.1   Distribution of SBHCs by School Setting.

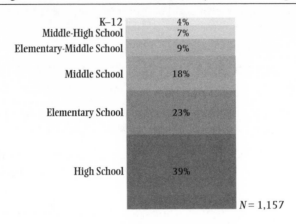

N = 1,157

Figure 14.2   Distribution of SBHCs by Sponsor Agency Type.

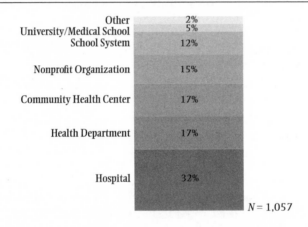

N = 1,057

is in rural schools. One in ten is in suburban school districts (see Figure 14.2).

Sponsorship of SBHCs is most typically by a local health care organization, such as a hospital, health department, or community health center. Other community partners include universities and mental health agencies.

Figure 14.3   Ethnic Profile of Student Population in Schools with SBHCs.

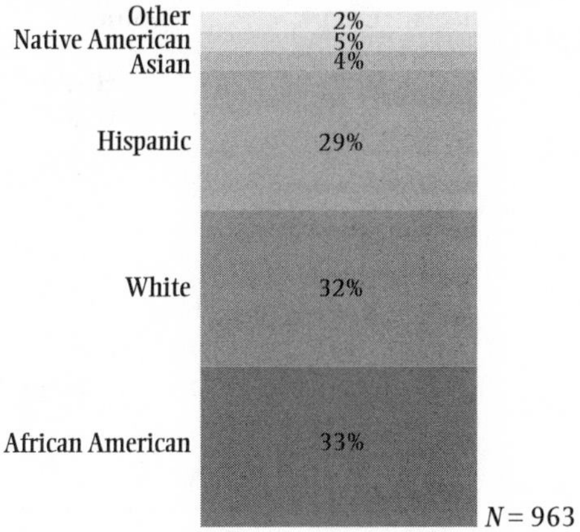

Other 2%
Native American 5%
Asian 4%
Hispanic 29%
White 32%
African American 33%

N = 963

Eighty-four programs had opened since 2001 and 71% had been open five years or more.

Students

Students in schools with SBHCs are largely minority and ethnic populations that have historically experienced health care access disparities (see Figure 14.3).

Four in ten SBHCs report that 50% or more of the SBHC users had no other source of primary care.

Community needs assessment of young people's health care access was most often identified (68%) as the primary reason for placing health centers in schools.

STAFFING PATTERNS

Staffing patterns in America's SBHCs are varied and can range from an on-site provider in a school four hours a week to six full-time equivalents from multiple disciplines operating in a center that is open

Table 14.1

SBHC Staff	Primary Care		Primary Care Mental Health		Primary Care Mental Health PLUS	
	%	Hrs/Week	%	Hrs/Week	%	Hrs/Week
Primary Care	100	23	100	25	100	35
Nursing/ Clinical Support	83	35	91	49	92	58
Mental Health	0	0	100	32	100	37
Health Educator	7	18	0	0	50	22
Social Services	8	29	0	0	39	28
Nutritionist	6	7	0	0	32	6
Dental	6	28	0	0	28	16

more than 40 hours each week. While there are many health care staffing configurations within SBHCs, the presence of primary care providers—in any combination of physician, nurse practitioner or physician assistant—is the common denominator. Three SBHC staffing patterns described here illustrate different approaches to school-based health care (see Table 14.1 and Figure 14.4).

Figure 14.4

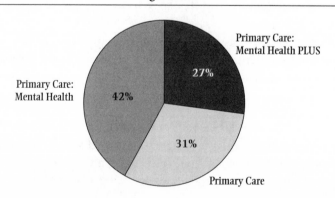

Primary Care

The primary care SBHC staff typically comprises a nurse practitioner or physician assistant with medical supervision by a physician. Clinical support is provided by a registered or licensed practical nurse with assistance from a medical clerk or health aide. In a small percentage of these SBHCs, staff may be augmented by social service, health education or dental professionals. The characteristic that distinguishes this staffing model from others is what it lacks: a mental health professional.

Primary Care: Mental Health

The largest group of SBHCs is staffed by primary care providers in partnership with a mental health professional—whether licensed clinical social worker, psychologist, or substance abuse counselor. Clinical and administrative support is similar to the primary care model.

Primary Care: Mental Health PLUS

The third model is the most comprehensive. Primary care and mental health staff are joined by other disciplines to complement the health care team. The most common addition is a health educator, followed by social services case manager, and nutritionist. Dental professionals—either a hygienist or dentist—were found in 28% of the PLUS health centers.

SCOPE OF SERVICES

Physical Health Services

The majority of SBHCs provide the basic tools of primary preventive care. The most common components in the SBHC scope of service are comprehensive health assessments, anticipatory guidance, vision and hearing screenings, immunizations, treatment of acute illness, laboratory services, and prescription services (see Figure 14.5).

The most frequently cited immunizations provided were Hepatitis B, measles-mumps-rubella, diptheria and tetanus toxoids, poliovirus, and influenza.

Figure 14.5

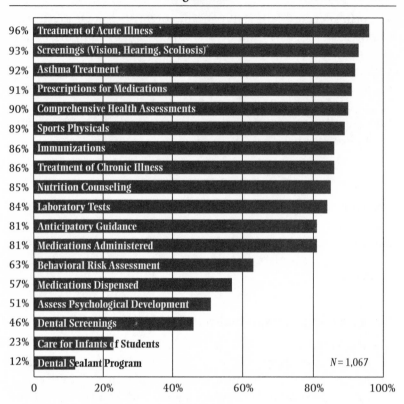

96%	Treatment of Acute Illness
93%	Screenings (Vision, Hearing, Scoliosis)
92%	Asthma Treatment
91%	Prescriptions for Medications
90%	Comprehensive Health Assessments
89%	Sports Physicals
86%	Immunizations
86%	Treatment of Chronic Illness
85%	Nutrition Counseling
84%	Laboratory Tests
81%	Anticipatory Guidance
81%	Medications Administered
63%	Behavioral Risk Assessment
57%	Medications Dispensed
51%	Assess Psychological Development
46%	Dental Screenings
23%	Care for Infants of Students
12%	Dental Sealant Program

$N = 1,067$

Figure 14.6

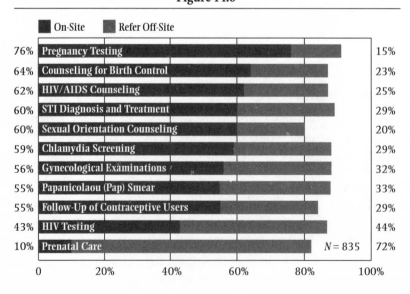

On-Site   Refer Off-Site

76%	Pregnancy Testing	15%
64%	Counseling for Birth Control	23%
62%	HIV/AIDS Counseling	25%
60%	STI Diagnosis and Treatment	29%
60%	Sexual Orientation Counseling	20%
59%	Chlamydia Screening	29%
56%	Gynecological Examinations	32%
55%	Papanicolaou (Pap) Smear	33%
55%	Follow-Up of Contraceptive Users	29%
43%	HIV Testing	44%
10%	Prenatal Care	72%

$N = 835$

Reproductive Health Services

Health centers serving middle- and high-school–aged students were more likely to provide on-site treatment for sexually transmitted diseases (60%), HIV/AIDS counseling (62%), and diagnostic services such as pregnancy testing (76%) than contraceptive services. Family planning services most often encompassed birth control counseling (64%) and follow up (55%). A minority of health centers neither provided on-site nor referred to an off-site provider for any sexual health services (see Figure 14.6).

Three of four school-based health centers serving middle and high school grades reported that contraception was not dispensed on-site.

Mental Health Services

School-based health centers offer a variety of on-site mental health and counseling services through several modalities, including individual, one-on-one counseling, student group counseling, family therapy, consultation and case management (see Figure 14.7). Most

Figure 14.7

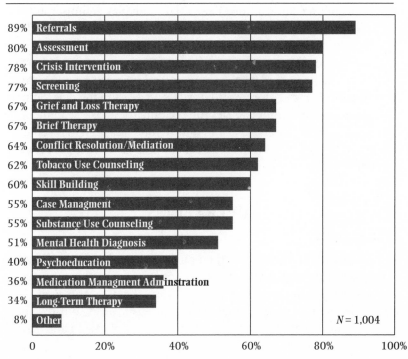

89%	Referrals
80%	Assessment
78%	Crisis Intervention
77%	Screening
67%	Grief and Loss Therapy
67%	Brief Therapy
64%	Conflict Resolution/Mediation
62%	Tobacco Use Counseling
60%	Skill Building
55%	Case Managment
55%	Substance Use Counseling
51%	Mental Health Diagnosis
40%	Psychoeducation
36%	Medication Managment Administration
34%	Long-Term Therapy
8%	Other

N = 1,004

0   20%   40%   60%   80%   100%

frequent of these include referrals (89%), assessment (80%), crisis intervention (78%), and screening (77%).

- SBHCs most frequently estimated that 50% of the mental health professional's time was spent in one-on-one service. The remaining 50% of their time is divided among student groups, case management, consultation, family therapy, and classroom presentations.

- 110 programs reported an alcohol and drug counselor and 67 programs report a psychiatrist in their staffing configuration.

- 33% of rural programs and 29% of suburban and urban SBHCs offer small groups for tobacco cessation.

- One in three health centers serving elementary-aged students conduct schoolwide health promotion activities focused on injury prevention.

Prevention/Early Intervention

Because of their unique setting, public health orientation, and proximity to children and youth at risk, SBHCs can play an important role in influencing the small number of risk behaviors that present the greatest threats to health (see Figure 14.8).

Interpersonal connections in the clinical setting and small group support enable providers to ask the questions young people rarely hear, assess their risks for health threats, and assist in the development of social skills and competencies for avoiding these risks. Augmenting these services with the classroom and schoolwide activities reported here reinforces the community values and norms that support student wellness beyond the clinic walls.

OPERATIONS

Hours Open

The majority of SBHCs are open during normal school hours and typically more than 30 hours a week (58%). One in five reported to be open eight hours or less a week. Some health centers provide expanded hours enabling students to make visits during out-of-school time, including after school (58%), before school (45%) and during the summer (38%)(see Figure 14.9).

Figure 14.8

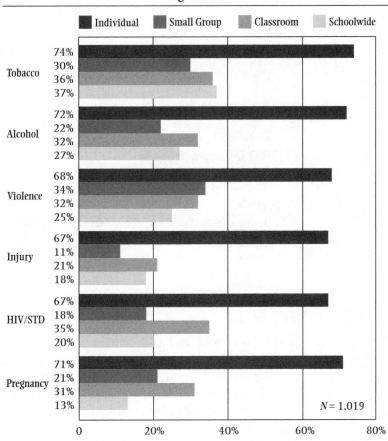

Figure 14.9   SBCH Hours of Operation by Community Characteristic.

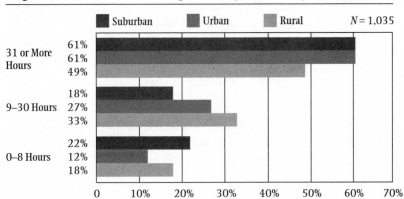

Figure 14.10   Age of SBHCs and Other Populations Served.

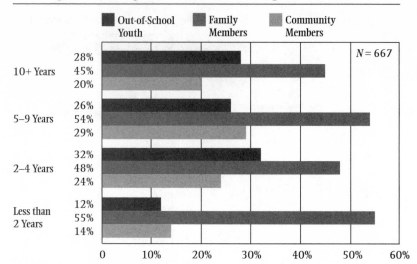

Other Populations Served

Although the school population is the health center's primary target, many SBHCs (65%) provide services to patients other than enrolled students. These populations include students from other schools in the community (38%), family members of students (33%), faculty and school personnel (31%), out-of-school youth (18%), and other community members (16%) (see Figure 14.10).

Third-Party Billing

Most SBHCs (69%) collect revenue for health center visits, predominantly from third-party payers such as Medicaid (68%), SCHIP (43%) and private insurance (45%). Twenty-three percent of SBHCs assess fees directly from the student or family (see Figure 14.11).

On-Site Training

Nearly eighty percent of SBHCs serve as training sites for health professionals. The percentages by profession include: nurse practitioners (73%), physicians (48%), mental health providers (34%) and nutritionists (10%).

Figure 14.11   Billing Practices of SBHCs by School Type.

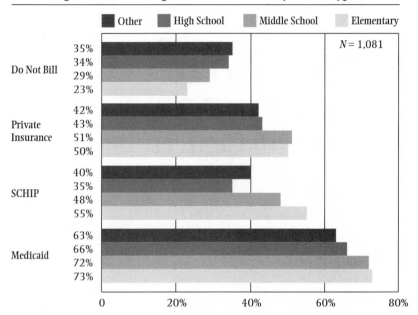

Evaluation

SBHCs use evaluation tools to assess students' health knowledge and stakeholders' satisfaction with services. Specific tools include: paper or computer student health assessments (70%), surveys of parents (50%), surveys of teachers (45%), and student questionnaires in classroom (33%).

Quality Assuranace

SBHCs employ a variety of mechanisms to assure high-quality health care: staff credentialing and training (92%), medical records reviews (91%), policies and procedures (89%), measures of patient satisfaction (74%), standards for physical environment (70%) and laboratory certification (69%).

CHAPTER 15

Managed Care and School-Based Health Centers

Use of Health Services

David W. Kaplan, B. Ned Calonge, Bruce P. Guernsey, Maureen B. Hanrahan, 1998

Providing effective and comprehensive physical, mental, and preventive health care for adolescents has been a complicated issue for health care providers and delivery systems, parents, school systems, and adolescents. During the last 2 decades, as the array of adolescent health problems has increased, the barriers adolescents face in accessing physical and mental health services have emerged in sharp focus.[1-7] Prominent obstacles include the availability and accessibility of physical and mental health services, confidentiality, and insurance coverage. Indeed, 9.8 million children and adolescents younger than 18 years had no health insurance at any time in 1995. During a 28-month period in 1992, 1993, and 1994, 30% of all children and adolescents younger than 18 years lacked health insurance for at least 1 of the 28 months (20.4 million).[8] Many more adolescents are underinsured, with health insur-

---

The chapter originally appeared as Kaplan DW, Calonge BN, Guernsey BP, Hanrahan MB. Managed care and school-based health centers: use of health services. *Arch Pediatr Adolesc Med*. 1998;152:25–33.

ance that does not include preventive care, counseling, substance abuse treatment, or other needed services.[9]

In response to the troubling physical and mental health status of many adolescents in the United States, and because of the desire to establish effective prevention and early intervention programs, there has been a resurgence of interest in the school as a focal point for integrating comprehensive health education with the provision of basic primary and preventive health and mental health services. Many of the most significant and costly national health problems are in large part caused by behaviors established during youth, including lifestyles, activities, and behaviors that cause unintentional and intentional injuries; drug and alcohol abuse; sexual behaviors that cause sexually transmitted diseases (STDs), including infection with the human immunodeficiency virus (HIV) and unintended pregnancy; tobacco use; inadequate physical activity; and dietary patterns that cause disease.[10] Focusing on preventing these behaviors has become increasingly important.

An emerging approach to these issues has been the development of school-based health centers (SBHCs) structured to provide basic physical and mental health services in the school. This model has several compelling features as a delivery system for adolescents: it reduces physical barriers to access,[11] improves compliance and follow-up,[12] offers self-initiated confidential care,[13] focuses on early identification of high-risk problems,[14] provides an array of services that can be customized for the adolescent population,[11] integrates health promotion into the school environment,[15] and uses midlevel practitioners to reduce health care costs.

The number of SBHCs has increased substantially during the last decade, from 40 in 1985 to 900 in 1995.[16] These health centers, most often supported by mixtures of grant money and local agency in-kind resources, have the potential for addressing the major issues facing health care of adolescents by having health and mental health care services available at a location where most teens spend substantial amounts of time.

However, the most important issue facing SBHCs is that of sustainable funding. The prospect of long-term funding from school district budgets is poor; health care is not a core business function of public schools, and our tax-averse environment seems unlikely to support expansion into this area. Foundation grants are not intended as long-term funding streams, and local youth-serving agencies have difficulty sustaining these expanded services on existing budgets. This gap leaves health insurance entities and public health funds as the most logical and perhaps only viable funding sources for these programs. Given the competitive health economic environment, insurance payers are not looking for additional areas in which to spend purchasers' dollars; yet, an increasing number of adolescents served by SBHCs are insured through managed care. The proliferation of SBHCs has coincided with the growth in managed care. An estimated 149 million Americans received their health care through health maintenance organizations (HMOs) and preferred provider organizations in 1995.[17] Thus, to encourage reimbursement of SBHCs, the value of these programs must be documented for insurers, managed care organizations, and health care consumers.

PARTICIPANTS AND METHODS
THE SCHOOL-BASED HEALTH CENTERS

The Denver SBHCs began providing health services in April 1988. The 3 high school SBHCs included in the study have a combined student body size of 3900 and serve an urban, inner-city student population in grades 9 through 12. By academic year 1990–1991, medical and mental health services were stable and fully operational. Primary health and mental health services are provided at each clinic by a pediatric nurse practitioner or physician assistant, clinical social worker, and substance abuse counselor, all with additional training in working with adolescents. Supervision of the nurse practitioners is provided by physicians who spend some time on-site and are available on-call. After-hours coverage is shared by the pediatric nurse practitioners and physician assistants by pager.

The SBHCs offer a broad array of basic primary physical and mental health services. Physical health services include health supervision examinations, including health screening, psychosocial histories, immunizations, and health guidance; diagnosis and treatment of acute illnesses and injuries; acute management of chronic conditions, such as asthma, diabetes, and epilepsy (the management of chronic conditions is usually coordinated with the student's medical home); treatment of common adolescent concerns, such as acne and weight management; gynecological examinations; pregnancy testing; and diagnosis and treatment of STDs, including HIV testing and counseling. Basic mental health services include mental health assessment and consultation; individual, group and family counseling; and crisis intervention. Substance abuse services include assessment and intervention for use of illicit drugs, mainly alcohol and marijuana. A few students were found to be abusing hallucinogens and other illegal drugs, and a small number were found to be abusing licit drugs. Tobacco use was not identified by substance abuse providers as warranting referral for their services. Student referrals to the substance abuse treatment provider originated from the medical and mental health providers, who, during an examination, identified substance abuse as a problem.

(continued)

Referrals also were made by school disciplinary staff when a student violated the school's substance abuse policy, which required a referral for counseling.

Health promotion services include one-on-one patient education, as well as classroom and community health education on a broad range of age-appropriate topics, such as the prevention of HIV infection and acquired immunodeficiency syndrome, other STDs, substance abuse, pregnancy, interpersonal violence, unintentional injury, and treatment of chronic diseases. Social services include identification of basic needs and referrals for food, shelter, clothing, legal and employment services, and public assistance.

All students attending a school with an SBHC are eligible to enroll and use services. Enrollment requires signed parental consent. No fees are charged to students, parents, or health care insurers for care delivered through the SBHC. During the study, SBHC and KPC had no fiscal or administrative relationship. The SBHCs are closed during winter and spring breaks and for 6 weeks during the summer.

KAISER PERMANENTE OF COLORADO

Kaiser Permanente is a national group model, closed-panel, nonprofit HMO. Providing care since 1969, KPC currently has approximately 320,000 members in the Denver metropolitan area, representing about 15% of the population and is the third largest health plan in the state. In 1993, KPC had approximately 20,000 members between the ages of 14 and 18 years. A KPC outpatient facility is located within 1 mile of each of the 3 SBHCs. The range of benefits provided by the health plan includes all medically necessary outpatient, physician, diagnostic, treatment, home health, preventive, and short-term rehabilitation services; medical detoxification and assessment of the need for chemical dependency treatment or referral; and up to 20 outpatient mental health care visits and 45 days of inpatient mental health per calendar year. Data about the average household income of families insured with KPC are not collected; however, the subscribers are uniformly employed. Office visit copayments range from $0 to $15, although the provider may waive the copayment for special situations, for example, when a teenager who is unable to pay requests a confidential service. The KPC pediatricians, family physicians, and nurse practitioners have demonstrated a special interest in adolescent health by establishing an adolescent task force that meets monthly to address issues related to the provision of adolescent health care. The members of the task force support coordination of care with the SBHCs.

Screening for health risks in adolescent members at KPC occurs within the context of health supervision visits (e.g., well-teen visits, camp and sports physicals, immunization visits, routine gynecological visits for sexually active teens). Medical forms for these office visits include brief checklists of health behaviors to be assessed and documented by the health care provider. Adolescents are encouraged to make routine visits during regular office hours. After-hours calls are triaged by trained nursing staff and referred for emergency care, urgent after-hours care, next-day routine care, or telephone advice.

(continued)

STUDY DESIGN

A retrospective cohort design with matching of age, sex, and socioeconomic status was used to compare the use of health services of adolescent members of KPC who had access to SBHCs with those with no such access. Adolescents enrolled in KPC were selected as the study population for the following reasons: (1) KPC is a closed-panel HMO. Covered visits must be made to a KPC facility, allowing identification of all outpatient, emergency department, mental health, and substance abuse visits in the KPC system. (2) KPC has had a special interest in serving adolescents and reducing barriers to providing comprehensive and confidential services to this age group. As an HMO system of care, KPC had the least number of barriers to providing adolescent services. The SBHCs have successfully served adolescents who had no health insurance or who faced barriers such as distance, cost, lack of confidentiality, or restrictive mental health and substance abuse benefits. We believed this design would provide the greatest insight into the use of SBHC services for insured adolescents enrolled in an HMO.

All adolescents registered in the Denver SBHCs from August 1, 1990, through June 7, 1993, were matched to the KPC enrollment database. Matching was based on birth date, name, and sex. Race was not used to match because race is not part of the KPC enrollment database. To be included in the study, adolescents had to be enrolled and eligible to receive services from KPC continuously during the study. A control group of adolescents who did not match enrollment in an SBHC was selected from the KPC enrollment database. The control group was limited to adolescents who were at least 14 years old at the beginning of each academic year and not older than age 18 years at the end of each academic year. Family income data were not collected by the SBHC or KPC. Because of the influence of socioeconomic status on patterns of health care use, a control group was selected by zip code from a geographic area in the city without access to an SBHC and with the same census tract median family income as the census tracts for the adolescents with access to an SBHC. To assure that adolescents were accurately classified as attending a school with an SBHC or not having access to an SBHC, the combined data set of study adolescents and control adolescents was matched to the Denver Public Schools pupil database. The school in which the student was enrolled, if any, was entered into the data set for each of the 3 academic years in the study period as follows: year 1, August 1, 1990, through June 7, 1991; year 2, August 1, 1991, through June 7, 1992; and year 3, August 1, 1992, through June 7, 1993. Adolescents who made at least 1 visit during the study period to the SBHC or KPC were included in the study. A total of 342 adolescents were enrolled in the study, accounting for 3394 visits.

Because students' use of health services and school of enrollment could change from one academic year to the next, most of the analyses were performed and reported for the individual academic year. For example, an adolescent attending an SBHC school could transfer to a school without access to

(continued)

a SBHC the following academic year or could drop out of school. Analysis on a yearly academic basis was used as a safeguard to avoid misclassification.

Use of services at the SBHC was obtained from audits of the SBHC medical records. The visit encounter forms are highly structured with checklists for the assessment of risk factors. The most common outpatient *International Classification of Diseases, Ninth Revision (ICD-9)*18 diagnoses are printed on the back of the encounter form to facilitate diagnostic coding. The forms are used at each SBHC visit. For visits at KPC, the medical records for each subject were reviewed. These records use a structured encounter form for health supervision visits but not for other types of visits. The assessment of health risks at KPC is not as formalized as that conducted at the SBHC sites. In addition, *ICD-9* diagnoses are not printed on the encounter form as they are in the SBHCs. Mental health and chemical dependency records at KPC and the SBHCs are kept separate from the medical record. These also were audited for the study participants.

Visit rates were compared for the KPC members with and without access to an SBHC. Visit type (ie, routine ambulatory, emergent or urgent care, mental health, or chemical dependency), diagnosis, and risk factor assessment were also examined. Fisher exact and 3 tests were used for categorical data comparisons, and the Student *t* test (2-tailed) was used to compare continuous data. Direct age standardization to the Colorado population was used to examine any effect of the differential age distribution that arose after confirmation of the study participants through school records.

To explore the potential value of SBHC services in the current health care environment, Kaiser Permanente of Colorado, Denver (KPC) and the University of Colorado Health Sciences Center Department of Pediatrics, Denver, undertook a collaborative study of the use and utility of SBHCs. The study was designed to compare the use of primary and subspecialty physical and mental health services for adolescents who were enrolled in managed care and had access to an SBHC with that of adolescents enrolled in managed care without access to an SBHC. Specifically, patterns of use were analyzed for physical health, mental health, and substance abuse services; preventive health services; and after hours (emergent or urgent) care services.

RESULTS

A total of 342 adolescents were included in the study, resulting in 3,394 visits occurring during the 3 academic years when the SBHCs were open. Of the adolescents, 194 (56.7%) were female and 148 (43.3%) were male.

Of the visits, 63% were by females and 37% by males. Table 15.1 gives the age and sex distribution for adolescents using KPC and an SBHC and adolescents using KPC without access to an SBHC. In each of the 3 academic years, there was no significant difference in the composition of the population by sex or age for adolescents using an SBHC and KPC compared with adolescents using KPC without access to an SBHC. During at least 1 of the 3 academic years, 240 adolescents attended a school with an SBHC, resulting in 2599 visits. The mean number of combined KPC and SBHC visits per adolescent during each of the academic years for adolescents who attended a school with an SBHC was 5.3 during year 1990–1991, 5.3 during year 1991–1992, and 5.7 during year 1992–1993. For adolescents not attending a school with an SBHC, the mean number of KPC visits per adolescent was 3.9 during year 1990–1991, 3.8 during year 1991–1992, and 3.4 during year 1992–1993. For the adolescents who attended a school with an SBHC and used the SBHC, the mean number of visits per individual was 7.6 during year 1990–1991, 6.7 during year 1991–1992, and 8.2 during year 1992–1993. For the adolescents attending a school with an SBHC who did not use the SBHC, the mean number of visits per adolescent was 2.8 during year 1990–1991, 4.1 during year 1991–1992, and 3.7 during year 1992–1993.

Table 15.2 gives data about the health, mental health, and substance abuse visits for adolescents using an SBHC and KPC compared with adolescents making KPC visits without access to an SBHC. The difference in utilization of mental health and substance abuse visits was significant for the adolescents with access to an SBHC: 96.5% of the 314 mental health visits occurred in the group with access to the SBHC ($P < .001$), and all of the 120 substance abuse visits occurred in the SBHC ($P < .001$).

The differential use of the SBHCs for mental health and substance abuse treatment is striking. Of the adolescents actually using the SBHC, 31% used mental health services. Eight percent used substance abuse services, and 36% used mental health or substance abuse services. These figures compare with only 3% of adolescents without access to an SBHC who visited KPC for mental health or substance abuse treatment ($P < .001$). Table 15.3 lists the frequency of mental health and substance abuse primary diagnoses for adolescents using the SBHC mental health and substance abuse services.

Because of the large difference in the number of mental health and substance abuse visits between the SBHC and KPC, the mean annual visit rate for adolescents using the SBHC for medical, mental health,

Table 15.1 Age and Sex Distribution for Adolescents Using KPC and an SBHC and Adolescents Using KPC Without Access to an SBHC.*

| | Academic Year | | | | | | | | | | | |
| | 1990–1991 | | | | 1991–1992 | | | | 1992–1993 | | | |
	SBHC and KPC†	KPC Only‡	Total	P	SBHC and KPC†	KPC Only‡	Total	P	SBHC and KPC†	KPC Only‡	Total	P
Female	42 (65)	27 (51)	69		51 (66)	39 (60)	90		45 (58)	44 (56)	89	
Male	23 (35)	26 (49)	49	.13	26 (34)	26 (40)	52	.44	32 (42)	36 (45)	68	.66
Total	65	53	118		77	65	142		77	80	157	
Age at visit, y												
14	8 (12)	4 (8)	12		8 (10)	3 (5)	11		1 (1)	5 (6)	6	
15	24 (37)	26 (49)	50		16 (21)	12 (18)	28		12 (16)	21 (26)	33	
16	28 (43)	20 (38)	48	.56	23 (35)	23 (35)	46	.41	22 (29)	14 (18)	36	.15
17	5 (8)	3 (6)	8		27 (30)	20 (31)	47		26 (34)	23 (29)	49	
18	0	0	0		3 (4)	7 (11)	10		16 (21)	17 (21)	33	
Total	65	53	118		77	65	142		77	80	157	

*SBHC indicates school-based health center; KPC, Kaiser Permanente of Colorado, Denver. Percentages do not always total 100 because of rounding.

†Number (percentage) of SBHC visits and KPC visits for adolescents attending an SBHC school.

‡Number (percentage) of KPC visits for adolescents not attending an SBHC school.

Table 15.2 Health, Mental Health, and Substance Abuse Visits for Adolescents Using KPC and an SBHC vs KPC Without Access to an SBHC.*

	Medical	Mental Health	Substance Abuse
SBHC and KPC visits	1236 (56.1)	303 (96.5)	120 (100)
KPC visits, not attending an SBHC school	968 (43.9)	11 (3.5)	0 (0)
Total	**2204 (100)**	**314 (100)**	**120 (100)**

*SBHC indicates school-based health center; KPC, Kaiser Permanente of Colorado, Denver. Data are given as number (percentage).

and substance abuse treatment services is greater than that for adolescents using KPC. If all the mental health and substance abuse visits are ignored, the use for adolescents using KPC *and* the SBHC for medical care only is much closer to the rate of use for adolescents using KPC without access to an SBHC (see Table 15.4). In each of the 3 academic years, the rates of use range from 4.4 to 4.7 medical visits per adolescent using the SBHCs and KPC and from 3.4 to 3.7 visits per adolescent using KPC without access to an SBHC. The difference in the rate of use of medical services was statistically significant only during the academic year 1992–1993.

Table 15.3 Frequency of Mental Health and Substance Abuse Primary Diagnoses for Adolescents Using an SBHC.*

	No. (%) of Visits
Adolescent or parent problem	115 (27.2)
Adolescent adjustment	67 (15.8)
Marijuana abuse	63 (14.9)
Depression	50 (11.8)
Other mental disorder	41 (9.7)
Alcohol abuse	38 (9.0)
Anxiety, stress, or phobia	22 (5.2)
Posttraumatic stress	17 (4.0)
Oppositional disorder	6 (1.4)
Other drug abuse	4 (0.9)
Total	**423 (99.9)**

*SBHC indicates school-based health center. Percentages do not total 100 because of rounding.

Table 15.4   Medical Visits Only.*

Academic Year	SBHC and KPC Visits per Adolescent Attending an SBHC School	KPC Visits per Adolescent Not Attending an SBHC School	P
1990–1991	4.4	3.7	.24
1991–1992	4.5	3.8	.10
1992–1993	4.7	3.4	.01

*SBHC indicates school-based health center; KPC, Kaiser Permanente of Colorado, Denver.

Figure 15.1 shows the frequency of primary medical diagnoses for SBHC visits and visits to KPC for the adolescents who used an SBHC. Table 15.5 gives further analysis of the primary medical diagnoses seen in higher frequency at KPC than at the SBHCs, grouping the diagnosis by the site of care. The grouping of diagnosis by site of care within KPC offers some insight into how adolescents used the 2 systems of care. For example, there was greater use of KPC for musculoskeletal problems, but 26.0% of the visits were to occupational and physical therapy and 48.0% to after hours (emergent or urgent) care, services not available at the SBHC. Similarly, 80.2% of visits for injuries and poisonings occurred after hours.

Table 15.5   Site of Care by Primary Diagnosis for Visits at KPC Seen in Higher Frequency Than in the SBHC.*

	Primary Diagnosis Category			
	Injuries or Respiratory	Poisonings	Infections	Musculo-skeletal
Site of care at KPC				
Primary care	76 (60.3)	12 (9.9)	34 (74)	12 (26.0)
After hours (emergent or urgent)	36 (28.5)	97 (80.2)	11 (24)	22 (48.0)
Medical specialties	14 (11.1)	5 (4.1)	1 (2)	
Occupational or physical therapy		7 (5.8)		12 (26.0)
Total	**126**	**121**	**46**	**46**

*SBHC indicates school-based health center; KPC, Kaiser Permanente of Colorado, Denver. Data are given as number (percentage). Percentages do not all total 100 because of rounding.

Figure 15.1 Primary Medical Diagnostic Categories, School-Based Health Center (SBHC) Visits vs. Kaiser Permanente of Colorado, Denver.

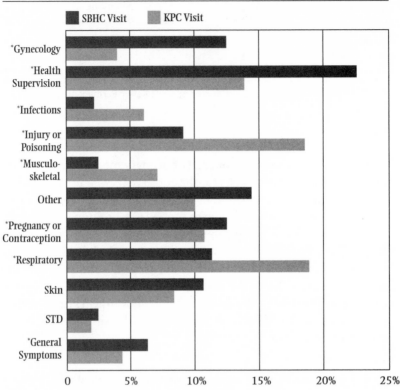

•An asterisk indicates a significant difference in the frequency of the primary diagnostic category between the SBJC and KPC (P = <.01). STD indicates sexually transmitted disease.

As shown in Figure 15.1, there was higher use of the SBHC for health supervision visits. During the 3-year study period, 80.2% of adolescents using the SBHC and KPC had at least 1 comprehensive health supervision visit compared with 68.8% of adolescents without access to an SBHC (P = .04). The rate of documentation of screening was much higher for high-risk health behaviors and anticipatory guidance during the comprehensive health supervision visits in the SBHCs compared with visits to KPC (see Table 15.6).

Table 15.7 compares the use of after-hours (emergent or urgent) services for adolescents using KPC and an SBHC with adolescents

Table 15.6   Documented Screening for High-Risk Behaviors and
Anticipatory Guidance During Comprehensive Health
Supervision Visits.*

Screening	SBHC Visits	KPC Visits	P
Abuse	51 (42.1)	4 (0.9)	<.001
Alcohol use	57 (47.1)	72 (16.3)	<.001
Drug use	57 (47.1)	76 (17.2)	<.001
Emotional health	58 (47.9)	13 (2.9)	<.001
Family relationships	59 (48.7)	153 (34.6)	<.005
Nutrition	57 (47.1)	173 (39.1)	.14
Peer relationships	60 (49.6)	19 (4.3)	<.001
Pregnancy risk	68 (56.2)	71 (16.1)	<.001
School problems	59 (48.7)	195 (44.1)	.36
Seatbelt use	58 (47.9)	81 (18.3)	<.001
Self-care	58 (47.9)	108 (24.4)	<.001
Sexual activity	74 (61.2)	135 (30.5)	<.001
Sleep problems	56 (46.3)	162 (36.7)	.05
STD risk	66 (54.5)	51 (11.5)	<.001
Tobacco use	57 (47.1)	76 (17.2)	<.001
Violence	52 (43.0)	1 (0.2)	<.001
Vocational plans	55 (44.5)	22 (4.9)	<.001
Total	**121**	**442**	

*SBHC indicates school-based health center; KPC, Kaiser Permanente of Colorado,
Denver; and STD, sexually transmitted disease. Data are given as number (percentage).

Table 15.7   After Hours (Emergent or Urgent) Use for Adolescents
Using KPC and an SBHC vs Adolescents Using KPC
Without Access to an SBHC.*

	KPC After Hours Visits for Adolescents Attending an SBHC School		KPC After Hours Visits for Adolescents Not Attending an SBHC School	
Academic Year	Visits per Adolescent	Adolescents Using ED, %	Visits per Adolescent	Adolescent Using ED, %
1990–1991	0.42	...	0.94	...
	...	29.2	...	52.8
1991–1992	0.55	...	0.88	...
	...	39.0	...	60.0
1992–1993	0.57	...	0.93	...
	...	41.6	...	53.8

*SBHC indicates school-based health center; KPC, Kaiser Permanente of Colorado,
Denver; and ED, emergency department. Ellipses indicate data not applicable.

using KPC without access to an SBHC. In each of the 3 academic years, the rate of use by adolescents with access to an SBHC (0.42–0.55 visits per adolescent) was significantly lower compared with the rate of use by adolescents without access (0.88–0.94 visits per adolescent). In 2 of the 3 academic years, the percentage of adolescents making after-hours visits if they had access to an SBHC (29.2%–41.6%) was also significantly lower compared with those who did not (52.8%–60.0%).

COMMENT

Use by Diagnosis

This study provides a first look at the patterns of use of health, mental health, and substance abuse treatment services for an insured population of adolescents with and without access to an SBHC. Overall, adolescents with access to SBHCs made nearly 1 additional medical visit, but fewer after-hours visits, than did adolescents without access to an SBHC. The annual rate of medical visits for adolescents using an SBHC compares favorably with the rates reported in other studies of the use of other SBHCs.[19]

The study provides some insight into whether provision of a similar array of basic primary health services in an SBHC for a population of insured adolescents is additive to or duplicative of services available through KPC. Figure 15.1 and Table 15.5 display statistically different primary medical diagnoses for the SBHC and KPC for adolescents using an SBHC. The greater proportion of health supervision visits in SBHCs could reflect easier access, program emphasis, or a means of circumventing the KPC copayment for a physical examination. It may be that the availability of an SBHC attracts a harder-to-reach segment of the population into preventive health care. Whatever the factor(s), the combination of KPC with an SBHC results in a higher health supervision rate for adolescents with access to an SBHC (80.2%) than for those without access (68.8%; $P = .04$). Further research is necessary to better understand the difference in use of preventive health care.

Other differences in use by diagnosis were found. A much greater proportion of gynecological care occurred at the SBHCs. This may be attributed to easier access, an understanding by the users that the

SBHC provided confidential services, a programmatic emphasis on early detection of STDs and pregnancy testing, or staff visiting the classrooms to encourage students to visit the health center if they thought they might be pregnant or have an STD. The higher rate of primary diagnosis at KPC related to pregnancy and contraception is because these services are not provided at the SBHC.

A greater proportion of diagnoses for injury and poisonings occurred at KPC. Because 80.2% of the visits for injury and poisonings occurred in the after-hours (emergent or urgent) clinics, these visits may reflect appropriate use for acute injuries. Similarly, KPC had a greater proportion of musculoskeletal primary diagnoses. Three quarters of these visits occurred in the after-hours clinics or to occupational or physical therapy. These services are not available in the SBHC.

Mental Health and Substance Abuse Services

Clearly, one of the most important findings of the study is the differential use of mental health and substance abuse services. Adolescents with access to an SBHC were 10 times more likely to make a mental health or substance abuse visit, with 96.5% of the mental health and all of the substance abuse visits occurring at the SBHC. Of the adolescents using the SBHC, 31.4% were seen by a mental health provider and 8.3% received substance abuse counseling. Emotional problems accounted for 29% of all diagnoses made in the Denver SBHCs.[11] The frequency of emotional problems treated is similar to that found in a study of the use by high school seniors of an SBHC in Los Angeles, Calif, where 26% of students who used the clinic had counseling about mental health and psychosocial problems.[20] Estimates of the prevalence of mental health disorders among adolescents living in the United States range from 12% to 22%.[3,21,22] Although rough estimates suggest that one fourth to one third of adolescents who need mental health services actually receive them,[3] few national data exist on the use of mental health services by adolescents.

The difference in use of mental health services could be due to a number of factors: differences in mental health "screening," identification, and referral by primary care providers; differences in availability of or access to mental health services; differences in the manner in which mental health services are delivered or the style or personality of the providers; or availability of other referral sources, such as teachers, administrators, school counselors, nurses, and social workers. A combination of factors may explain the stark contrast in use. Providers in the SBHCs received specific training in the identification of common emotional problems in the age group. Many of the adolescents seeking care because of physical symptoms that could have an underlying emotional basis were introduced to the on-site clinical social worker (mental health provider). This on-site multidisciplinary team approach resulted in effective mental health referrals and helped reduce perceived stigma attached to "going to counseling." No outcome data were collected for the adolescents receiving mental health treatment. However, because continued participation was usually voluntary and the mean number of mental health visits was between 5.4 and 6.4 per adolescent per year, the continuation in treatment seems to be perceived as beneficial by the students.

The difference in use for substance abuse treatment was similarly striking. Adolescent use of substance abuse treatment services in the SBHCs is consistent with epidemiologic studies of substance abuse: about 8% of students using the SBHCs made at least 1 visit, and 6% made at least 2 visits to substance abuse counselors.[11] Of the students who had initial visits to substance abuse counselors, 76% continued in counseling, and 84% of students who made at least 2 visits continued. Slightly more than half (51%) of students having any contact with substance abuse counselors also had contact with mental health counselors.[11] Engaging adolescents with substance abuse disorders into treatment is important, not only because this age group is difficult to draw into treatment, but also because of the high national prevalence of substance use. The most recent national data document that 51.3% of seniors and 38.8% of sophomores drank alcohol during the preceding month. Almost 21.9% of high school seniors and 20.4% of sophomores have used marijuana during the past month. Of high school seniors, 39% report having used an illicit drug during the preceding 12 months.[23]

In addition to the aforementioned possible factors for increasing use of mental health services in the SBHC, an important factor contributing to the use of substance abuse treatment was the institution of a school policy that gave students caught drinking alcohol or using other illegal drugs at school a choice between suspension or compulsory substance abuse treatment through the SBHC. For students selecting treatment, the treatment process began with an assessment of the extent, duration, and type of abuse, as well as contributing and enabling factors, such as family and peer relationships. Treatment modalities included small closed-ended groups, which met weekly for about 12 weeks, and adolescent counseling. Aftercare groups were available for students needing a longer period of support to remain substance free. Telephone contacts were made with parents as appropriate and necessary.

The success of the SBHCs in engaging adolescents into mental health and substance abuse services may be the program's coordination between physical and mental health providers, which has been a long-standing challenge in traditional health care settings.[24] Almost one fourth of adolescents in the Denver SBHCs had contact with more than 1 category of service provider. The increased access to mental health and substance abuse services seems to meet an important need in this population.

Health Supervision

The higher rate of documented screening for high-risk health behaviors and anticipatory guidance during the comprehensive health supervision visits in the SBHCs (Table 15.6) may be a result of 3 factors. First, the SBHC used an encounter form for the provider to comment on each risk behavior that was raised and addressed during any preventive health visit. Except for preventive visits, a more limited form was used in KPC. The documented difference thus may be related primarily to a recording artifact. Protocols and forms have been found to improve provider behavior.[25] Second, SBHC providers spend more time during each preventive health visit, with a mean visit time of 45 minutes compared with 20 minutes at KPC. Thus, there was more time available to cover a broader array of subjects. Third, providing comprehensive and prevention-oriented care was a major objective of the SBHC program.

After-Hours (Emergent or Urgent) Services

This study confirms the findings of the study by Santelli et al[26] that documented a self-reported reduction in emergency department use by students who had attended a school with an SBHC for more than 1 year compared with students in comparable schools without SBHCs. Both of these studies contrast an evaluation of the SHBCs funded by the Robert Wood Johnson Foundation, Princeton, NJ. The evaluation found a nonsignificant increase in emergency department use among adolescents relative to a comparison group of urban adolescents interviewed by telephone.[15] However, that study had a number of methodological limitations, including the choice of comparison group. Our finding that in each of the academic years there was a significantly lower rate of visits to the after-hours (emergent or urgent) services by adolescents with access to an SBHC compared with adolescents without access is strengthened by the study design to identify all emergent and urgent care. Adolescents enrolled in KPC must use a KPC facility for all routine and emergency care for the care to be compensated. If the study population were not limited to a KPC facility, documenting all emergency department and after-hours care in a large metropolitan area with various sources of care would have been extremely complicated.

We believe that the availability of acute care services at the school has decreased the rate of after-hours (emergent or urgent) visits at KPC. In addition, this may improve continuity of care because after-hours care is seldom provided by the patient's primary care provider and, provision is more expensive. This is a potential opportunity for managed care to improve the comprehensiveness and quality of care provided to adolescents while reducing costs, and it may prompt discussion of formal relationships with SBHC programs.

The study was limited by restriction to adolescents insured by KPC only, and the results may not be generalizable to uninsured teens or to those insured through other types of plans.

CONCLUSIONS

This comparison of the use of health services by adolescents enrolled in a closed-panel nonprofit HMO (KPC) who had access to an SBHC with adolescents without access to an SBHC found that adolescents with access to an SBHC were more than 10 times more likely to make a mental health or substance abuse visit, with 98% of these visits occurring at the SBHC. Adolescents with access to an SBHC had between 38% and 55% fewer after-hours (emergent or urgent) visits than did adolescents without access to an SBHC, and a significantly lower percentage of adolescents used after-hours (emergent or urgent) services if they had access to an SBHC compared with those who did not. A greater percentage, 80.2%, of adolescents with access to SBHCs had at least 1 comprehensive health supervision visit compared with 68.8% of adolescents without access. Furthermore, there was a much higher rate of documentation of screening for high-risk health behaviors in the SBHC.

School-based health centers providing comprehensive primary physical and mental health services seem to have a synergistic effect for adolescents enrolled in KPC. Adolescents seem to use both systems of care appropriately, and the significant improvement in access to mental health and substance abuse treatment may be an important finding in improving adolescent health services. A decrease in the number of after-hours (emergent or urgent) visits may be an area of potential savings for insurers.

Notes

1. National Center for Health Statistics. Table 1-27. Deaths from 282 selected causes, by 5–year age groups, race, and sex: United States, 1993. Hyattsville, Md: US Department of Health and Human Services; 1993.

2. Youth Risk Behavior Surveillance—United States, 1995. *MMWR Surveill Summ.* 1996;45(SS-4):2–83.

3. US Congress, Office of Technology Assessment. Mental health problems: prevention and services. In: *Adolescent Health Background and the Effectiveness of Selected Prevention and Treatment Services.* Washington, DC: US GPO; 1991;2:433–496. Office of Technology Assessment Publication OTA-H-466.

4. US Department of Health and Human Services, Public Health Service, Division of STD Prevention. *Sexually Transmitted Disease Surveillance, 1995.* Atlanta, Ga: Centers for Disease Control and Prevention; September 1996.

5. Centers for Disease Control and Prevention. *HIV/AIDS Surveillance Report.* Atlanta, Ga: Centers for Disease Control and Prevention; 1996;8(2):1–33.

6. Child Trends Inc. *Facts at a Glance: 1995 Teen Birth Rate in the United States.* Washington, DC: Child Trends Inc; October 1996.

7. Substance Abuse and Mental Health Services Administration. *1995 National Household Survey on Drug Abuse.* Washington, DC: US Department of Health and Human Services, Public Health Service; 1996.

8. US Bureau of the Census. *Current Population Reports, Health Insurance Coverage: 1996.* Washington, DC: US Bureau of the Census; March 1997.

9. McManus P, Newacheck PW. Health insurance status of adolescents and young adults: fact sheets. San Francisco, Calif: Institute for Health Policy Studies; 1991.

10. Kolbe LJ. An essential strategy to improve the health and education of Americans. *Prev Med.* 1992;22:1–17.

11. Anglin TM, Naylor KE, Kaplan DW. Comprehensive school-based health care: high school students' use of medical, mental health, and substance abuse services. *Pediatrics.* 1996;97:318–330.

12. Bearss N, Santelli JS, Papa P. A pilot program of contraceptive continuation in six school-based clinics. *J Adolesc Health.* 1995;17:178–183.

13. Santelli JS, Kouzis A, Newcomer S. Student attitudes toward school-based health centers. *J Adolesc Health.* 1996;18:349–356.

14. Walter HJ, Vaughan RD, Armstrong B, et al. Characteristics of users and nonusers of health clinics in inner-city junior high schools. *J Adolesc Health.* 1996;18:344–348.

15. Kisker EE, Brown RS. Do school-based health centers improve adolescents' access to health care, health status, and risk-taking behavior? *J Adolesc Health.* 1996;18:335–343.

16. Lear JG, Schlitt JJ. School-based health centers continue to grow. In: *Access to Comprehensive School-Based Health Services to Children and Youth.* Washington, DC: George Washington University School of Public Health and Health Services; 1997.

17. White D. *HMO and PPO Trends Report, 1997.* Washington, DC: American Association of Health Plans; 1996.

18. World Health Organization. *International Classification of Diseases, Ninth Revision (ICD-9).* Geneva, Switzerland: World Health Organization; 1977.

19. Lear JG, Gleicher HB, St Germaine A, Porter PJ. Reorganizing health care for adolescents: the experience of the school-based adolescent health care programs. *J Adolesc Health.* 1991;12:450–458.

20. Adelman HS, Barker LA, Nelson P. A study of a school-based clinic: who uses it and who doesn't? *J Clin Child Psychol.* 1993;22:52–59.

21. Coiro MJ, Zill N, Bloom B. *Health of Our Nation's Children.* Vital Health Stat. 1994;10(191):1–61.

22. Costello EJ. Introduction to developments in child psychiatric epidemiology. *J Am Acad Child Adolesc Psychiatry.* 1989;28:836–841.

23. National Institute on Drug Abuse. *National Survey Results on Drug Use: Monitoring the Future Study.* Rockville, Md: US Department of Health and Human Services; 1996.

24. Tuma JM. Mental health services for children: the state of the art. *Am Psychol.* 1989;44:188–199.

25. Baron ME, Zanga JR. Use of structured clinical forms in child abuse. *Pediatrics.* 1996;98(pt 1):429–433.

26. Santelli JJ, Kouzis A, Newcomer S. School-based health centers and adolescent use of primary care and hospital care. *J Adolesc Health.* 1996;19:267–275.

CHAPTER 16

Burden of Asthma in Inner-City Elementary Schoolchildren

Do School-Based Health Centers Make a Difference?

*Mayris P. Webber, Kelly E. Carpiniello, Tosan Oruwariye,
Yungtai Lo, William B. Burton, David K. Appel, 2003*

In the past decade, the number of school-based health centers (SBHCs) nationwide has increased from 150 to about 1,400, offering health care to approximately 1.1 million children.[1] The SBHCs are designed to provide primary, preventive, and acute care for school-aged children and are equipped to treat chronic conditions and educate both parents and children about health concerns.[2] Despite the intuitive appeal of putting children's health services where the children are, questions remain about the fundamental mission of SBHCs. If the sole mission of SBHCs is to improve access to health care, there is no doubt that SBHCs succeed.[3] However, in this era of evidence-based medicine, for SBHCs to survive financially, they must demonstrate that improved access is accompanied by improved outcomes. Previous studies of SBHCs have primarily focused either on access or on cost-effectiveness, demonstrating better coverage for vaccination programs,[4,5] an increase in the number of students using reproductive and mental health services,[6,7] and the cost-effectiveness of school-based tobacco control programs.[8] Fewer evaluative studies have been published, and to our knowledge, none using a quasi-experimental design, to assess the effect of SBHCs on the health and well-being of elementary school children.

During the 1999–2000 school year, we undertook a 3-year project to evaluate whether the availability of SBHCs *measurably* affected the health and school performance of children with asthma attending 6 Bronx, NY, elementary schools. We selected asthma as our indicator condition because it is the most common chronic illness affecting US children[9] and is costly; children with asthma struggle with adherence to strict medication regimens[10] and frequent hospital and emergency department (ED) visits. Asthma is also the leading medical cause of school absenteeism,[11] which may have educational and social consequences,[9] especially in inner-city children.

This study reports asthma symptoms and illness-related burden and examines differences in ED visits; hospitalizations; medication use by sex, race, or ethnicity; health insurance coverage; and availability of SBHCs. School absenteeism according to availability of SBHCs is also reported.

METHODS

Data were obtained from surveys completed by the parents or guardians of kindergartners through fifth graders attending 6 elementary schools in the Bronx. Four of the schools have SBHCs in which, on average, 86% of children are enrolled. These SBHCs provide comprehensive services by a pediatrician or a nurse practitioner during the school day with backup services after hours provided by 2 community health centers affiliated with Montefiore Medical Center in the Bronx. Two of the schools ("comparison schools") do not provide comprehensive services, but provide some acute care via the services of a traditional school nurse. The comparison schools were selected based on the cooperation of the school principals and the demographic and socioeconomic similarities to students attending schools with SBHCs. For example, 86% and 90% of students at the 2 comparison schools were eligible for the free lunch program compared with 82%, 84%, 97%, and 99% at the 4 schools with SBHCs.[12]

During the 1999–2000 school year, bilingual Spanish and English surveys were sent home with the children. At least 3 attempts were made to obtain responses from parents by distributing the surveys to children during different weeks. Small prizes (pencils or stickers) were given on return of completed surveys. Survey information included the following: demographic information (with race or ethnicity noted as optional), asking if the child has asthma, and asking about the presence of specific asthmatic symptoms in the last year. In addition, we collected information on ED visits, hospitalizations, and medication use during the last year. Additional details of the survey are described elsewhere.[13]

DEFINITION

The present analysis is based on information from children we identified as having "probable asthma" from the parent survey. Criteria for probable asthma were checking off "yes" to the question inquiring if the child has ever had asthma and reporting that 1 or more of the following was true during the past 12 months: (1) that he or she had taken asthma medication; (2) that he or she had experienced sleep disturbance due to wheezing, coughing, or tightness in the chest; (3) that he or she coughed after or during exercise when he or she did not have a cold; (4) that he or she had weather-related breathing problems; or (5) that he or she wheezed in the presence of pets, mold, strong odors, or cigarette smoke.

INDEPENDENT VARIABLES

Parents classified the race or ethnicity of the schoolchildren as Puerto Rican, other Latino, African American, White, Asian, Arabic, mixed, or "other" ethnic group. Respondents could check off as many categories as they chose, and children with 2 or more selections were considered mixed. Analyses combined children of White, Asian, Arabic, other, and mixed race or ethnicity into a single group labeled "other" because of the small number of study participants. Analyses by race or ethnicity excluded 69 children whose parents did not specify one. We used the proportion of children eligible for the free lunch program in each school (range, 82%–99%) as our proxy measure of socioeconomic status (SES). Individual data on SES or free lunch eligibility were unavailable.

All schools, with the exception of 1 comparison school, provided absenteeism data. Analyses of absenteeism records excluded children who had attended this comparison school, as well as children who attended any of the participating schools for fewer than 90 days of the

180-day school year. As per school policy, no information on school attendance was available for children who were discharged or transferred or left school for any reason before the end of the school year. In addition, once children were graduated, their attendance records were removed from the system.

The study was approved by the institutional review board of Montefiore Medical Center for schools with an on-site Montefiore-affiliated SBHC and by the Office for Protection from Research Risks, now known as the Office for Human Research Protections, for schools with no on-site services.

DATA ANALYSIS

Univariate analyses were performed using rate ratios (RRs) with 95% confidence intervals (CIs) to assess the association between ED use, hospitalization, and other categorical variables. We used the t test to assess differences in the mean number of school days missed by children attending schools with SBHCs, compared with a comparison school. $P < .05$ was considered statistically significant. Multivariate analyses were conducted using Poisson regression (SAS statistical software, Version 8.1; SAS Institute Inc, Cary, NC) to examine the effect of SBHCs on hospitalization. We created 2 dummy variables, one for SES by grouping schools by the proportion of children eligible for the free lunch program, either 80% to 90% (high SES) or > 90% (low SES). The other represented the presence or absence of an SBHC. We started with a full model including sex, age (in years), and race or ethnicity as potential confounders. Variables with $P > .10$ or those having less than a 10% effect on parameter estimates of variables already in the model were removed from the model. Interaction between the covariates was tested using the same criteria.

RESULTS

Of the 6433 families surveyed, 74.2% (4,775/6,433) returned completed questionnaires. The response rate for schools with and without SBHCs was 72.6% (3,419/4,709) and 78.7% (1,356/1,724), respectively. We identified 949 children (19.9%) as having probable asthma as previously defined. The prevalence of asthma was 18.9% at schools with an SBHC and 22.4% at schools without an SBHC. Characteristics of children with asthma by school type are given in Table 16.1.

Table 16.1   **Characteristics of 949 Asthmatic Children at Schools with and Without School-Based Health Centers (SBHCs).***

Variable	4 Schools with an SBHC ($n = 645$)	2 Schools without an SBHC ($n = 304$)
Sex		
Male	343 (53.2)	166 (54.6)
Female	302 (46.8)	137 (45.1)
Not specified	. . .	1 (<1)
Age group, *y*		
<5	16 (2.5)	6 (2.0)
5–9	515 (79.8)	240 (78.9)
≥10	112 (17.4)	52 (17.1)
Not specified	2 (0.1)	6 (0.1)
Race or ethnicity		
Puerto Rican	266 (41.2)	132 (43.4)
Other Latino	117 (18.1)	48 (15.8)
African American	109 (16.9)	60 (19.7)
Other†	101 (15.7)	47 (15.5)
Not specified	52 (8.1)	17 (5.6)
ED visits in the last year		
≥1	303 (47.0)	135 (44.4)
Hospitalizations in the last year		
≥1	68 (10.5)	52 (17.1)
Health insurance coverage		
Yes	565 (87.6)	265 (87.2)
No	60 (9.3)	26 (8.6)
Not specified	20 (3.1)	13 (4.3)

Abbreviation: ED, emergency department.

*Data are given as the number (percentage) of schoolchildren. Ellipses indicate not applicable.

†Other includes children of white, Asian, Arabic, mixed, and other specified races or ethnicities.

Asthma Symptoms and Medication Use

Table 16.2 lists the percentages of children whose parents answered the questions and reported the symptoms targeted by the survey. Only 34 children (3.6%) had no symptoms within the past year. When we asked parents about the frequency of symptoms, specifically how often their child wheezed, coughed excessively, or felt tightness in his or her chest in the past year, 15.8% (134/847) reported that their child wheezed at

Table 16.2   Percentage of Children Reporting Asthmatic Symptoms by Attendance at Schools With and Without School-Based Health Centers (SBHCs).

Variable	4 Schools with an SBHC ($n = 645$)	2 Schools without an SBHC ($n = 304$)
In the last 12 months, has your child's sleep been disturbed due to wheezing, coughing, or tightness in the chest?	80.2	76.8
In the last 12 months, has your child coughed during or after exercise when she or he did not have a cold?	67.5	66.2
In the last 12 months, did a change in the weather cause your child to have difficulty breathing?	73.1	81.1
In the last 12 months, did your child wheeze, cough, or feel tight in the chest after being near cigarette smoke, pets, mold, or strong odors?	63.5	66.4

least once per week, and only 10.7% (91/847) reported no wheezing at all. Most of the frequent wheezers (64.1% [84/131]) were taking daily medications, compared with 27.7% (191/689) of the less frequent and nonwheezer groups (RR, 3.5; 95% CI, 2.6–4.9). There were no statistically significant differences in symptom frequency by sex, race or ethnicity, or health insurance coverage. Children attending comparison schools were less likely to report wheezing symptoms (i.e., to answer that they experience no symptoms at all) than children attending schools with an SBHC (14.0% [38/271] vs 9.2% [53/576], respectively; RR, 1.5; 95% CI, 1.0–2.3). No statistically significant associations were noted between daily medication use and sex, health insurance coverage, or availability of a SBHC, but African American children were more likely than others to take daily asthma medications (43.4% [72/166] vs 30.7% [209/680], respectively; RR, 1.4; 95% CI, 1.1–1.7).

Activity Limitation

Parents were asked how much asthma limits their child's activities and were given response options of "not at all," "a little," "moderately," and "a lot." Eight hundred sixty-five (91.1%) of the 949 respondents answered this question. Two hundred thirty-four (27.1%) of the 865 respondents reported at least a moderate amount of limitation, while 293 (33.9%) of the same respondents reported that their child did not experience any limitation in activity. No statistically significant differences were noted in activity limitation by sex, race or ethnicity, health insurance coverage, or availability of an SBHC.

Hospitalization

One hundred twenty (12.6%) of the 949 children had been hospitalized for asthma at least once in the past year. In bivariate analyses, children attending the comparison schools were more likely than those in schools with SBHCs to have been hospitalized for asthma (17.1% [52/304] vs 10.5% [68/645], respectively; RR, 1.6; 95% CI, 1.2–2.3). No statistically significant associations were noted between hospitalization and sex, race or ethnicity, and health insurance coverage.

Emergency Department

Four hundred thirty-eight (46.2%) of the 949 parents responded that their child had been treated in the ED at least once for asthma in the past year. No statistically significant differences were noted in ED use by sex, race or ethnicity, health insurance coverage, or availability of an SBHC.

Absenteeism

Absenteeism data were available for 602 (63.4%) of the 949 asthmatic children and 2,305 (60.2%) of the 3,826 nonasthmatic children. Of the 602 asthmatic children with available absenteeism data, 25.1% (151/602) attended a comparison school and 74.9% (451/602) attended schools with an SBHC. Overall, students in the comparison school missed more days of school than those with an SBHC (mean [SD] 16.4 [12.9] days vs 14.5 [11.2] days, respectively; $P < .001$). This difference appears partly because of the asthmatic children. Among asthmatic children, those attending the comparison school missed, on average, 3 more school days than those attending schools with an SBHC (i.e., mean [SD] days absent, 21.3 [15.4] vs 18.2 [13.0], respectively; $P = .02$).

Multivariate Analyses

The final Poisson regression model identified attendance at schools without an SBHC as the only statistically significant factor associated with hospitalization for asthma in the last year (RR, 1.5; 95% CI,

1.1–1.9). Sex, race or ethnicity, age (in years), and our SES indicator (proportion of children receiving a free lunch) failed to remain in the final model.

COMMENT

This study reports a strikingly lower asthma-related hospitalization rate in children who attend schools with SBHCs compared with those attending comparison schools. In addition to reduced hospitalization rates, we also document a gain of 3 days of school for asthmatic children attending schools with an SBHC compared with asthmatic children attending a comparison school. These findings, from different data sources, reinforce and support each other: it is logical that fewer hospitalizations among asthmatic children would result in fewer missed days of school. Since hospitalizations account for a high proportion of the direct costs of asthma,[14,15] and school absenteeism a high proportion of the indirect costs, our data suggest that SBHCs may reduce asthma-associated costs while increasing access to health care. Further, while schools have an obvious interest in reducing barriers to learning, high absenteeism presents them with a double burden: it is harder for students to keep up with the pace of learning if they miss a lot of school, and New York City and other urban districts provide incentives to schools based, in part, on good student attendance.

While we documented 2 outcomes in which SBHCs make important contributions to the health and well-being of inner-city schoolchildren, significant challenges remain. For example, we did not find an influence of SBHCs on ED use. Our findings are consistent with a study from an SBHC serving elementary schoolchildren in Minneapolis, Minn, which also documented reduced hospitalization but unchanged rates of ED use after a brief asthma intervention.[16] The lack of effect on ED use in both of these studies underscores the importance of improving asthma management skills in parents of young children. Working with families of children with asthma to improve knowledge, compliance with preventive medications, and early detection and response to symptoms promises benefit in both health and cost outcomes.

Recognition of our findings that access to school-based services contributes toward improved outcomes in asthmatic children is dependent on evidence that children attending comparison schools are otherwise comparable. We acknowledge that different schools and children are never strictly comparable and note that SBHCs and comparison schools differed somewhat in survey response rates and in the prevalence of asthma. However, we offer the following as support. First, Bronx parents do not select an elementary school for their child to attend. Rather, children are assigned to schools based on their home address. Second, the racial or ethnic composition of schools with an SBHC and comparison schools is similar, and, using eligibility for the free lunch program as a marker of SES, our 2 comparison schools ranked exactly midrange (ranks 3 and 4) of the 6 schools studied. Third, the higher frequency of symptoms we reported among children attending schools with SBHCs would argue against the theory that children attending schools with SBHCs have less severe disease. Fourth, in contrast with others,[17] we found that health insurance coverage was similar and high among asthmatic children in all schools. Fifth, one motivation we had for constructing a regression model of factors related to hospitalization was to assess whether the observed bivariate association between schools with SBHCs and reduced hospitalization could be explained by SES or other potential confounders. We found that the variable for SES was not statistically significant, while the protective relation between schools with SBHCs and hospitalization for asthma was undiminished. Thus, we suggest that our findings are not explainable by better family or financial resources in schools with SBHCs but were likely due, at least in part, to improved access to asthma care.

On an additional methodological note, we compared outcomes in *all* asthmatic children in schools with and without SBHCs to assess the effect of school-based services.[18] We chose this comparison as opposed to comparing outcomes in SBHC users to outcomes in children attending comparison schools because we expect that students with moderate to severe asthma might be more likely to use SBHCs than children with milder disease. Therefore, children using the SBHCs might overrepresent children with more serious asthma relative to the population of all children with asthma. To avoid this potential bias, we compared outcomes in all asthmatic children with and without SBHCs to estimate the effect of on-site health services. Utilization analyses attest to frequent SBHC use for asthma. During the period under study, 13.5% (2,816/20,902) of all visits at the 4 schools with SBHCs were for asthma care, with a mean annual frequency of 4.9 visits per child. In addition, half of the asthmatic children (320/645) identified by the parent survey in this study used the SBHCs for asthma care during this 1-year period.

As a final note, the analyses presented were carried out on baseline data collected before our intervention to better engage students and their families. The asthma services provided were predominantly focused on treatment of acute exacerbations with rescue medications and short-course steroid treatment. Daily nebulizer treatments were given if prescribed by a community medical provider. It remains to be demonstrated whether the outreach and intervention strategy we are using can further affect the health and well-being of these families. In either case, our findings support the efficacy of SBHCs for inner-city schoolchildren with asthma and have implications for access to and funding of school-based primary care.[18]

Notes

1. Health in Schools. Moving forward: Making the Grade becomes the Center for Health and Health Care in Schools. Available at: http://www.healthin-schools.org/pubs/access/Winter2001.asp. Accessed January 17, 2002.

2. Morone JA, Kilbreth EH, Langwell KM. Back to school: a health care strategy for youth. *Health Aff.* 2001;20:122–136.

3. Kaplan DW, Brindis CD, Phibbs SL, Melinkovich P, Naylor K, Ahlstrand K. A comparison study of an elementary school-based health center: effects on health care access and use. *Arch Pediatr Adolesc Med.* 1999;153:235–243.

4. Lancman H, Pastore DR, Steed N, Maresca A. Adolescent hepatitis B vaccination: comparison among 2 high school-based health centers and an adolescent clinic. *Arch Pediatr Adolesc Med.* 2000;154:1085–1088.

5. Hall S, Galil K, Watson B, Seward J. The use of school-based vaccination clinics to control varicella outbreaks in two schools. *Pediatrics* [serial online]. 2000;105:e17. Available at: http://www.pediatrics.org. Accessed February 4, 2002.

6. Anglin TM, Naylor KE, Kaplan DW. Comprehensive school-based health care: high school students' use of medical, mental health, and substance abuse services. *Pediatrics.* 1996;97:318–330.

7. Fothergill K, Ballard E. The school-linked health center: a promising model of community-based care for adolescents. *J Adolesc Health.* 1998;23:29–38.

8. Wang LY, Crossett LS, Lowry R, Sussman S, Dent CW. Cost-effectiveness of a school-based tobacco-use prevention program. *Arch Pediatr Adolesc Med.* 2001;155:1043–1050.

9. Lenney W. The burden of pediatric asthma [review]. *Pediatr Pulmonol Suppl.* 1997;15:13–16.

10. Brito A, Wurm G, Delamater AM, et al. School-based identification of asthma in a low-income population. *Pediatr Pulmonol.* 2000;30:297–301.

11. Newacheck PW, Halfon N. Prevalence, impact, and trends in childhood disability due to asthma. *Arch Pediatr Adolesc Med.* 2000;154:287–293.

12. New York City Department of Education [home page]. Available at: http://www.nycenet.edu.

13. Webber MP, Carpiniello KE, Oruwariye T, Appel DK. Prevalence of asthma and asthma-like symptoms in inner-city elementary schoolchildren. *Pediatr Pulmonol.* 2002;34:105–111.

14. Weiss KB, Sullivan SD. The health economics of asthma and rhinitis, I: assessing the economic impact [review]. *J Allergy Clin Immunol.* 2001;107:3–8.

15. Smith DH, Malone DC, Lawson KA, Okamoto LJ, Battista C, Saunders WB. A national estimate of the economic costs of asthma. *Am J Respir Crit Care Med.* 1997;156:787–793.

16. Lurie N, Bauer EJ, Brady C. Asthma outcomes at an inner-city school-based health center. *J Sch Health.* 2001;71(1):9–16.

17. Stroupe KT, Gaskins D, Murray MD. Health-care costs of inner-city patients with asthma. *J Asthma.* 1999;36:645–655.

18. Santelli JS, Kouzis A, Newcomer S. School-based health centers and adolescent use of primary care and hospital care. *J Adolesc Health.* 1996;19:267–275.

Reprint from *To Improve Health and Health Care 2000: The Robert Wood Johnson Foundation Anthology*

CHAPTER 17

School-Based Health Clinics

Paul Brodeur, 1999

At an elementary school in Connecticut, an eight-year-old third-grader who has seen his father beat his mother and has a history of violent behavior tells a lie in class and is given detention. Soon afterward, he tries to hang himself when his parents, who are getting a divorce, seek to punish him for the infraction by refusing to let him play on a Little League baseball team. After being treated as an outpatient at a local hospital, he returns to school and starts seeing a social worker at the school health center. The social worker tries to help him recognize the kind of emotionally charged incidents—such as when he sees his brother hit his sister—that trigger violence and depression in him. The idea is that by so learning he will be able to cope with stressful situations and take charge of his life as he grows older.

In California, a suicidal fifteen-year-old tenth-grader tells a therapist at her school health center something she has never revealed to anyone:

---

at the age of three she was raped by an uncle and two cousins who were living in her parents' home. At first she is deeply reluctant to disclose the names of her abusers, out of fear that she will get them in trouble and thus incur the wrath of her mother and father, both of whom have beaten her over the years. After talking with the therapist, however, she is persuaded, to her great relief, to identify her attackers. She then decides to join one of the health center's sexual-abuse therapy groups, where, in the company of girls who have experienced similar trauma, she comes to understand that what was done to her was wrong and not in any way her fault. As a result, she gains self-respect and self-esteem.

Intervention in psychological problems of such magnitude may come as a something of a shock to those who remember health care in school as amounting to little more than the school nurse excusing feverish kids from gym and advising them to see their family doctor. The fact is, however, that school-based health centers equipped to diagnose and deal with mental health problems, as well as with drug abuse, teenage pregnancy, sexually transmitted diseases, and myriad ordinary physical afflictions are springing up across the nation. During the past twelve years, more than eleven hundred health centers have been established in high schools and elementary schools in forty-five states and the District of Columbia. Approximately one in ten of them either have been supported or are being supported with the aid of grants from the Robert Wood Johnson Foundation, which has been a pioneering force behind the idea that health care can be delivered to children and adolescents most effectively where they most easily can be found—in the nation's schools.

ROOTS OF SCHOOL-BASED HEALTH CLINICS

National awareness that school-age children in America were a medically underserved population came into focus during the mid-1960s when President Lyndon B. Johnson's War on Poverty identified serious health problems in youngsters coming from poor families. The advent of Medicaid in 1965 highlighted the need for better health care for low-income children. In 1967, physician and pediatrician Philip J. Porter, head of pediatrics at Cambridge City Hospital in Massachusetts and director of Maternal and Child Health for the city's health department, assigned a nurse practitioner to work in an elementary school and deliver primary medical care to the children enrolled there. Four additional health clinics were opened in Cambridge schools in the years that followed.

During the early 1970s, school-based health centers staffed by nurse practitioners, part-time physicians, and mental health professionals were established in Dallas and St. Paul. In 1972, the newly founded Robert Wood Johnson Foundation entered the field by funding several school health programs and by setting up a health center for children from impoverished families in Posen and Robbins—neighboring steel-mill towns near Chicago. Two years later, the Foundation supported a National School Health Conference in Galveston, Texas, which was attended by pediatricians and health professionals who were seeking to improve the quality and scope of medical care for school children.

In 1978, the Robert Wood Johnson Foundation underwrote an ambitious five-year School Health Services Program, which brought nurse practitioners into elementary schools attended by 150,000 children in Colorado, New York, North Dakota, and Utah. The program, which was directed by Catherine DeAngelis, a physician and pediatrician with the Department of Pediatrics at The Johns Hopkins University School of Medicine in Baltimore, demonstrated that nurse practitioners backed by community-based primary care physicians could deliver adequate health care to children in elementary schools. The project was not considered a success, however, because officials of most of the school districts in which the health centers operated concluded that the cost of maintaining them without Foundation funding would pose too great a financial burden.

As a result, officials of the Robert Wood Johnson Foundation came to the conclusion that if health centers serving the needs of the poor were to succeed, responsibility for their organization and financing would have to be shared by institutions within the community at large, such as community hospitals and health centers, state and city health departments, schools of public health, corporate foundations, and school districts. So, in 1981, the Foundation launched its Community Care Funding Partners Program—an initiative designed to encourage local corporations, foundations, and other organizations to support community health centers that would serve the medically indigent.

Under the Community Care Funding Partners Program, the Robert Wood Johnson Foundation committed half a million dollars over an eight-year period to each of eight cities in which broad-based community support for health centers existed and in which local partners and, in some cases, national foundations could be brought together to sponsor the centers and help share in the cost of staffing and maintaining them. Between 1981 and 1989, under the auspices of the program, community health centers for families and children were established in Chicago, Dallas, Houston, Kansas City, New York, and Philadelphia, as well as in Flint, Michigan, and Wilmington, Delaware.

A striking aspect of the Community Care Funding Partners Program was the decision of officials in five of the eight cities to situate the community health centers in secondary schools. This decision reflected a growing concern across the nation about the deteriorating health status of American teenagers; according to a report issued by the Surgeon General in 1979, people between fifteen and twenty-four years old were the only age group in the nation whose mortality rate rose between 1960 and 1979.[1(pp43–82)]

By the mid-1980s, it was estimated that six million adolescents in the United States had at least one serious health problem.[2(p1)] Five million adolescents had no health insurance, more than one in ten had no regular source of health care, and approximately one in three had not been seen by a physician during the previous year.[3] Increased drug and alcohol abuse on the part of teenagers was causing a steep rise in deaths and injuries from motor vehicle accidents. Increased sexual activity was creating a plethora of unplanned pregnancies among teenage girls. Statistics compiled by the Children's Defense Fund showed that the number of babies born to single adolescent mothers between 1950 and 1988 rose from just under sixty thousand to well over three hundred thousand.[4] In addition, high-risk sexual behavior was resulting in a dramatic increase in the rate of sexually transmitted diseases among teenagers.

Other problems were less obvious but highly disturbing. Relatively few of an estimated five million emotionally disturbed youngsters in the nation were receiving treatment. Nearly 20 percent of boys twelve to seventeen years old were reported as having emotional or behavioral problems. One in three adolescents had considered suicide. One in seven had attempted it.[2(p1)]

THE SCHOOL-BASED ADOLESCENT HEALTH CARE PROGRAM

In 1986, spurred by the distressing state of teenage health and having had experience with secondary school health centers through the Community Care Funding Partners Program, the Robert Wood Johnson Foundation launched its School-Based Adolescent Health Care Program—a large-scale demonstration project that was designed to determine whether health centers in secondary schools could deliver comprehensive medical and mental health care to teenage students across the nation, and whether communities and local institutions could be persuaded to provide long-term support for school-based health centers. The program was directed by Philip Porter, who had become a senior program consultant to the Foundation. The codirector was Julia Graham Lear, also a senior program consultant as well as an assistant professor of child health and development at George Washington University's School of Medicine and Health Sciences in Washington, D.C.

In 1987, the Foundation awarded 19 six-year grants of up to $600,000 to public and private institutions to set up adolescent health centers. As a result, health centers were established in twenty-four high schools in fourteen cities across the nation, including Baton Rouge, Denver, Detroit, Greensboro, North Carolina, Jersey City, Los Angeles, Memphis, Miami, Minneapolis, New Orleans, New York, St. Paul, San Jose, and San Fernando.

Thanks to experience gained from previous programs, the Foundation had developed strict criteria governing how the new adolescent centers were to be set up, how they should function, and how they were to be financed. Thus they were alike in many respects. Each center was

- Operated by a local hospital, city health department, or other qualified health provider, either directly or under contract..

- Staffed by one or more part-time physicians, a nurse practitioner, a full-time or part-time social worker, and a medical office assistant.

- Planned in consultation with broad-based community groups, whose membership might include parents, school administrators, school board members, faculty, churches, youth and family-service agencies, local health and welfare departments, and representatives of local business and industrial firms.

- Required to cooperate with the existing school nurses, teachers, coaches, counselors, and school principals and their staffs.

- Set up to function in coordination with a community advisory committee whose members were required to generate funds to help support the center during the initial six-year period of its development, and, more important, to maintain it after the Robert Wood Johnson Foundation's grant had expired.

• Financed from the outset by a coalition of public and private
institutions—city and state health and welfare agencies, for
example, as well as local corporations and foundations—that
joined the Robert Wood Johnson Foundation in underwriting
the project for the first six years, and then worked with the community advisory committee to build a long-term funding base.

To further ensure the economic stability of the health centers, the
Foundation required their administrators to submit financial management plans that included projected operating costs for the six-year
start-up period and evidence that patient revenues and funds from
public and private institutions would be available to make up expenses
not covered by the Foundation grant. The administrators were also
required to present plans for financing the centers after the Foundation grants ended.

To be eligible for a Robert Wood Johnson Foundation grant, an
adolescent health care center had to be located in a city with a population of 100,000 or more and to be housed in one or more secondary
schools with a combined enrollment of at least 1,000 students. Once
established, the centers were required to provide a comprehensive
range of services, including the following:

• Treatment for common illnesses and minor injuries

• Referral and follow-up for serious illnesses and emergencies

• On-site care and consultation, as well as referral and follow-up
for pregnancy and chronic diseases

• Counseling and referral for drug and alcohol abuse, sexual
abuse, anxiety, depression, and thoughts about suicide

• On-site care and referrals for sexually-transmitted diseases

• Counseling aimed at preventing high-risk behavior that leads to
pregnancy, sexually-transmitted diseases, and drug and alcohol
abuse

• Sports and employment physicals

• Immunizations

Parents and guardians were required to sign consent forms before
their children could receive any of the services provided by the health
centers. The consent forms listed the services available at the center,

and parents and guardians were free to indicate any services they did not want their children to receive.

When the Robert Wood Johnson Foundation determined that the school-based centers established under its School-Based Adolescent Health Program should be planned in consultation with parents and parents groups, as well as with local civic, religious, and business groups, it hoped to avoid objections that might be raised to some of the services that would be offered, such as those dealing with the prevention of pregnancy and of sexually-transmitted diseases. From the beginning, however, many school-based health centers became the targets of protests mounted by religious and political groups.

Some objected that health care should be the prerogative of parents, not schools. Others said that counseling adolescents on the use of contraceptives to prevent pregnancy and sexually-transmitted diseases would encourage sexual activity and promiscuity. Still others feared that school-based health centers were little more than camouflage for abortion clinics.

Overt political opposition to the School-Based Adolescent Health Care Program occurred in Florida in 1987, when Governor Bob Martinez, a pro-life advocate, turned down a Robert Wood Johnson Foundation grant that had been awarded to the Dade County Health Department for a health center at Miami's Northwestern High School. It soon became apparent that the governor had taken a minority position. A survey of 619 parents conducted by the Miami Herald showed that two-thirds favored a health clinic that supplies contraceptives with parental approval to students in their neighborhood high schools. Moreover, community support for the proposed health center at Northwestern High was especially strong among the parents of students enrolled there, as well as among members of the Miami-Dade County School Board, who, in spite of bomb threats, voted in favor of it.

A health center was finally established at Northwestern High in 1988, after the Robert Wood Johnson Foundation awarded its grant to Dade County's Public Health Trust—an organization that sponsored Miami's Jackson Memorial Hospital and a number of community clinics. This had the effect of moving the project from state to local control. Today, the center at Northwestern High serves 2,500 of the 3,000 students who are enrolled there, and fifteen additional school-based health centers have been established in Dade County schools.

In the 1980s, religious opposition to school-based health centers came for the most part from conservative Christian groups such as the

Moral Majority and from the Catholic Church. Some of it originated in high places. In 1986, Archbishop (now Cardinal) Roger M. Mahoney, of the Los Angeles Diocese, issued a pastoral letter criticizing the decision of the Los Angeles Unified School District to establish health centers supported by Robert Wood Johnson Foundation grants at three high schools in the Los Angeles area. The Archbishop was particularly concerned about moral issues posed by the distribution of contraceptives to teenagers, and by referrals for abortion for pregnant teenage girls. In his letter, he declared that the Catholic Church viewed abortion as an unacceptable solution to pregnancy and warned that "by making contraceptives readily available, the clinics' personnel will tacitly promote sexual relations outside of marriage." He went on to say that the clinics would "destroy the partnership between parents and school upon which responsible education is founded."[5]

In spite of such opposition, adolescent health centers were established in 1987 with the help of Robert Wood Johnson Foundation grants at the three high schools selected by the Los Angeles Unified School District. The three high schools had a combined enrollment of some seven thousand students. Within two years, 85 percent of the parents of students attending two of the schools and nearly 60 percent of the parents of students at the third had signed consent forms allowing their children to use the centers. Today, adolescent health centers are flourishing in more than two dozen high schools and elementary schools in the greater Los Angeles area.

By 1990, consent forms had been signed by more than 70 percent of the parents of some thirty-four thousand students who were enrolled in twenty-four schools across the nation in which health centers had been established with grants from the Robert Wood Johnson Foundation. Largely as a result of parental support, none of them were forced to close because of controversy. Support for school health centers had by then been voiced by the U.S. Public Health Service, the American Medical Association, the American Academy of Pediatrics, and the American School Health Association, as well as by the American Nurses Association and a number of other organizations that represented nurses and nurse practitioners. Further evidence that opposition to the centers was waning came in 1991, when President Bush's Advisory Commission on Social Security recommended that federally funded health centers be established in the nation's elementary schools. By the end of the following year, the number of school-based health centers in the United States had risen from fewer than fifty in 1986 to almost three hundred.

EVALUATION OF THE PROGRAM

In 1992, outside consultants to the Robert Wood Johnson Foundation evaluated the twenty-four school-based health centers supported by grants from the Foundation.[6] To no one's surprise, the evaluation determined that the centers had increased the access of adolescents to health care. Indeed, more than half of the students who were enrolled in schools with health centers were receiving health care from them. Approximately one in four of their visits was to obtain treatment for acute illness and injury and about one in six to obtain mental health care.

According to the evaluation, most teenagers who sought psychosocial counseling were suffering from depression caused by basic adolescent concerns about relationships with peers and family members. However, a significant amount of depression was found to be caused by serious emotional problems, such as those produced by family violence, excessive drinking by family members, drug use, and physical and sexual child abuse.

The evaluators found that requests for mental health care had risen sharply during the five years that the school-based health centers had been in operation. At first, students had been reluctant to avail themselves of the psychosocial services that were being offered, but as they came to realize that their problems would be held in strict confidence by health center staff members, they began to use the counseling services in greater numbers. Because of financial considerations, clinically trained social workers provided the bulk of this counseling. Only two of the twenty-four adolescent centers were found to have a staff psychologist; none had a psychiatrist. According to the evaluation report, the heavy reliance on social workers meant that some students with severe mental and emotional problems might not be receiving adequate treatment.

The report, issued in 1993, found that school-based health centers had had little effect on high-risk behavior, such as drug use and unprotected sexual activity, or on teenage pregnancy rates. Indeed, the report estimated that one in four female students at the schools under study would become pregnant by their senior year, and that about half of the pregnant girls would bear children. As a result, the authors of the report suggested that earlier and more intensive intervention to reduce unprotected sexual activity among adolescents might be appropriate.

The authors also noted that dental facilities were lacking at most of the centers. In addition, they found that many centers either had not tried or had not been able to recover significant portions of their operating expenditures from third-party insurers such as Medicaid. In fact, Medicaid was found to be contributing less than 5 percent of the operating costs of the school-based health centers. For this reason, the evaluators warned that long-range financing for the centers could become a critical issue, especially in light of health care reforms that were being proposed and adopted across the nation.

The evaluation found that the School-Based Adolescent Health Program, despite its shortcomings, demonstrated that health care focusing on both physical and emotional needs could be provided in school-based settings to thousands of adolescents, especially those living in low-income communities who had previously gone without adequate medical and mental health attention. Nowhere was this stated more dramatically than in the frontispiece of the evaluation report, which quoted testimony given to the U.S. Senate Committee on Labor and Human Resources in July of 1992 by Laura Secord, a nurse practitioner who had gone to work at a health center established with Robert Wood Johnson Foundation funding at Ensley High School in Birmingham, Alabama. Secord described her first patient and her first weeks at Ensley High:

> She was a 17-year-old with a severe kidney infection. She was also six months pregnant and had been starving herself to keep her pregnancy a secret. She was severely depressed. Her pregnancy was a result of sexual abuse by an older family friend. By the end of the first month, I had treated kids with a wide range of problems, including strep throat, fractured femur, diabetes, high blood pressure, severe depression, dental disease, anemia, epilepsy, and gonorrhea.

THE MAKING THE GRADE PROGRAM

Through the early 1990s, school-based health centers had been supported largely by private foundations, local health departments, and Maternal and Child Health block grants provided by the U.S. Department of Health and Human Services. Only a few states—Arkansas, Connecticut, Delaware, Maryland, Michigan, New York, and Oregon—had initiated state funding for school health centers. By 1992, it was apparent that if health centers were to become established in the nation's schools, their long-term financial stability must be secured through state and community involvement. As a result, in July of that year, the trustees of the Robert Wood Johnson Foundation authorized $25.2 million for a new program called Making the Grade: State and Local Partnerships to Establish School-Based Health Centers.

The goal of Making the Grade was to increase the availability of comprehensive health care for school-age children by reorganizing state and local funding policies. Under the program, the state partners were asked to reduce funding barriers for school-based health centers—for example, by making it easier for the centers to receive reimbursement from state-controlled Medicaid funds. Community partners were asked to mount a collaborative effort in which school districts, parents' groups, community groups, and a health provider—a local hospital, perhaps, or a municipal health department—would commit themselves to establishing health centers at two or more high schools, middle schools, or elementary schools in at least two communities.

This program was launched in the spring of 1993, and it has been directed since then by Julia Graham Lear, who works out of a National Program Office located within the George Washington University Medical Center's School of Public Health and Health Services. (Lear is now an associate research professor in the school's Department of Health Services Management and Policy.) During the first phase of the program, which was completed in early 1994, the Foundation awarded $100,000 grants to twelve states to develop new policies for financing school health centers and for planning the establishment of at least two new school health centers in each of two communities. In the second phase, in 1995 and 1996, the Foundation awarded implementation grants of up to $2.3 million each to nine of these states to develop policies that would guarantee long-term financing for the centers and to help support them during their first four years of operation. The states were Colorado, Connecticut, Louisiana, Maryland, New York, North Carolina, Oregon, Rhode Island, and Vermont.

In 1993, most of the states participating in the program were planning to pay for new school-based health centers by augmenting state grant commitments with money from President Clinton's ill-fated Health Security Act, which included $300 million for health care in schools. However, the collapse of federal health care reform the following year, together with mounting opposition to government-sponsored programs in general, persuaded many states to abandon this strategy and to search for alternative funding. As a result, with the exception of Louisiana, the states with Making the Grade grants shelved plans to increase their grants to school health centers and shifted their attention to contractual arrangements that would integrate the centers into Medicaid managed care.

A major flaw in this strategy, however, was that Medicaid did not reimburse many of the mental health, health education, and preventive services that were being provided by school-based health centers. For example, group therapy and consultation with teachers and parents regarding health matters were not covered by Medicaid. As a result, officials of Medicaid managed-care plans were reluctant to negotiate contracts with school health centers. Although some centers began to contract with Medicaid managed care plans, Medicaid revenues in many cases covered only a small fraction of the school-based health center's operating costs.

This problem notwithstanding, most states have tried to encourage and facilitate negotiations between school-based health centers and Medicaid managed care plans. As might be expected, state strategies for allowing the health centers to tap into Medicaid managed care dollars have varied widely. Some states confer preferential status on school-based centers by a so-called "carve-out" process that provides special treatment for children and adolescents or for certain services, such as those dealing with family planning, substance abuse, and mental health. Other states—among them Connecticut, Delaware, Maryland, Massachusetts, Michigan, and New York—require managed care plans serving Medicaid beneficiaries to enter into contracts with school-based health centers. Still others, such as Colorado, have tried to encourage school-based health centers and Medicaid managed care plans to enter into voluntary partnerships.

What has resulted is a hodgepodge of different relationships and a maze of varying contractual arrangements. For example, in Connecticut—a state that is considered to have one of the best school health programs in the nation—the sponsors of fourteen school-based health center programs and officials of eleven Medicaid managed care health plans have had to negotiate 125 separate contracts. A major reason for this is that all of the state's managed care plans contract separately for dental services, and most of them subcontract for mental health services. In New York City, where 150,000 children rely on ninety-nine school-based health centers for primary health care and no fewer than twenty-five Medicaid managed care plans are in operation, the task has been even more daunting. Small wonder that no one knows just how many of the nation's 1,200 or so school-based health centers have made agreements with Medicaid managed care plans! What is known is that some school-based health centers that were billing Medicaid under fee-for-service arrangements have reported a decline in revenue since the Medicaid managed care plans were introduced.

One way the financial plight of school health centers could change for the better is if states decide to finance them with part of the money they will receive under the 1998 agreement that settled their litigation against the tobacco industry. Another funding source could be the State Children's Health Insurance Program, which was passed by Congress in 1997. Under this program, Congress has authorized $48 billion over ten years for states to buy health insurance for an estimated three million uninsured children who come from low-income families. As many of these uninsured children are enrolled in school-based health centers, it is hoped that the Children's Health Insurance Program will reimburse the centers for the services they are providing. Depending upon decisions yet to be made, school-based health centers may also be eligible to receive some of the $4 billion that Congress has set aside under the program for what are described as "related purposes," which could include safety-net providers such as school-based health centers.

Unfortunately, many congressional and state legislators appear to be laboring under the assumption that an adequate provider system already exists for the delivery of medical attention to uninsured and underprivileged children. This assumption is, of course, questionable for many communities. Indeed, the fact that an adequate provider network does not exist for millions of poor children is precisely the problem that the Robert Wood Johnson Foundation has been trying to remedy for more than twenty years.

The School-Based Health Center in Bridgeport, Connecticut

Today, the Robert Wood Johnson Foundation is contributing to the support and development of forty-four school-based health centers serving poor children in low-income areas across the nation. One is at the Read Elementary and Middle School in Bridgeport, Connecticut. Once a thriving steel-fabricating and textile center, Bridgeport has fallen on hard times in recent years and is struggling to rebound from bankruptcy. Despite the city's economic woes, the Bridgeport Health Department has been a strong supporter of health care programs in the city's schools since the mid-1980s. The department currently operates nine of the city's ten school-based health centers, including the one at Read, which it opened in November of 1996 using funds awarded to the state of Connecticut under the Making the Grade Program.

About half of the kindergarten-through-eighth-grade children who attend Read are African-American. More than a third are Hispanic and come from homes in which English is not the primary language.

Three out of four qualify for free or reduced-price meals because they come from low-income families. Many of them have parents who are unemployed or who receive vocational training.

Sixty-four percent of the children at Read are enrolled in the health center, which is staffed by a full-time nurse practitioner, a social worker, an outreach worker, and a medical assistant. These full-time staff members are assisted by a physician from a local pediatrics group, who visits the school once a week, and by a dentist and dental hygienist, who pay weekly visits to provide dental treatment.

As at most school-based health centers, the nurse practitioner and the back-up physician at Read provide diagnosis and on-site treatment for acute illnesses, such as sore throats, earaches, headaches, and stomach upsets. They also deliver reproductive health care, including pregnancy testing, Pap smears, diagnosis and treatment for sexually transmitted diseases, and education and referral for birth control, if necessary.

A master's level social worker at Read provides individual, group, and family counseling for psychosocial problems. She and the nurse practitioner also give classroom presentations on topics such as reproductive health, conflict resolution, and substance abuse. In addition, the social worker leads special counseling groups that deal with gender issues, life skills, asthma (about fifty children at Read suffer from this disease), anger management, and self-esteem.

Health center staff teach first-graders about stranger danger and how to distinguish good touch from bad touch; third- and fourth-graders are taught how to resolve conflicts and control their behavior; seventh-graders discuss dating, marriage, sex, drugs, and violence; and eighth-graders learn about the consequences of early sexual activity and the importance of abstinence. At the request of teachers, the social worker holds special sessions on depression and sadness. Nearly half of the diagnoses are for emotional problems, including depression, anxiety, behavioral disorders, parent-child problems, and family problems.

On a midweek afternoon in October of 1998, a visitor to the Read School Health Society—the name the children at Read have picked for the center—is invited to attend an impromptu meeting of its staff members. That morning, in addition to dealing with the usual colds and sore throats, the nurse practitioner has examined a wheezing fourteen-year-old boy who suffers from asthma but is not taking his asthma medicine. The social worker, who has seen the boy because he has been sleeping in class and often behaves in disruptive fashion, points out that he has a history of truancy, is smoking marijuana, and is using LSD. According to the outreach worker, the boy's mother works evenings and exercises little control over him. The social worker reminds her colleagues that when the boy was suspended for disorderly behavior, he showed up at school, claiming he didn't have any other place to go. The staff members agree that they should discuss with school authorities whether this boy's problems can be dealt with at Read or whether he should be transferred to a special education school with a modified curriculum that can better meet his needs.

That same morning, the social worker at the health center counseled a fourteen-year-old girl who feels that some of her teachers have been nagging her unfairly. The social worker knows that the girl's father is dead, that she has great difficulty in dealing with an alcoholic mother, and that she has run away from home on several occasions. The outreach worker, who recently visited the home, found the girl's mother to be inappropriately dressed, apparently drinking, and unreceptive to dealing with her daughter's problems. According to the nurse practitioner, the girl has acknowledged having sex with a boyfriend. In counseling sessions, the social worker has found that the girl wants desperately to talk about her feelings and problems. As a result, she referred the girl to an outside support group that works with adolescents who must deal with alcohol and substance abuse by family members. Meanwhile, she is trying to provide the girl with some of the approval and acceptance that are obviously lacking in her home, and is acting as an advocate for the girl to help resolve her problems with her teachers.

The School-Based Health Center in San Fernando, California

One of the first school-based health centers to be financed by the Robert Wood Johnson Foundation was at San Fernando High School, about twenty-five miles north of Los Angeles. More than 90 percent of the students at the school come from Latino families, including old and new immigrants from Mexico and refugees from war-torn countries in Central America such as El Salvador, Guatemala, and Nicaragua. About 40 percent of the residents of the area have incomes below the federal poverty line. During the 1980s, the region had one of the worst teenage birth, teen prenatal care, and teen homicide records in all of California.

In 1987, San Fernando High School was one of three schools in the Los Angeles Unified School District to be selected as the site for a health center funded by the Robert Wood Johnson Foundation's School-Based Adolescent Health Program. At the time, the need for a health center at San Fernando High seemed great. More than one in three of the 2,500 students who were then enrolled at the school had not seen a physician in three years. More than half had not seen a physician in two years or more, and many had never seen a physician at all. In addition, two out of three sexually active female students at the school said they never used birth control, and one in eight said they used them only rarely.

Even before it opened, Archbishop Mahoney voiced opposition to the establishment of a health center at San Fernando High in his pastoral letter of November, 1986. Protest marches, candlelight vigils, and petition drives were subsequently organized by antiabortion and anti–birth control groups, as well as by a priest from a Catholic church near the school. Much of the opposition appeared to originate outside the local community. During one protest meeting, a plane flew over the school towing a sign that read "RWJ Go Home." This prompted the principal of San Fernando High to observe that the parents of his students didn't have enough money to hire airplanes.

Criticism of the health center, which opened in November of 1987, soon dissipated, thanks to strong support from parents, students, faculty, and the Northeast Valley Health Corporation, which operates the center in cooperation with the University of California at Los Angeles Medical Center. Today, 60 percent of the 4,500 students currently enrolled at San Fernando High make regular use of the center, which handles about ten thousand patient visits during the school year. Roughly five thousand of these visits are for the treatment of illness and injury or for physical examinations, immunizations, health education, pregnancy tests, and family-planning counseling. These services are handled by a full-time nurse practitioner and two assistant nurses, with the help of a physician from the UCLA Department of Pediatrics, who visits the center twice a week. (The health center's services do not include abortion counseling and referral.)

The other five thousand visits are occasioned by mental health problems, such as depression, anxiety, grief, suicidal tendencies, and emotional trauma caused by violence, abusive families, substance abuse, sexual abuse, and child abuse. Students with such problems are treated by a ten-member staff that includes a clinical psychologist, three licensed therapists, and six UCLA graduate students who are training to be psychotherapists.

The clinical psychologist at San Fernando High is José Cárdenas, who has worked at the health center since it opened. A graduate of San Fernando High himself, he is familiar with the neighborhood and its predominantly Hispanic school population, and the students trust him. Cárdenas says that depression is the most common diagnosis he makes at San Fernando High. He points out that a large percentage of students at the school come from families that have recently emigrated from Mexico or Central America. These students are often made fun of and discriminated against by students whose families have been in the United States longer, and they need counseling to help them adjust to new surroundings, new customs, and a new language. Bilingual therapists at the center provide such counseling in a group that meets once a week. Other therapy groups have been formed to help students who feel isolated because they are African-American or gay.

Additional therapy groups at San Fernando High help students deal with sexual abuse, psychological abuse, suicide, grief, and domestic violence. Over the years, patients have ranged from a sixteen-year-old girl who was suffering from severe depression and suicidal thoughts because she had been raped by her mother's boyfriend at the age of twelve and subjected to repeated beatings by her mother and her grandmother to a boy of seventeen who, suffering from shock after learning of his cousin's murder on the evening television news, was about to join a gang to avenge his cousin's death. Therapists at the health center helped the girl to feel her anguish without thinking of suicide, and to regain her self-esteem and well-being by asserting herself when she felt in danger. Grief therapy in the form of individual and group counseling helped the boy to realize that he was not alone in his loss and sadness and to seek support by forming new friendships. The school performance of both students improved markedly following therapy, and both went on to graduate from San Fernando High.

Cárdenas believes that early intervention in such cases is crucial. He points out that if children and adolescents who have been traumatized by sexual abuse and domestic violence are not diagnosed and treated at an early age, they are going to lead troubled lives and have an adverse impact on society later on. He is a strong advocate of group therapy, because he feels that it is important for children to be able to empathize with their peers and show compassion. "Kids have to learn to talk about their problems with other kids," he says. "What better place is there for them to do that than in school?"

Notes

1. Surgeon General of the United States. *Healthy People: The Surgeon General's Report on Health Promotion and Disease Prevention.* Washington, DC: US GPO; 1979.

2. Marks EL, Marzke, CH. *Healthy Caring: A Process Evaluation of the Robert Wood Johnson Foundation's School-Based Adolescent Health Care Program.* Princeton, NJ: MathTech Inc; 1993.

3. Lear JG, Gleicher HB, St Germaine A, Porter PJ. Reorganizing health care for adolescents: the experience of the School-Based Health Care Program. *J Adolesc Health.* 1991;12:450–458.

4. Lear JG. *The Answer Is at School: Bringing Health Care to Students.* Washington, DC: School-Based Health Care Program; 1993.

5. Mahoney R. A pastoral letter. *Tidings.* November 7, 1986.

6. The consultant team consisted of experts from Mathematica Policy Research Inc. and MathTech Inc. The project director was William A. Morrill. See the final evaluation report: Kisker EL, Brown RS, Hill J. *Healthy Caring: Outcomes of the Robert Wood Johnson Foundation's School-Based Adolescent Health Care Program.* Princeton, NJ: Mathematica Policy Research Inc; 1994.

Grant Report Summaries from the Robert Wood Johnson Foundation

ASSISTING COMMUNITY-OWNED HOSPITALS TO DEVELOP AND SUSTAIN SCHOOL-BASED HEALTH CENTERS

(last updated January 2001)

This grant from the Robert Wood Johnson Foundation (RWJF) supported the Voluntary Hospitals of America (VHA) Health Foundation in providing technical assistance on the design, implementation, and sustainability of school-based health centers (SBHCs) to health care organizations across the country. The VHA Health Foundation is a national not-for-profit foundation created to encourage community health leadership and innovation across the larger health care community through practical research and demonstration projects. VHA convened a nine-member advisory group that met three times during the grant period; developed a list of 50 peer advisers available to confer with others in the health care field interested in developing SBHCs; produced a 314-page workbook, *Making the Healthy Connection: Establishing and Sustaining the Hospital-Sponsored School-Based Health Center;* and disseminated the workbook and adviser list through direct mail and at professional meetings. To date, nearly 1,200 workbooks and adviser lists have been distributed to health care organizations, professional organizations, and schools of public health, as well as to other groups. VHA Health Foundation also conducted a $1\frac{1}{2}$-day national miniconference, "Making the Healthy Connection," in Philadelphia October 29–30, 1999, which attracted 110 participants. Project staff continues to promote partnerships between health organizations and schools by disseminating the workbook and making presentations at national conferences.

MANAGEMENT INFORMATION SYSTEM FOR SCHOOL-BASED HEALTH CENTERS

(last updated March 2003)

The Project

The Children's Hospital in Denver has developed and implemented a management information system (MIS) for school-based health centers (SBHCs). The Robert Wood Johnson Foundation (RWJF) supported this work with three grants, from August 1991 to August 2000, totaling $836,598.

The Context

Having made significant investments in promoting and expanding SBHCs, RWJF determined that development of an MIS that included medical case management and third-party billing was crucial to SBHCs' long-term viability.

Results

With the first grant, the project team expanded the existing software applications and provided two technical training sessions for SBHC staff from other locations throughout the country. The second grant established the National Center for School-Based Health Systems. The center's staff continued to refine the SBHC MIS and responded to 300 to 400 calls per month for technical assistance from software users. It also provided 33 training sessions for SBHCs and technical assistance to 22 state health departments on how to integrate SBHC data with their own systems, as well as how to conduct evaluations of their SBHCs. The U.S. Public Health Service chose this software for use in its SBHC programs. Under the third grant, project staff upgraded the software to a Windows-based system.

Communications

Project staff developed a Web site (htpp://www.clinicalfusion.org) to facilitate the distribution of software updates and provide online technical assistance. They also published a number of articles in professional journals that used data collected with the software developed under these grants.

Postgrant

There are now 800 to 900 sites using the software. The project charges an annual maintenance fee of $150 to $250 to support activities without continued RWJF grant funding. In addition, staff are working on a pilot project with a national health care billing service to help SBHCs use the software to process bills and payments.

MAKING THE GRADE: STATE AND LOCAL PARTNERSHIPS TO ESTABLISH SCHOOL-BASED HEALTH CENTERS

(last updated November 2003)

Making the Grade: State and Local Partnerships to Establish School-Based Health Centers was a national program of the Robert Wood Johnson Foundation (RWJF) that supported state-local collaborations designed to expand comprehensive school-based health services for children and adolescents. First authorized by the board of trustees in 1992, the program, which operated from 1994 to 2001, helped states and their local partners establish new school-based health centers (SBHCs) and promote policies to sustain the centers over the long term.

Although SBHCs vary from place to place, their basic mission is to provide children and adolescents with comprehensive primary, acute, and preventive care for physical and mental health conditions in school settings. The centers, which have interdisciplinary staffs, not only deliver routine primary health care—physical exams, screening and treatment for physical and mental health problems—but also teach students how to manage their own health.

The Problem

Millions of school-age children in the United States are without health insurance, and multiple barriers keep many who are insured from getting the care and preventive health services they need. Projects funded by RWJF under two previous national programs, the School Health Services Program, which ran from 1977 through 1984, and the School-Based Adolescent Health Care program, which ran from 1986 to 1993, have shown that using school-based health centers to increase children's use of needed health services can be an effective public health strategy. These projects also demonstrated, however, that SBHCs need stable, ongoing funding to be viable once foundation funding ends. Building financial and political stability for SBHCs through supportive state policies was a major objective of Making the Grade.

The Program

The Making the Grade National Program Office Grade was affiliated with the George Washington University in Washington. Through a competitive process, 12 states (Colorado, Connecticut, Delaware, Hawaii, Louisiana, Maryland, New York, North Carolina, Oregon, Rhode Island, Tennessee, and Vermont) received 12- to 18-month planning grants to develop a plan for expanding the number of SBHCs in their respective states and improving the conditions for sustaining them. Each state set up a Making the Grade office within state government. State project directors, who headed these offices, worked with other government officials responsible for child health to develop financing strategies and remove barriers to SBHC stability, such as eligibility for Medicaid reimbursement. In addition, the state Making the Grade office partnered with providers and school districts in at least two communities to create at least two new SBHCs in each community. Local partners were responsible for building local political and financial support and for operating the centers.

At the start of the program, states like Connecticut and New York already had significant numbers of SBHCs. Others, such as Rhode Island and Vermont, were just beginning to develop school-based health care. After the planning period, nine states (Colorado, Connecticut, Louisiana, Maryland, New York, North Carolina, Oregon, Rhode Island, and Vermont) received 4-year implementation grants to undertake their projects. Six of these states first required a second planning grant to complete laying the groundwork for implementation.

Results

According to the National Program Office, Making the Grade achieved the following results:

> The program helped expand the total number of school-based health centers in the nine states from 278 in 1994 to 442 in 2000, an increase of 59%.

> It brought about more stable state financing, primarily from state general funds.

> It stimulated more favorable state policies, including expanding centers' eligibility to participate in Medicaid and managed care programs.

> It strengthened quality improvement practices in SBHCs and created a specialized continuous quality improvement tool.

> It established the comprehensive SBHC model as the gold standard for school-based health care.

It helped launch the National Assembly on School-Based Health Care (http://www.nasbhc.org), with state chapters in eight Making the Grade states and many others.

Evaluation of Findings

The Barents Group of KPMG Consulting in Washington conducted an evaluation of the program. Among its key findings are these:

School-based health centers have become an established, permanent, and respected part of the publicly supported health system infrastructure.

Although school-based health centers have not achieved widespread penetration through the public school systems of this country, there is continued momentum toward program growth, even in states nurturing new and fragile programs.

School-based health centers need mixed financing strategies involving federal, state, and local sources in both the private and public sectors.

Political support is of fundamental importance to the long-run sustainability of SBHCs.

Postprogram

In February 2001, the Making the Grade National Program Office became the Center for Health and Health Care in Schools under a RWJF grant program authorized by the board of trustees for up to $6 million. The first grant under this authorization supports the Center to serve as a resource for school-based health care, to provide technical and communications assistance and funding to school-based health centers and school health programs, and to develop approaches to include mental and dental health care in the services they provide. Through the grant, the Center started a multisite national program, Caring for Kids: Expanding Dental and Mental Health Services Through School-Based Health Centers, which funds eight mental health and seven dental health demonstration SBHCs. The program is described on the Center's Web site, http://www.healthinschools.org/dental.asp.

Mental Health and Teenage Pregnancy Prevention Programs

Reprints of Key Reports and Articles

CHAPTER 18

School-Based Mental Health Services

A Research Review

Michelle Rones, Kimberly Hoagwood, 2000

I t is now well documented that insofar as children receive any mental health services, schools are the major providers.[1–4] However, precisely what is provided by schools under the rubric of mental health services and whether those services are effective are largely unknown. The inattention in the scientific literature, even at a descriptive level, to identifying types, intensities, dose, or quality of preventive or treatment services in schools is surprising when one considers the quantity of rigorous educational science on topics such as learning disabilities, cognitive curriculum, and the development of psychological tests and strategies. In fact, given the disproportion of educational expenditures for children who meet criteria for having emotional disorders,[5] it is surprising that so little attention has been given to the effectiveness of school programs targeted toward prevention, reduction, or treatment of mental health problems.

Until recently, it would have been difficult to describe in any detail school-based mental health services, because basic instruments were lacking. However, since 1994, three major instruments that assess mental health services across a variety of settings, including schools, have been developed, tested, and applied in both community epidemiologic studies and clinical trials.

The availability of these instruments in concert with household-based psychiatric interviews has generated growing national awareness of the levels of unmet need for mental health services for children in this country.[2,6] These data indicate that although one-fifth of children in the United States have a diagnosable mental disorder, only a small percentage ever receive intervention or treatment services.[1,7] In addition, between 5% and 9% of children can be classified as seriously emotionally disturbed and are served in multiple, separate systems that often provide uncoordinated and redundant services.[8] Furthermore, although only 16% of children receive any mental health services, the overwhelming majority (70% to 80%) receive them within the school setting. In fact, for the majority of these children, the school system provides the only source of mental health service.[1]

The system of care is a conceptual model of community care that includes school-based services. Typically, preventive services have not been included in the concept of the system of care; however, there have been suggestions for their inclusion.[9] The system of care was developed as a strategy for improving the services and outcomes for seriously emotionally disturbed children and adolescents.[10,11] The concept of a system of care is that services should be child centered, family focused, community based, and culturally competent. Furthermore, in the system of care framework, children should have access to a wide variety of services (e.g., outpatient treatment, home-based services, day treatment, case management, crisis services, therapeutic foster care, residential treatment centers, health services, school services, social services) tailored to their individual physical, emotional, social, and educational needs.[12] The system of care serves as the foundation for effective, comprehensive mental health services within communities. Schools and the health care sector are pivotal to these systems.

Although the provision of mental health services in the schools appears necessary for the fulfillment of the schools' mandate to educate all children, and although schools are clearly providing such services,[13] it is not known whether the programs being implemented are based on scientific knowledge of their effectiveness or are simply built into the curriculum because of tradition or whim. To date, most studies that have assessed the impact of mental health services delivered in community clinics have determined that such interventions are ineffective and, in some cases, harmful.[14,15] One first step in assessing the base of knowledge about the effectiveness of school-delivered mental health programs is to review the scientific evidence about those programs.

In 1999, there were several major synthetic reviews or consensus statements that have provided a framework for establishing evidence about the effectiveness of mental health services. Reviews of the evidence based on psychosocial and medication treatments,[16,17] psychopharmacology for specific psychiatric disorders,[18] mental health services and preventive interventions,[19,20] risk and protective factors for socioemotional development of young children,[21] programs for juvenile delinquency,[22] and diagnosis and treatment for attention deficit hyperactivity disorder (ADHD)[23] have all been published since 1998. This remarkable event probably reflects an awareness by policy makers, the scientific community, and family advocates of an explosion of information and a need for informational frameworks to separate strong and important findings from background noise. This body of research reviews may be meeting a need to harness knowledge in policy-relevant areas so that program development can be built on a surer basis.

The purpose of the present paper is to do the same for school-based mental health services. Specifically, this paper seeks to provide a synthetic review of the evidence base for services delivered in schools by reviewing the published literature, applying scientific criteria to this literature, and identifying major strengths and weaknesses in the knowledge base. Given the significant role schools play in providing mental health services to children and adolescents, the fragmentation and inconsistencies in the existing literature, the growing numbers of children with unmet needs, and the overwhelming number of programs being used that have no evidence of impact, it was believed that such a review would be timely.

The time frame of 1985 to 1999 was selected because it represents a period in which the sheer quantity of school mental health services grew exponentially. School-based mental health services were defined as any program, intervention, or strategy applied in a school setting that was specifically designed to influence students' emotional, behavioral, or social functioning. Recommendations for school-based mental health services research in the future and for wider implementation of evidence-based programs are also provided.

METHOD

A computerized search of references identified from ERIC, PSYCH LIT, or MEDLINE and published between 1985 and 1999 was used to identify studies of school-based mental health services for children. Services was defined to include prevention, risk reduction, and intervention/treatment. Key words for identifying the original pool of studies included terms such as schools, children, mental health, services, prevention, outcomes, effectiveness, and specific syndromes (e.g., ADHD, depression), among others.

Of 5128 entries identified by the computer search, 337 were program evaluations. The majority of these entries were either descriptive or opinion papers. Of the 337 program evaluations, 130 used designs that contained a control group and standardized outcome measures. However, the majority of these studies used only pre- and/or postdesigns, imperfect for drawing inferences about effectiveness. The final pool of studies included only those that used one of three designs that included a control group, standardized outcome measures, and assessed outcomes at baseline and postintervention. The three designs allowed into the final pool were (1) randomized designs to achieve greatest control over threats to validity; (2) quasi-experimental designs that used matched samples to minimize selection biases; and (3) multiple baseline designs using sample cohorts as their own controls. Although randomized controlled designs minimize validation threats better than the other designs, ethical considerations may preclude a true random assignment. Therefore, quasi-experimental designs that used multiple sites and demographically matched comparison schools or multiple baseline designs were also included. Of the 130 evaluations, only 47 met these criteria and were selected into the final pool of studies for this review. This group contained 36 randomized controlled trials, 9 quasi-experimental designs, and 2 multiple baseline designs.

RESULTS

The school-based programs reviewed targeted a range of maladaptive behaviors at varying levels of development. Within each problem category, programs fell along a continuum, ranging from universal preventive interventions, designed to enhance the social and problem-solving skills of all students, to selective preventive interventions, targeted to individuals at higher risk for developing a particular emotional or behavioral problem than the general population, to indicated preventive interventions, targeted toward students who manifest signs and symptoms of behavioral and emotional difficulties but do not meet diagnostic criteria for a specific disorder.[24] Programs differed in scope (e.g., emotional and behavioral problems to depression), intensity (e.g., target child to child and his or her parents, teacher, and classmates), duration, and modality (e.g., school policy change to informational presentation). This review is organized around the type of problem for which the service was targeted. For example, child maladjustment, depression, and conduct problems are among the problems identified for specific types of school interventions. Within each category of the targeted problem, the types of programs are described. Universal prevention programs are discussed first, followed by selective and indicated prevention programs. The review includes both programs that were effective and those with mixed or negative effects (see Table 18.1). The implications of these results are described in the Discussion section.

EMOTIONAL AND BEHAVIORAL PROBLEMS

Epidemiologic studies conducted throughout the 1990s suggest that approximately 20% of children and adolescents meet diagnostic criteria for a mental disorder currently or in the past 6 months,[27,25,26] and 5–9% meet criteria for serious emotional disturbance.[8] The most common disorders are depression, anxiety, oppositional defiant disorder, conduct disorder, and ADHD.[12,27] Case complexity is increased by comorbid disorders[28–30]; deficits in educational, social, and adaptive functioning[8,31]; experience of major life losses (e.g., death, divorce, separation); and exposure to domestic, community, and media violence.[32]

Universal Prevention

A number of classroom-based, teacher-implemented programs have been developed to prevent the development of emotional, behavioral, and social problems among youth. The Promoting Alternative Thinking Strategies (PATHS) curriculum aims to increase children's ability to discuss and understand emotions, facilitate the development of self-control, promote a positive peer climate, and enhance interpersonal

Table 18.1   School-Based Mental Health Service Evaluation Results.

Study	Target Problem	Outcome Domain	Results	Detailed Results
Catron & Weiss (1994)[35]	Emotional and behavioral problems	Services/systems	Effective	1. Increased service use
Catron et al. (1998)[36]	Emotional and behavioral problems	1. Services/systems 2. Functioning	Mixed	2. Both the SBS and AT groups improved; not significantly different from each other
Greenberg et al. (1995)[33]	Emotional and behavioral problems	Functioning	Mixed	1. Improvements in children's ability to label and discuss feelings 2. No significant differences in knowledge of emotional cues or simultaneous feelings 3. Differential improvements related to psychopathology
Hawkins et al. (1999)[88]	Emotional and behavioral problems	Functioning	Effective	
Knoff & Batsche (1995)[34]	Emotional and behavioral problems	1. Services/systems 2. Functioning	Effective	
Clarke et al. (1993)[41]	Depression	1. Symptom reduction 2. Functioning	Not effective	
Clarke et al. (1995)[43]	Depression	Symptom reduction	Effective	1. Significant reductions on IIPS in exp. group
Gillham et al. (1995)[44]	Depression	Symptom reduction	Effective	2. No significant effect on Loneliness or Empathy scales
Klingman & Hochdorf (1993)[42]	Depression	1. Symptom reduction 2. Functioning 3. Consumer perspectives	Mixed	3. Increased coping skills 4. Increased knowledge 5. High satisfaction reported
Reynolds & Coats (1986)[89]	Depression	Symptom reduction	Effective	1. Reductions in aggressive cognitive biases
Aber et al. (1998)[50]	Conduct problems	Functioning	Mixed	2. Increases in negotiation strategies 3. Outcomes differed by the number of program sessions received 4. No significant between group differences in aggressive fantasies or conduct disorder symptoms

Table 18.1 School-Based Mental Health Service Evaluation Results (Continued).

Study	Target Problem	Outcome Domain	Results	Detailed Results
Battistich et al. (1996)[87]	Conduct problems	Functioning	Effective	1. Initiated fewer negative behaviors
Bierman et al. (1987)[63]	Conduct problems	Functioning	Mixed	2. Targets of fewer negative behaviors
				3. Positive peer interactions
				4. No significant effects for aggression or sociometric ratings
Braswell et al. (1997)[38]	Conduct problems	1. Symptom reduction 2. Functioning	Not effective	
Conduct Problems Research and Prevention Group (1992)[55]	Conduct problems	1. Functioning 2. Services/systems	Effective	
Cunningham et al. 1988)[51]	Conduct problems	1. Functioning 2. Consumer perspectives	Effective	
Dolan et al. (1993)[52]	Conduct problems	Functioning	Effective	
Dupper & Krishef (1993)[78]	Conduct problems	Functioning	Not effective	
Fuchs et al. (1990)[62]	Conduct problems	1. Functioning 2. Services/systems	Effective	
Gottfredson et al. (1993)[48]	Conduct problems	1. Environment 2. Functioning	Mixed	1. Schools improved significantly if program was well implemented
Grossman et al. (1997)[54]	Conduct problems	1. Symptom reduction 2. Functioning	Mixed	1. No significant differences on parent and teacher behavior rating scales 2. Lower levels of observed aggressive behavior 3. Higher levels of observed prosocial behavior
Hudley & Graham (1993)[65]	Conduct problems	1. Symptom reduction 2. Functioning	Effective	
Kellam et al. (1993)[53]	Conduct problems	1. Symptom reduction 2. Functioning	Mixed	1. No main effects 2. Intervention effective for children who were highly aggressive in the first grade

(Continued)

373

Table 18.1 School-Based Mental Health Service Evaluation Results (*Continued*).

Study	Target Problem	Outcome Domain	Results	Detailed Results
King & Kirschenbaum (1990)[39]	Conduct problems	1. Symptom reduction 2. Functioning	Mixed	1. Decreased depressed mood 2. No differences on teacher rated behavior 3. Parent reported improvement 4. Group leaders reported improvement
Lochman (1993)[66]	Conduct problems	Functioning	Mixed	
Lochman & Curry (1986)[67]	Conduct problems	1. Symptom reduction	Effective	1. Decreased teacher report of externalizing problems
Pepler et al. (1995)[59]	Conduct problems	1. Symptom reduction 2. Functioning	Mixed	2. No significant differences for parent or peer ratings
Reid et al. (1999)[49]	Conduct problems	1. Functioning 2. Services/systems	Effective	
Rosal (1993)[68]	Conduct problems	1. Symptom reduction 2. Functioning	Not effective	
Suter & Kehle (1989)[69]	Conduct problems	Functioning	Not effective	1. Decreased grade retentions until age 13 2. No differences in teacher rate disruptiveness 3. Decreased self-reported juvenile delinquency 4. No differences in juvenile court records
Tremblay et al. (1995)[60]	Conduct problems	Functioning	Mixed	
Vitaro & Tremblay (1994)[61]	Conduct problems	Functioning	Mixed	1. Decreased teacher-rated aggression 2. No differences on self-reported delinquency 3. No differences for number of friends or having a best friend 4. Best friends rated as less disruptive
Cecil & Forman (1990)[71]	Stress management	Functioning	Effective	1. Decreased cigarette smoking 2. Decreased marijuana use 3. No significant effects for alcohol use 4. Increased knowledge 5. Increased communication skills 6. No differences on self-efficacy, self-esteem, or social anxiety
Henderson et al. (1992)[70]	Stress management	Functioning	Effective	
Botvin et al. (1990)[73] Life Skills Training (LST)	Substance use		Mixed	

Table 18.1 School-Based Mental Health Service Evaluation Results (*Continued*).

Study	Target Problem	Outcome Domain	Results	Detailed Results
Botvin et al. (1995)[75] LST	Substance use	Functioning	Effective	1. Lower intentions to use alcohol, marijuana and other drugs
Botvin et al. (1994)[74] LST and Culturally Focused Intervention (CFI)	Substance use	Functioning	Mixed	2. No differences in knowledge 3. Increased negative attitudes toward drinking and drugs
Botvin et al. (1995)[76] LST and CFI	Substance use	Functioning	Mixed	1. Lower alcohol use 2. No differences in marijuana use 3. Lower intentions to use alcohol or drugs
Dent et al. (1995)[84]	Substance use	Functioning	Effective	1. Increased knowledge
Dielman et al. (1986)[79]	Substance use	Functioning	Mixed	2. No change in alcohol use
Ellickson et al. (1993)[78]	Substance use	Functioning	Mixed	1. Lower marijuana and tobacco use among students who had never used and experimenters
	Substance use	Functioning		2. Increased smoking among early users 3. No effects on alcohol use 4. By end of 12th grade, no significant effects on drug, alcohol, or tobacco use 5. Increased knowledge and beliefs
Hostetler & Fisher (1997)[85]	Substance use	Functioning	Not effective	1. Decreased alcohol use
Perry et al. (1996)[77]	Substance use	Functioning	Mixed	2. No differences for tobacco and marijuana use 3. Increased knowledge and attitudes
Rosenbaum et al. (1994)[80]	Substance use	Functioning	Not effective	
Rosenbaum & Hanson (1998)[82]	Substance use	Functioning	Not effective	
Sussman et al. (1993)[83]	Substance use	Functioning	Effective	

problem-solving skills.[33] Program evaluation was based on a sample of 286 second- and third-grade children in regular education (67%) and special education (33%) classrooms, randomly assigned by school or classroom to treatment and control groups. Sample children were not selected based on the presence of psychopathology. Approximately 1 month following the intervention, PATHS participation was associated with significantly higher emotional vocabularies, greater ease discussing emotional experiences, and greater understanding of others' feelings. The PATHS curriculum demonstrated effectiveness in modifying child cognitions, beliefs, and behaviors that may increase the risk of adjustment problems.

Programs may intervene on multiple levels through modification of school policy, implementation of classroom management strategies, development of curricular changes, and facilitation of parent-school communication. Multiple-level approaches are exemplified by Project ACHIEVE, a school reform process designed to reduce the risk of educational and social failure among at-risk and underachieving students.[34] Project ACHIEVE aims to facilitate the development of classroom interventions for students with academic and behavioral problems; enhance teachers' classroom management skills to optimize class time and improve student behavior; increase support services to students with academic difficulties in the regular education classroom; and create a positive school climate.

Program evaluation, using both a matched-comparison school and a single-school multiple baseline method, revealed that 3 years after the initiation of Project ACHIEVE there were significant declines in special education referral (75%) and placement (67%), disciplinary referrals (28%), suspensions (64%), and grade retention (90%). In addition, the Project ACHIEVE school demonstrated markedly lower rates of these variables than the comparison school. For example, special education referral and placement rates were 333% and 350%, respectively, greater at the comparison school.[34] Results suggest that school-wide, multicomponent intervention strategies can reduce child discipline problems and promote student achievement.

Indicated Prevention

The provision of accessible mental health services has also been attempted as a strategy for treating adolescents who demonstrate symptoms of psychopathology. Programs aim to dispel the attitudinal and logistic barriers to service use. The Vanderbilt School-Based Counseling Program provides referred students with appropriate services from trained and licensed mental health clinicians.[35–37] On-site services include individual therapy, group therapy, family therapy, parent training, parent education, consultation, preventive interventions, and case management. Service modality, intensity, and duration vary according to individual need.

Student referrals to the program were made based on grade-wide assessments using teacher, peer, and self-report. Children were randomly assigned to either school-based counseling or academic tutoring. A matched group of children from comparison schools was referred to local community mental health centers (CMHC) for services. In the first 6 months of program implementation, 98% of children referred to the school-based counseling program entered services whereas 17% of children referred to CMHCs entered treatment. This finding suggests that service accessibility and use were significantly increased by the presence of school-based counseling services. Students in both the school-based counseling and academic tutoring groups improved significantly in their level of functioning,[36] but there were no significant differences between the groups, thus calling into question the added value of school-based counseling services.[37]

Program factors associated with mixed or nonsignificant effects included short duration and limited focus.[38,39]

DEPRESSION

Major depressive disorder is a serious clinical problem among children and adolescents, affecting between 2% and 5% of adolescents in community samples.[6] Serious deficits in emotional, behavioral, social, and academic functioning are associated with depression, and depressed children are at increased risk for depressive episodes in adulthood.[40] Burns, Hoagwood, and Mrazek concluded that "early clinical intervention is critical to alleviate distress and to prevent further functional impairment, relapse, and potentially, suicide."[19(p227)]

Universal Prevention

Cognitive-behavioral programs aimed to prevent the development of depressive symptoms and suicidal behaviors among youth have resulted in varying levels of success.[41,42] Coping with Distress and Self-Harm, a 12-session education program, taught adolescents about the nature and universality of distress, responses to distress, the role of cognitions and emotions, and strategies for reframing distress.[42] Students also learned coping skills, such as positive self-talk, empathy, help seeking, and refuting irrational beliefs. In addition, students were taught to identify peer distress and warning signs of suicide. Skills were applied through behavioral homework assignments and in-class feedback.

Program evaluation used a sample of 237 eighth-grade students randomly assigned to the treatment and control groups within classrooms. Students in the treatment condition obtained lower scores on the Israeli Index of Potential Suicide (IIPS) and demonstrated more positive coping skills than students in the control group. There was also a significant increase in knowledge of suicide facts and help resources among students in the treatment group. The findings suggest that students can benefit from a cognitive-behavioral intervention aimed at reducing distress and self-harming behaviors and increasing knowledge and coping skills.

The majority of depression prevention programs reviewed did not achieve such positive results. Clarke et al. evaluated the effectiveness of an educational intervention and a behavioral-skill training intervention, both designed to prevent the development of depressive symptoms in high school students.[41] Both of the programs consisted of five 50-minute lessons presented on consecutive days to ninth- and tenth-grade students. Both studies used large samples ($n = 622$ and $n = 380$, respectively) and randomized controlled designs. Neither intervention demonstrated any significant effect on depressive symptoms, knowledge of depression, or attitudes toward treatment seeking immediately after the intervention or at 12-month follow-up. The results suggest that depression prevention programs of short duration and limited focus may not achieve their intended goals among the general population of students.

Indicated Prevention

In addition to the prevention of depression among all students, many programs target students who report elevated levels of depressive symptoms. The Coping with Stress Course is a group cognitive-behavioral intervention lead by trained school psychologists and counselors. The group teaches at-risk adolescents cognitive skills to identify and challenge negative or irrational thoughts and beliefs that may contribute to the development of depression.

Students were eligible for program participation following a two-stage screening process. All 1,652 ninth- and tenth-grade students in three high schools were screened for depressive symptoms using the Center for Epidemiologic Studies—Depression Scale (CES-D). Students with high CES-D scores participated in a diagnostic interview, and students who did not meet criteria for an affective disorder were randomly assigned to the cognitive intervention or the usual care control condition (students with a diagnosis were referred for mental health assistance). Results indicated that there were significantly fewer cases of major depression or dysthymia across the follow-up period among students in the intervention group compared to students in the control group. The total incidence of unipolar depressive disorder in the treatment group was approximately half of that in the control group. Postintervention assessment indicated that the intervention group scored lower than the control group on measures of depressive symptoms and obtained higher Global Assessment of Functioning scores. Thus, programs that teach at-risk adolescents cognitive skills for modifying depressive thinking styles may be effective for reducing the risk for developing depression.

Elementary school children may also benefit from cognitive interventions for depression. Program effectiveness was demonstrated in a cognitive and social problem-solving intervention targeted to fourth- and fifth-grade students who reported elevated levels of depressive symptoms.[44] Over the course of the 12-week, manualized program, a graduate student in clinical psychology taught students cognitive and social problem-solving skills. Program evaluation used 118 children who obtained elevated scores on the Children's Depression Inventory (CDI) and the Children's Perceptions Questionnaire.

Students in the treatment group reported significantly fewer depressive symptoms at follow-up than students in the control condition. At 12-month follow-up, 29% of students in the control group reported depressive symptoms at or above the moderate range (CDI score ≥ 15), whereas only 7.4% of children in the prevention group had CDI scores at or above this level. Significant between-group differences persisted at the 24-month follow-up. This suggests that cognitive-behavioral interventions for at-risk preadolescents may be effective in reducing the risk for depression.

CONDUCT PROBLEMS

Conduct disorder is a severe, persistent, and costly societal problem, affecting between 2% and 6% of children and adolescents.[15] Conduct-disordered behaviors, such as consistent stealing, fighting, and non-compliance, represent the most frequent reason for referral to treatment services (i.e., up to 50% of all referrals).[46] In addition to the pattern of behavior that violates the basic rights of others, children with conduct disorder are also likely to exhibit academic difficulties, poor interpersonal relationships, and deficits in cognitive problem solving.[45] Conduct disorder is resistant to treatment because it is complex and pervasive. The frequent lack of resources in the families and communities of youth with conduct disorder further complicates treatment.[47]

Universal Prevention

School programs that aim to prevent the development of conduct disorder in children have used a range of strategies that have demonstrated varying degrees of effectiveness. These programs range from those that seek to increase children's social and problem-solving skills to those that aim to alter the school, classroom, and peer contexts in which aggressive behaviors occur.

Mixed program effects were demonstrated for programs that sought to increase the clarity of school rules, improve the consistency of rule enforcement, enhance classroom organization and management, increase home–school communication, and reinforce students' appropriate behaviors.[48] These school policy and classroom management changes were used to create a school environment that minimized the development and expression of violent, aggressive behavior. Results were mixed in reducing student problem behaviors. However, in schools where the program was well implemented, student behavior was reported to improve significantly. The results suggest that the changes in school policy and classroom management strategies do not necessarily lead to reductions in student behavior problems. In addition, appropriate and consistent implementation may be necessary to realize the benefits of certain school-based programs.

Program effectiveness was demonstrated for Linking the Interests of Families and Teachers (LIFT), a program designed to prevent the development of aggressive and antisocial behaviors in elementary school–age children who reside in high-crime neighborhoods.[49] The LIFT program is a multicomponent intervention that includes parent training, social skills training, a playground behavioral program, and regular communication between teachers and parents.

Program evaluation was based on a sample of 671 first- and fifth-grade students from 12 schools randomly assigned to the treatment or control conditions. Following program participation, students engaged in significantly less aggressive behaviors on the playground, parents demonstrated fewer negative behaviors during family problem-solving activities, and teachers reported improved student social behaviors and peer interactions. Three years following the intervention, students who participated in the program were less likely to engage in consistent alcohol use, less likely to have troublesome friends, and were less likely to be arrested for the first time than students who did not participate in the program. Students were also less likely to demonstrate inattentive, impulsive, overactive, and disruptive behaviors in the classroom.[49]

Other multifaceted programs aim to alter the school climate to minimize student aggression. The Resolving Conflicts Creatively Program (RCCP) aimed to facilitate the development of a classroom, peer group, and social context that supports nonviolent conflict resolution.[50]

Program evaluation used a sample of 5,053 second- through sixth-grade children from 11 elementary schools in New York City. Schools were divided into four groups at varying levels of program implementation. Program participation was associated with significantly lower aggressive cognitive biases and use of more competent interpersonal negotiation strategies. Among students enrolled in intervention schools, students exposed to a low number of program sessions demonstrated high levels of hostile attributional bias and a pattern of aggressive interpersonal negotiation strategies compared to students who did not receive any sessions at all. This suggests that inappropriately delivered interventions may be harmful to children, exacerbating the problems they are intended to prevent.

Single-component peer mediation and classroom management strategies have demonstrated effectiveness in reducing playground aggression among elementary school children. The Student-Mediated Conflict Resolution Program trains, uses, and supports fifth-grade students in peer mediation and conflict resolution.[51] Teams of eight mediators monitor the playground during each recess period, attempt to intervene in potential conflict situations, and use the mediation and conflict resolution processes.

The Student-Mediated Conflict Resolution Program was evaluated using a multiple baseline design used in three elementary schools.

Student mediators monitored the playground during each recess, approached individuals who appeared to be at the start of a conflict, and conducted the mediation process in accordance with a standard protocol. The program resulted in a significant reduction in aggressive playground behavior. Aggressive behavior dropped from 57% of the weekly baseline observations to 28% of the observations in school 1. Similar declines were observed in schools 2 and 3. At 1-year follow-up, treatment effects were maintained. Physical aggression decreased 57% in school 1, 75% in school 2, and 70% in school 3 compared to baseline levels measured the previous year.

Classroom management techniques have also been used to reduce children's aggression. The Good Behavior Game (GBG), a classroom-based behavior management strategy for first-grade students, promoted positive behaviors by rewarding teams of students for their lack of negative, disruptive behaviors during specific time periods.[52,53] Game duration, reward delay, and unannounced game times increased throughout the year to promote skill generalization. The major evaluation to date of GBG consisted of an analysis of 19 schools matched on student achievement, family socioeconomic status, and ethnicity and then randomly assigned to the intervention or control condition. Within intervention schools, first-grade classrooms were randomly assigned to the intervention or control condition (GBG internal controls). Results demonstrated that teachers rated boys and girls who participated in the GBG as having lower levels of aggressive behavior than children who did not participate. In fact, although teacher-rated aggressive behavior declined in the GBG classrooms between fall and spring of the academic year, it increased in the control classrooms. One significant feature of this study is that at 6-year follow-up, continued program effects were observed in boys who had high levels of aggression at baseline. Among boys who attended the same school, aggressive boys who participated in the GBG in first grade demonstrated significantly less aggressive behavior immediately after the intervention and at 6-year follow-up than aggressive boys who did not participate.[53] This suggests that the effects of classroom-based interventions can persist for high-risk students.

Finally, educational materials and informational presentations have been used for violence prevention. These programs have demonstrated mixed levels of effectiveness and seem to work best when delivered in conjunction with additional program components, such as peer mediation.[54]

Indicated Prevention

In addition to the primary prevention of conduct problems, programs have been developed and targeted to children who display aggressive and antisocial behaviors. Specific programs range from those that intervene with the child, parent, teacher, and peers to those that provide behavioral consultation services, social skills training, or cognitive-behavioral therapy. Several strong, multifaceted programs that aim to prevent the development of severe and persistent conduct problems in children have had positive effects on student outcomes.[39,55,56] Early intervention with aggressive children is imperative because children who exhibit conduct disordered behaviors (e.g., persistent physical fighting, stealing, noncompliance) prior to or during early adolescence are at the highest risk for the future commitment of repeated delinquent and antisocial acts.[55]

The Family and Schools Together (FAST) Track Program is a multifaceted, multiyear intervention that targets aggressive kindergarten children. The intervention consists of parent training, home visiting and case management activities, social skills training, academic tutoring, and teacher-based classroom interventions to improve classroom management. An evaluation of the FAST Track Program ($n = 891$) indicated that by the third grade, students enrolled in the FAST Track Program displayed less oppositional and aggressive behavior and were less likely to require special education services than students who were not enrolled in the program. The program is hypothesized to influence special education placement through both parent (discipline style, warmth, parenting behavior, attitude toward the child, and attitude toward education) and child (emotional regulation, coping, social problem solving, reading comprehension, and peer relations) factors.[56–58]

Several interventions train aggressive children in social and problem-solving skills while training their parents in behavior management techniques.[59–61] However, program effectiveness has been limited when parent groups were optional.[59]

Programs that combine school-based social skills training with home-based parent training for boys have demonstrated little short-term effectiveness.[60] In a bimodal preventive intervention for aggressive boys, interventions were targeted toward boys rated at or above the 70th percentile for disruptive behavior on the Social Behavior Questionnaire (SBQ) by their kindergarten teachers. Parents learned techniques for child monitoring, positive reinforcement, effective discipline, and crisis management. Children participated in social skills groups that included the target child and teacher-nominated prosocial peers. Students learned prosocial skills, problem-solving skills, and strategies for maintaining self-control.

Other interventions have focused on teachers who participated in behavioral consultation services to attempt to accommodate difficult students in the classroom prior to special education referral.[62] Mainstream Assistance Teams (MAT), a consultant driven prereferral intervention program that seeks to reduce the number of special education referrals and placements were found to effectively reduce the number of special education referrals and improve teacher ratings of the student's target behavior problem.

Additional interventions target aggressive and peer-rejected children's social and problem-solving skills.[63–69] Bierman et al. evaluated a social skills training program for peer-rejected boys.[63] Target children engaged in cooperative activities with prosocial peers in the context of the instructions condition (students are taught a skill and reinforced for appropriate skill use), the prohibitions condition (students are presented with a set of rules and are not rewarded for specific skill demonstration), or a combined condition (children are instructed in target skills and prohibitive rules are presented).

According to the behavioral observations, boys in the prohibitions condition initiated fewer negative behaviors post-treatment and at 6-week follow-up than did boys in the instructions and no-treatment conditions. Boys in the instructions and combination conditions were targets of fewer negative behaviors and demonstrated higher levels of positive peer interactions than boys in the no-treatment condition. Boys in the treatment conditions also demonstrated lower levels of negative peer interaction than boys in the no-treatment condition. This suggests that interventions targeted to the child and delivered in the school setting may be effective in producing positive changes in that setting.

Additional examples of child-focused programs are the School Survival Program,[64] anger-coping intervention,[67] attributional retraining,[65] social activities,[69] and cognitive-behavioral art therapy.[68] The School Survival Program is a social cognitive skills training program for middle school students with school behavior problems. The program seeks to increase awareness of provocative situations, teach a sequential problem-solving process, and provide the opportunity to discuss and practice specific skills. Students in the treatment group improved on the self-control and locus of control measures relative to themselves. However, there were no significant differences on these measures between the treatment and control groups. Cognitive-behavioral interventions such as the anger-coping intervention[67] and the attributional change intervention[69] were found to be effective in reducing aggressive behaviors. Significant differences in terms of level of conduct problems between treatment and control groups were not found for social activities or cognitive-behavioral art therapy.

STRESS

Children and adolescents must cope with an increasingly complex set of environmental and social issues, placing them at risk for the development of emotional, behavioral, and health difficulties.[27] In addition, teachers today face the challenges of educating youth in the face of dwindling resources, increased class size, and low amounts of support. Programs that aid both students and teachers in coping with their daily stresses and anxieties have been developed. Several projects have demonstrated effective outcomes in reducing stress among school children.

Universal Prevention

The Coping with Kids Program, a cognitive-behavioral stress control and relaxation training program, demonstrated effectiveness among third-grade students.[70] The program consisted of nine 45-minute sessions in which students were taught methods for coping with stress, anger management, friendship development, and problem solving. Program evaluation using 65 predominantly African-American students from inner-city schools, revealed that students who participated in the program demonstrated higher locus of control, self-concept, and use of appropriate coping strategies than students in a no-treatment control group.

Stress Inoculation Training groups appeared to reduce levels of self-reported stress and increase the use of appropriate coping skills among elementary and middle schoolteachers.[71] The Stress Inoculation Training group consisted of six 90-minute sessions. The group used a cognitive-behavioral approach to educating teachers about stress and teaching skills such as relaxation training and cognitive restructuring to cope with stress. Program evaluation, using 54 classroom teachers from nine elementary schools, revealed that Stress Inoculation Training was superior to a coworker support group and a no-treatment control group.

SUBSTANCE USE

Alcohol, tobacco, and drug use among youth are significant and pervasive problems, associated with a range of immediate and long-term health and social consequences.[72] Among teenagers, rates of alcohol, tobacco, and drug use have been steadily increasing since 1992. Alcohol continues to be the most commonly used substance among adolescents and is associated with motor vehicle accidents, injuries, and deaths; social, academic, and vocational problems; and aggressive and delinquent behavior. In addition, heavy drinking (i.e., having five or more drinks in a row in the previous 2 weeks) greatly increases the risk of these negative consequences. In 1997, almost 1 in 3 12th graders, 1 in 4 10th graders, and more than 1 in 10 8th graders reported heavy drinking.[72]

Universal Prevention

Several programs have been implemented that seek to prevent use of alcohol, drugs, and tobacco among children and adolescents. Cognitive-behavioral techniques and social skills training have been the main intervention components.[73–78] Botvin et al. used a cognitive-behavioral approach to prevent alcohol, tobacco, and drug use among early adolescents.[73–76] The Life Skills Training (LST) Program has been evaluated using randomized controlled trials, long-term follow-ups, and samples of white and minority youth from varying socioeconomic strata. The LST program is both a substance abuse prevention and a competency enhancement program, designed to facilitate the development of personal and social skills in youth. The program emphasizes the development of skills for coping with social influences to smoke, drink, or use drugs. LST teaches students skills for building self-esteem, anxiety management, effective communication, relationship development, assertiveness, and resisting advertising pressure. In addition, information and skills specific to resistance to the use of alcohol and drugs are taught. The program includes booster sessions, 1 year (10 class sessions) and two years (5 class sessions) following the intervention. Students who participated in LST demonstrated lower levels of cigarette smoking and marijuana use and higher levels of knowledge about drug and alcohol use, interpersonal skills, and communication skills than students who did not participate in LST. Treatment effects were maintained at 6-year follow-up, where LST students reported significantly lower monthly and weekly cigarette use, heavy smoking, problem drinking, marijuana use, and weekly polydrug use than information-only control students.

Other programs use multilevel approaches to prevent alcohol use, involving parents, teachers, and community members. Project Northland is a multiyear, multilevel program designed to prevent adolescent alcohol use.[77] The program includes parent involvement and education programs, behavioral curricula, peer participation, and community task force activities. Interventions occur during students' sixth-, seventh-, and eighth-grade years. During the sixth grade, students learn skills to communicate with their parents about alcohol; during the seventh grade, students engage in a program that focuses on strategies to resist alcohol use; and in the eighth grade, students become involved with groups that influence adolescent alcohol use and availability and teach community action skills.

Program evaluation used 20 school districts, blocked by size and randomly assigned to the intervention (10) or the reference (10) condition. Students were in sixth grade at baseline ($n = 2,351$). At the end of the eighth grade, the sample included 1901 students. Students in the intervention condition reported significantly lower tendencies to use alcohol, less alcohol use in the previous month, and less alcohol use in the previous week than students in the reference condition. These rates were even lower among baseline nonusers in the intervention condition. There were no significant differences between groups in terms of cigarette, smokeless tobacco, and marijuana use. Students in the intervention condition also endorsed significantly more reasons for not using alcohol than students in the reference condition. Although no significant differences were found between groups on the self-efficacy, peer influence, and perceived access items, students in the intervention condition were significantly more likely to report that they could resist alcohol at a party or when it was offered by a boyfriend or girlfriend.

Social learning and/or skill training approaches have also been used for the prevention of alcohol, tobacco, and drug use among children.[78,79]

Ellickson et al. evaluated Project Alert, a curriculum designed to help students develop the motivation and skills to resist drug use.[78] After participation, students reported more negative beliefs about drug use, less marijuana use, less smoking initiation, and a reduction in current, weekly, and daily smoking among experimental smokers. However, the program had a negative effect on the smoking behavior of early smokers, and by the end of high school, the program did not have any significant effect on smoking, alcohol use, or drug use. Program effects on cognitive risk factors (knowledge and beliefs about drug use) persisted.

Programs that use informational presentations and skills training have demonstrated mixed effectiveness.[79–81] Alcohol Misuse Prevention (AMP) is a curriculum that teaches students about the effects of alcohol, consequences of alcohol misuse, the situations or social pressures to misuse alcohol, and skills to deal with these pressures.[79] Outcome assessments indicated that although treatment students demonstrated more knowledge than control students, the two groups were not significantly different in terms of alcohol use and misuse. Small and/or insignificant program effects have also been demonstrated in randomized controlled trials and a meta-analysis of Project DARE, a drug resistance education and skill training program delivered in the classroom setting by police officers.[80–82]

Project Towards No Tobacco Use was a 5-year school-based tobacco use prevention and smoking cessation program that targeted junior high school students.[83] Program evaluation compared the effectiveness of four curricula (refusal skills, advertising tactics, consequences of tobacco use, and a combination of the three) that focused on the prevention of cigarette and smokeless tobacco (i.e., chewing tobacco and snuff) use, taught over a 10-day period.

Program evaluation used a randomized block design and used 48 junior high schools from 27 southern California school districts. Schools were recruited and randomly assigned within blocks to participate in either one of the four treatment conditions (32) or the standard curriculum control condition (16). Students in all program conditions except the advertiser tactics condition demonstrated lower rates of tobacco use initiation and weekly tobacco use compared with students in the control condition. The combined condition was associated with the lowest rate of weekly smokeless tobacco use compared to all other conditions. Program effects were maintained at 2-year follow-up.[84]

Indicated Prevention

Programs have also been developed and targeted toward students at high risk for drug and alcohol use. Botvin et al. evaluated a culturally focused intervention (CFI) targeted to high-risk students.[74,76] Professionally trained leaders and peers conducted the intervention in a group counseling format. Program content (cognitive, behavioral, and environmental components) and implementation (type of teaching medium) were informed by the characteristics of high-risk students. The program uses stories to model different skills through main characters that face alienation and hopelessness. Through these stories, students learn cognitive-behavioral skills for problem solving, decision making, self-esteem building, anxiety management, effective communication, assertiveness, and positive relationship development.

Program evaluation was based on 639 students randomly assigned by school to LST, CFI, or information-only control (IOC) groups. Behavioral intentions to use alcohol and illicit drugs were lower in both the LST and CFI groups relative to the controls. LST and CFI students also reported more negative attitudes toward drinking, marijuana, cocaine, and other drug use and lower risk-taking behaviors relative to the control group. At 2-year follow-up, students who had participated in LST or CFI reported significantly less alcohol use than students in the control group. Drinking frequency, amount of alcohol consumed, and frequency of drunkenness were significantly lower in both treatment conditions compared to the control condition. In addition, the CFI students demonstrated lower scores on these variables compared to the students in LST.

Other targeted, multicomponent programs have not achieved such success. Project CARE, a substance abuse prevention program for high-risk youth, consisted of student groups (focused on issues such as building self-esteem, alcohol and drug education, the consequences of unhealthy behaviors, and decision-making and coping skills), student field trips (e.g., swimming, going on a picnic in the park, visiting a farm), in-home family meetings, parent group meetings, 1-week residential summer camp, and family activities (e.g., talent shows, pizza parties, field trips).[85]

The program was targeted toward at-risk fourth-grade students identified through teacher-completed student assessment forms. Children at highest risk were randomly assigned to the treatment or control group. Unexpectedly, program students reported significantly more negative behaviors and substance abuse than control students and significantly less participation in alternative activities than control students. It is unclear why treatment was associated with negative child outcomes. Program participation may have given children the opportunity to create a deviant peer group, where negative behaviors were reinforced and propagated.

DISCUSSION

Media reports make it clear that children and adolescents today must cope with a more complex set of social issues than a generation ago. The list of horrors is by now well known: substance use and abuse and related unintended injuries (e.g., car accidents); sexual risks (e.g., unintended pregnancy) and sexually transmitted diseases (e.g., HIV); suicide and self-mutilating behaviors; school, community, and domestic violence; physical and sexual abuse; eating disorders; and homelessness.[27] Each of these events has been found to place a child at risk for the development of emotional, behavioral, or developmental disorders. Although schools are not the only (and in some cases are not even the tertiary) social agency responsible for addressing these significant issues, they cannot ignore them if they hope to fulfill their mandate to educate all children.[86] Children whose emotional, behavioral, or social difficulties are not addressed have a diminished capacity to learn and benefit from the school environment. In addition, children who develop disruptive behavior patterns can have a negative influence on the social and academic environment for other children. As a significant part of the larger community where children live, as well as a critical component in the system of care, it would seem to be in the best interests of schools to facilitate children's functioning academically, socially, and emotionally.

This review identifies a robust group of school-based mental health programs as having evidence of an impact across a variety of emotional and behavioral problems in children. However, a lack of treatment studies, even among the most prevalent disorders of childhood (i.e., anxiety, ADHD, depression) was also identified. Despite the growing evidence of the significance of these disorders and their impact on child functioning, no studies that targeted particular clinical syndromes were identified. In addition to identifying those programs that have an evidence base in support of their impact, this review has also revealed several important features of the implementation process itself, features that increase the probability of service sustainability and maintenance. These key program components include (1) consistent program implementation; (2) inclusion of parents, teachers, or peers; (3) use of multiple modalities (e.g., the combination of informational presentations with cognitive and behavioral skill training); (4) integration of program content into general classroom curriculum; and (5) developmentally appropriate program components.

Past research suggests that implementation variation is associated with program outcomes. There are several components of implementation factors that have implications for program success, dissemination, and maintenance. These include the school culture and climate, the cooperation of school leadership, funding mechanism, and program fidelity. For example, in a school reform intervention that increased the clarity of school rules and consistency of rule enforcement, program success was found only in schools where the program was well implemented.[48] Strategies that facilitated appropriate program implementation included the communication of program goals, rationale, and components to school staff; the provision of feedback on program effects; the development of plans to overcome barriers to implementation; and the specification of individual responsibilities.[48] Successful program implementation was associated with clear, specific expectations (e.g., school rules, consequences, a reward system for appropriate student behavior described in the student handbook); creative involvement by individual schools (e.g., report card of appropriate behavior); and feedback, consultation, and support to teachers (e.g., refresher training sessions, classroom observation, small group discussions).

Although well-implemented programs can achieve previously demonstrated program effects, poor program implementation can mitigate program effects.[48,51,87] For example, in a student-mediated conflict resolution program, the level of aggressive playground behaviors increased to baseline levels when the size of the mediation team was reduced to two members instead of the recommended eight. When the school increased the number of peer mediators to eight, aggression declined markedly.[31]

Program effectiveness was also found to be associated with multicomponent programs that targeted the ecology of the child. For example, three of the effective preventive intervention programs targeted parents, teachers, and peers in the intervention process (e.g., FAST

Track, LIFT Program). These interventions included teacher training in classroom management techniques, parent training in child management, and child cognitive-social skills training.[88] Although these programs have been associated with successful outcomes, multilevel programs are not a panacea and do not guarantee program success.[38,85]

This review also reveals that those programs with the strongest evidence of an impact were those that were directed toward changing specific behaviors and skills associated with the intervention (e.g., depression, conduct problems, drug use), whereas extraneous activities, such as field trips, 1-week residential summer camps, or optional parenting groups, did not seem to offer any comparative advantage.

Inclusion of multiple approaches to changing behavior (e.g., informational presentation combined with skill training) was also associated with program success. It appears that these multiple modalities were successful because they focused on the change agents that were theoretically linked to the target problem. For example, the FAST Track program uses strategies designed to mitigate specific risk factors associated with the development of conduct disorder. All students receive the PATHS curriculum, which includes skills for emotional understanding and communication, friendship skills, self-control skills, and social problem-solving skills. High-risk children also participate in academic tutoring, their parents participate in parent training groups, and the family receives home visits.[56–58]

For other clinical problems of children, however, more unilateral approaches may be appropriate. For example, the Coping with Stress course teaches cognitive-behavioral skills to alter the cognitions and beliefs thought to underlie the development of depression to adolescents who are at risk for developing depression.[43]

A fourth element that was found in this review to be associated with program effectiveness was integration of the program into the general classroom curricula.[33,56–58,88] Insofar as the mental health service program was delivered as an integral part of the classroom curricula rather than as a separate and specialized lesson, it was associated with more positive outcomes.[41] This suggests that for services to be sustained beyond the tenure of the research study, inclusiveness of the service within the normal educational routine of the school is important to attain.

Finally, this review revealed that effectiveness was associated with those programs where the concepts and curricula were developmentally appropriate. For example, in an elementary school intervention aimed at preventing health risks, parent training classes were specifically designed to reflect the developmental level of the target children.[88] When children were in the first and second grades, parents were trained in behavior management strategies. In fifth and sixth grades, parents were taught skills to reduce their child's risk for drug use. These various sessions were created to address parental concerns about children's maturation and to complement their children's classroom-based social skills training.

FUTURE RESEARCH

Future research efforts must target several gaps that this review reveals. First, there is a severe paucity of programs that focus on special education students, particularly those classified as seriously emotionally disturbed (SED). Children with serious emotional disturbances represent the most severely impaired group of students in the schools and those most in need of comprehensive services. In addition, these students tend to be the most expensive for school systems to accommodate, as they may require more restrictive placements as their behavioral and emotional problems escalate.[5] Yet this review uncovers few studies specifically focused on this group of children. This is a major shortcoming in the knowledge base.

Second, although some variables related to the implementation process have been identified in the literature, there are still many questions yet unanswered about the active ingredients that lead to successful program implementation and dissemination. These must be identified. As the research base on effective programs continues to grow, it will be important to determine elements of replicability to identify how these programs can be transferred to different schools, school systems, and populations of students, and to identify barriers to successful implementation. In addition, it is important to identify malleable risk factors for poor implementation and develop appropriate strategies for addressing these.

Third, there are also gaps in the types of mental health and social problems targeted by current school-based mental health service programs. There is a need to develop conduct disorder interventions for middle and high school students and depression and sex education interventions for elementary school students. The bulk of the research base thus far has focused on preventive strategies to manage disruptive behaviors among younger children, or on interventions for mood disorders among high school youth. This imbalance impedes true system-of-care approaches that aim to include all levels of the school (with appropriate services calibrated to the needs of the children) in the continuum.

Surprisingly, we did not find any school-based anxiety prevention or intervention programs that met the criteria for entry into this review. Development and evaluation of such programs is greatly needed, as anxiety disorders are the most common mental disorder among children and adolescents. There are also important service implications associated with such disorders, as anxiety disorders have been found to lead to lost school days due to somatic complaints and school refusal.

Finally, evaluations of school-based mental health services have typically ignored or underemphasized school-relevant outcomes. Thus, the effects of mental health services for student achievement, attendance, and school-related behavior (as measured by disciplinary referrals, suspensions, and retention) have not been explored. This is a noteworthy omission, but one that can be corrected. As research moves more and more toward collaborative models that include administrators, practitioners (e.g., clinicians, teachers, physicians), and parents in its enterprise, the breadth, range, and relevancy of outcomes are likely to improve.

Notes

1. Burns BJ, Costello EJ, Angold A, et al. Children's mental health service use across service sectors. *Health Aff.* 1995;14:147–159.
2. Costello EJ, Angold A, Burns BJ, et al. The Great Smoky Mountains Study of Youth: goals, design, methods, and the prevalence of DSM-III-R disorders. *Arch Gen Psychiatry.* 1996;53:1129–1136.
3. Leaf PJ, Alegria M, Cohen P, et al. Mental health service use in the community and schools: results from the four-community MECA study. *J Am Acad Child Adolesc Psychiatry.* 1996;35:889–896.
4. Zahner G, Pawelkiewicz W, De Francesco JJ, Adnopoz J. Children's mental health service needs and utilization patterns in an urban community: an epidemiological assessment. *J Am Acad Child Adolesc Psychiatry.* 1992;31:951–960.
5. Parrish TB. Special education finance: past, present, and future. Policy Paper Number 8. Palo Alto, Calif: Center for Special Education Finance; 1996.
6. Shaffer D, Fisher P, Dulcan MK, et al. The NIMH Diagnostic Interview Schedule for Children Version 2.3 (DISC 2.3): description, acceptability, prevalence rates, and performance in the MECA study. *J Am Acad Child Adolesc Psychiatry.* 1996;35:865–877.

7. Roberts RE, Attkinsson CC, Rosenblatt A. Prevalence of psychopathology among children and adolescents. *Am J Psychiatry.* 1998;155:715–725.

8. Friedman RM, Katz-Leavy JW, Mandersheid RW, Sondheimer DL. Prevalence of serious emotional disturbance in children and adolescents. In: Manderscheid RW, Sonnenschein MA, eds. *Mental Health, United States, 1996.* Center for Mental Health Services. Washington, DC: US GPO; 1996:83.

9. Hoagwood K, Koretz D. Embedding prevention services within systems of care: strengthening the nexus for children. *Appl Prevent Psychol.* 1996;5:225–234.

10. Stroul BA, Friedman RM. *A System of Care for Severely Emotionally Disturbed Children and Youth.* Washington, DC: Georgetown University Child Development Center; 1986.

11. Stroul BA, Friedman RM. The system of care concept and philosophy. In: Stroul BA, ed. *Children's Mental Health: Creating Systems of Care in a Changing Society.* Baltimore, Md: Brookes; 1996:3–21.

12. Friedman RM. The practice of psychology with children, adolescents, and their families: a look to the future. In: Hughes J, Conoley JC, La Greco A, eds. *Handbook of Psychological Interventions for Children and Adolescents.* New York, NY: Oxford University Press; 1999:1–34.

13. Adelman HS, Taylor L. Mental health in schools and system restructuring. *Clin Psychol Rev.* 1999;19:137–163.

14. Bickman L. Practice makes perfect and other myths about mental health services. *Am Psychol.* 1999;54:965–979.

15. Weisz JR, Weiss B, Donenberg GR. The lab versus the clinic: effects of child and adolescent psychotherapy. *Annu Prog Child Psychiatry Child Dev.* 1993;47:1578–1585.

16. Weisz JR., Jensen PS. Efficacy and effectiveness of child and adolescent psychotherapy and pharmacotherapy. *Ment Health Serv Res.* 1999;1:125–158.

17. Weisz JR, Weersing VR. Psychotherapy with children and adolescents: efficacy, effectiveness, and developmental concerns. In: Cicchetti D, Toth DL, eds. *Developmental Approaches to Prevention and Intervention: Rochester Symposium on Developmental Psychopathology,* vol 9. Rochester, NY: University of Rochester Press; 1999.

18. Vitiello B, Bhatara VS, Jensen PS. Current knowledge and unmet needs in pediatric psychopharmacology. *J Am Acad Child Adolesc Psychiatry.* 1999;38:501–502.

19. Burns BJ, Hoagwood K, Mrazek P. Effective treatment for mental disorders in children and adolescents. *Clin Child Fam Psychol Rev.* 1999;2:199–254.

20. Empirically supported psychosocial interventions for children [special issue]. *J Clin Child Psychol.* 1998;27:138–226.

21. Huffman LC, Mehlinger SL, Kerivan AS. Risk factors for academic and behavioral problems at the beginning of school. In: FPG Child Development Center. *Off to a Good Start: Research on the Risk Factors for Early School Problems and Selected Federal Policies Affecting Children's Social and Emotional Development and Their Readiness for School.* Chapel Hill, NC: FPG Child Development Center, University of North Carolina; 2000.

22. Muller J, Mihalic S. *Blueprints: A Violence Prevention Initiative.* Washington, DC: Office of Juvenile Justice and Delinquency Prevention; 1999.

23. National Institutes of Health. Diagnosis and treatment of attention deficit hyperactivity disorder (ADHD). *NIH Consensus Statement,* 1998;16(2):1–37.

24. National Institutes of Health. *A Plan for Preventive Research for the National Institute of Mental Health.* Rockville, Md: National Institutes of Health; 1996.

25. Brandenburg NA, Friedman RM, Silver SE. The epidemiology of childhood psychiatric disorders: prevalence findings from recent studies. *J Am Acad Child Adolesc Psychiatry.* 1990;29:76–83.

26. Costello EJ. Developments in child psychiatric epidemiology: an epidemiological study of behavior characteristics in children. *J Am Acad Child Adolesc Psychiatry.* 1989;28:836–841.

27. Nastasi B. A model for mental health programming in schools and communities: introduction to the miniseries. *Sch Psychol Rev.* 1998;27:165–174.

28. Angold A, Costello EJ, Erkanli A. Comorbidity. *J Child Psychol Psychiatry.* 1999;40:57–87.

29. Kessler RC. The National Comorbidity Survey of the United States. *Int Rev Psychiatry.* 1994;6:365–376.

30. Greenbaum PE, Prange ME, Friedman RM, Silver SE. Substance abuse prevalence and comorbidity with other psychiatric disorders among adolescents with severe emotional disturbance. *J Am Acad Child Adolesc Psychiatry.* 1991;30:575–583.

31. Quinn KP, Epstein MH. Characteristics of children, youth, and families served by local interagency systems of care. In: Epstein MH, Kutash K, Duchnowski A, eds. *Outcomes for Children and Youth with Emotional and Behavioral Disorders and Their Families: Programs and Evaluation Best Practices.* Austin, Tex: Pro-Ed Inc; 1998:81–114.

32. Friedman RM. Mental health and substance use services for adolescents: clinical and service system issues. *Admin Policy Ment Health.* 1992;19:191–206.

33. Greenberg M, Kusche C, Cook E, Quamma J. Promoting emotional competence in school-aged children: the effects of the PATHS curriculum. *Dev Psychopathol.* 1995;7:117–136.

34. Knoff H, Batsche G. Project ACHIEVE: analyzing a school reform process for at-risk and underachieving students. *Sch Psychol Rev.* 1995;24:579–603.

35. Catron T, Weiss B. The Vanderbilt School-Based Counseling Program: An interagency, primary-care model of mental health services. *J Emotion Behav Disord.* 1994;2:247–253.

36. Catron T, Harris V, Weiss B. Posttreatment results after 2 years of services in the Vanderbilt School-Based Counseling Project. In: Epstein M, Kutash K, Duchnowski A, eds. *Outcomes for Children and Youth with Emotional and Behavioral Disorders and Their Families: Programs and Evaluation Best Practices.* Austin, Tex: Pro-Ed Inc; 1998:633–656.

37. Weiss B, Catron T, Harris V, Phung T. The effectiveness of traditional child psychotherapy. *J Consult Clin Psychol.* 1999;67:82–94.

38. Braswell L, August G, Bloomquist M, Realmuto G, Skare S, Crosby R. School-based secondary prevention for children with disruptive behavior: initial outcomes. *J Abnorm Child Psychol.* 1997;25:197–208.

39. King C, Kirschenbaum D. An experimental evaluation of a school-based program for children at risk: Wisconsin early intervention. *J Community Psychol.* 1990;18:167–177.

40. Lewinsohn PM, Clarke GN, Hops H, Seeley JR. A course in coping: a cognitive-behavioral approach to the treatment of adolescent depression. In: Hibbs ED, Jensen PS, eds. *Psychosocial Treatments for Child and Adolescent Disorders: Empirically Based Strategies for Clinical Practice.* Washington, DC: American Psychological Association; 1996:109–135.

41. Clarke G, Hawkins W, Murphy M, Sheeber L. School-based primary prevention of depressive symptomatology in adolescents: findings from two studies. *J Adolesc Res.* 1993;8:183–204.

42. Klingman A, Hochdorf Z. Coping with distress and self harm: the impact of a primary prevention program among adolescents. *J Adolesc.* 1993;16:121–140.

43. Clarke G, Hawkins W, Murphy M, Sheeber L, Lewinsohn P, Seeley J. Targeted prevention of unipolar depressive disorder in an at-risk sample of high school adolescents: a randomized trial of a group cognitive intervention. *J Am Acad Child Adolesc Psychiatry.* 1995;34:312–321.

44. Gillham J, Reivich K, Jaycox L, Seligman M. Prevention of depressive symptoms in schoolchildren: two-year follow-up. *Psychol Sci.* 1995;6:343–351.

45. Kazdin A. Practitioner review: psychosocial treatments for conduct disorder in children. *J Child Psychol Psychiatry.* 1997;38:161–178.

46. Robins LN. Epidemiological approaches to natural history research: antisocial disorders in children. *J Am Acad Child Adolesc Psychiatry.* 1981;20:566–680.

47. Practice parameters for the assessment and treatment of children and adolescents with conduct disorder. *J Am Acad Child Adolesc Psychiatry.* 1997; 36:122S-139S.

48. Gottfredson D, Gottfredson G, Hybl L. Managing adolescent behavior: a multiyear, multischool study. *Am Educ Res J.* 1993;30:179–215.

49. Reid J, Eddy M, Fetrow R, Stoolmiller M. Description and immediate impacts of a preventive intervention for conduct problems. *Am J Community Psychol.* 1999;27:483–517.

50. Aber J, Jones S, Brown J, Chaudry N, Samples F. Resolving conflicts creatively: evaluating the developmental effects of a school-based violence prevention program in neighborhood and classroom context. *Devel Psychopathol.* 1998;10:187–213.

51. Cunningham C, Cunningham L, Martorelli V, Tran A, Young J, Zacharias R. The effects of primary division, student-mediated conflict resolution programs on playground aggression. *J Child Psychol Psychiatry.* 1998;39: 653–662.

52. Dolan L, Kellam S, Brown C, et al. The short-term impact of two classroom-based preventive interventions on aggressive and shy behaviors and poor achievement. *J Appl Dev Psychol.* 1993;14:317–345.

53. Kellam SG, Rebok GW, Ialongo N, Mayer LS. The course and malleability of aggressive behavior from early first grade into middle school: results of a developmental epidemiologically based preventive trial. *J Child Psychol Psychiatry.* 1994;35:259–281.

54. Grossman D, Neckerman H, Koepsell T, et al. Effectiveness of a violence prevention curriculum among children in elementary school: a randomized controlled trial. *JAMA.* 1997;277:1605–1611.

55. Conduct Problems Prevention Research Group. A developmental and clinical model for the prevention of conduct disorder: The FAST Track Program. *Dev Psychopathol.* 1992;4:509–527.

56. Conduct Problems Prevention Research Group. *FAST Track Update.* Rockville, Md: National Institute of Mental Health, 1999.

57. Conduct Problems Prevention Research Group. Initial impact of the FAST Track prevention trial for conduct problems, I: the high-risk sample. *J Consult Clin Psychol.* 1999; 67:631–647.

58. Conduct Problems Prevention Research Group. Initial impact of the FAST Track prevention trial for conduct problems, II: classroom effects. *J Consult Clin Psychol.* 1999;67:648–657.

59. Pepler D, King G, Craig W, Byrd B, Bream L. The development and evaluation of a multisystem social skills group training program for aggressive children. *Child Youth Care Forum.* 1995;24:297–313.

60. Tremblay R, Pagani-Kurtz L, Masse L, Vitaro F, Pihl R. A bimodal preventive intervention for disruptive kindergarten boys: its impact through mid-adolescence. *J Consult Clin Psychol.* 1995;63:560–568.

61. Vitaro F, Tremblay R. Impact of a prevention program on aggressive children's friendships and social adjustment. *J Abnorm Child Psychol.* 1994;22:457–475.

62. Fuchs D, Fuchs L, Bahr M. Mainstream assistance teams: a scientific basis for the art of consultation. *Except Child.* 1990;57:128–139.

63. Bierman K, Miller C, Stabb S. Improving the social behavior and peer acceptance of rejected boys: effects of social skill training with instructions and prohibitions. *J Consult Clin Psychol.* 1987;55:194–200.

64. Dupper D, Krishef C. School-based social-cognitive skill training for middle school students with school behavior problems. *Child Youth Serv Rev.* 1993;15:131–142.

65. Hudley C, Graham S. An attributional intervention to reduce peer-directed aggression among African-American boys. *Child Dev.* 1993;64:124–138.

66. Lochman J, Coie J, Underwood M, Terry R. Effectiveness of a social relations intervention program for aggressive and nonaggressive rejected children. *J Consult Clin Psychol.* 1993;61:1053–1058.

67. Lochman J, Curry J. Effects of social problem solving training and self-instruction training with aggressive boys. *J Clin Child Psychol.* 1986;15:159–164.

68. Rosal M. Comparative group art therapy research to evaluate changes in locus of control in behavior disordered children. *Arts Psychother.* 1993;20:231–241.

69. Suter D, Kehle T. Evaluation of the Primary Mental Health Project model of early identification and prevention of school adjustment problems. *Spec Serv Sch.* 1988;4:89–107.

70. Henderson P, Kelbey T, Engerbreston K. Effects of a stress-control program on children's locus of control, self-concept, and coping behavior. *Sch Counselor.* 1992;40:125–130.

71. Cecil M, Forman S. Effects of stress inoculation training and coworker support groups on teacher's stress. *J Sch Psychol.* 1990;28:105–118.

72. Federal Interagency Forum on Child and Family Statistics. *America's Children: Key National Indicators of Well-Being.* Washington, DC: US GPO; 1998.

73. Botvin G, Baker E, Dusenbury L, Tortu S, Botvin E. Preventing adolescent drug abuse through a multimodal cognitive-behavioral approach: results of three studies. *J Consult Clin Psychol.* 1990;58:437–446.

74. Botvin G, Schinke S, Epstein J, Diaz T. Effectiveness of culturally focused and generic skills training approaches to alcohol and drug abuse prevention among minority youths. *Psychol Addict Behav.* 1994;8:116–127.

75. Botvin G, Baker E, Dusenbury L, Botvin E, Diaz T. Long-term follow-up results of a randomized drug abuse prevention trial in a white middle-class population. *JAMA.* 1995;273:1106–1112.

76. Botvin G, Schinke S, Epstein J, Diaz T, Botvin E. Effectiveness of culturally focused and generic skills training approaches to alcohol and drug abuse prevention among minority adolescents: two-year follow-up results. *Psychol Addict Behav.* 1995;9:183–194.

77. Perry C, Williams C, Veblen-Mortenson S, et al. Project Northland: outcomes of a community-wide alcohol use prevention program during early adolescence. *Am J Public Health.* 1996;86:956–965.

78. Ellickson P, Bell R, McGuigan K. Preventing adolescent drug use: long-term results of a junior high program. *Am J Public Health.* 1993;83:856–861.

79. Dielman T, Shope J, Butchart T, Campanelli P. Prevention of adolescent alcohol misuse: an elementary school program. *J Pediatr Psychol.* 1986;11:259–282.

80. Rosenbaum D, Flewelling R, Bailey S, Ringwalt C, Wilkinson D. Cops in the classroom: a longitudinal evaluation of Drug Abuse Resistance Education (DARE). *J Res Crime Delinquency* 1994;31:3–31.

81. Ennett S, Tobler N, Ringwalt C, Flewelling R. How effective is drug abuse resistance education? A meta-analysis of project DARE outcome evaluations. *Am J Public Health.* 1994;84:1394–1400.

82. Rosenbaum D, Hanson G. Assessing the effects of school-based drug education: a six-year multilevel analysis of project DARE. *J Res Crime Delinquency.* 1998;35:381–412.

83. Sussman S, Dent C, Stacy A, et al. Project Towards No Tobacco Use: 1–year behavioral outcomes. *Am J Public Health.* 1993;83:1245–1250.

84. Dent C, Sussman S, Stacy A, Craig S, Burton D, Flay B. Two-year behavior outcomes of a Project Towards No Tobacco Use. *J Consult Clin Psychol.* 1995;63:676–677.

85. Hostetler M, Fisher K. Project CARE substance abuse prevention program for high-risk youth: a longitudinal evaluation of program effectiveness. *J Community Psychol.* 1997;25:397–419.

86. Adelman HS, Taylor L. Mental health in schools: moving forward. *Sch Psychol Rev.* 1998;27:175–190.

87. Battistich V, Schaps E, Watson M, Solomon D. Prevention effects of the Child Development Project: early findings from an ongoing multisite demonstration trial. *J Adolesc Res.* 1996;11:12–35.

88. Hawkins JD, Catalano RF, Kosterman R, Abbott R, Hill K. Preventing adolescent health-risk behaviors by strengthening protection during childhood. *Arch Pediatr Adolesc Med.* 1999;153:226–234.

89. Reynolds WM, Coates KI. A comparison of cognitive-behavioral therapy and relaxation training for the treatment of depression in adolescents. *J Consult Clin Psychol.* 1986;54:653–660.

CHAPTER 19

Expanded School Mental Health Services

A National Movement in Progress

Mark Weist, 1997

In 1982, Knitzer's compelling *Unclaimed Children* underscored the tremendous gap between the mental health needs of children in the United States and services actually available to them.[1] Throughout the 1980s and into the 1990s, some progress has been made to improve the mental health system of care for youth, as exemplified by national reform efforts that improve the coordinated delivery of services (e.g., the Child and Adolescent Service Systems Program [CASSP]),[2] the growth of family preservation models of treatment,[3] and the development of "multisystemic" treatment approaches for youth with severe disturbances.[4] In spite of these improvements, a large gap between youth who need and receive services remains,[5] mental health services continue to be fragmented and

---

This chapter originally appeared as Weist MD. Expanded school mental health services: a national movement in progress. *Adv Clin Child Psychol.* 1997; 19:319–351. Copyright © 1997 Springer Science and Business Media. Reprinted with kind permission from Springer Science and Business Media.

uncoordinated,[6] and university-based applied research efforts have not been effectively integrated into communities on a wide scale.[7]

One method to significantly address gaps in mental health services for youth is to place more of them in schools. Each day during the school year, 40 million children attend one of the 82,000 public elementary and secondary schools in the United States.[8] By placing services in them, we are reaching youth "where they are," eliminating many of the barriers that exist for traditional child mental health services (e.g., as provided in community mental health centers and private offices).

Most school-based mental health services are limited to youth in special education.[9] However, a national movement is under way to place a full range of mental health services (from primary to tertiary preventive) for youth in schools. This movement is part of a broader effort, now around two decades old, to bring health services to schools. The movement to place "expanded" mental health services in schools offers considerable opportunities for mental health professionals for clinical service, program development, and research. The purpose of this chapter is to provide an overview of expanded school mental health services, with discussion of broad, systems issues, followed by review of challenges confronting individual clinicians working in schools.

LIMITATIONS IN THE MENTAL HEALTH SERVICE DELIVERY SYSTEM FOR YOUTH

Statistics indicate that many youth who need mental health services are not receiving them. In 1991, the Congressional Office of Technology Assessment (OTA) reported that up to 20% of youth under the age of 20 present emotional and behavioral disorders severe enough to warrant intervention, but less than one-third of these youth actually receive mental health services.[10] Zahner, Pawelkiewicz, Di Francesco, and Adnopoz (1992) conducted a survey of parents and teachers of 822 children (aged 6–11) who were attending public and private schools in a northeastern city.[21] Based on parent and teacher screening measures, 38.5% of the children were determined to be at risk for developing psychiatric disturbance. However, only 11% of the children determined to be at risk had received treatment in traditional mental health settings (i.e., community outpatient clinics and private offices). Goodwin, Goodwin, and Cantrill surveyed over 500 personnel from a Colorado school district on the mental health needs of elementary students.[12] Approximately 15% of the students were identified as needing, but not receiving, mental health services.

Dryfoos, a leading researcher on youth at risk, estimated that one in four U.S. youth aged 10 to 17 "do it all," that is, engage in early unprotected sexual activity, use drugs, skip school, and fall behind in their schoolwork.[8] With 40 million children attending U.S. public schools, 10 million could benefit from mental health services, based on her estimate of one in four being at risk.

Children and adolescents from the inner city are in particular need for mental health services, given the high life stress they contend with, including poverty,[13] exposure to crime and violence,[14,15] frequent abuse and neglect,[16] and commonly occurring family problems (e.g., absence of one parent, large family size, substance abuse in the home).[17] Related to these conditions, urban youth are evidencing rising rates of troubling problems such as teen pregnancy[18]; sexually transmitted diseases (including HIV infections)[19]; substance use [19]; drug trafficking[21]; depression, anxiety, and post-traumatic stress[22,23]; and school avoidance, poor school performance, and dropout).[24]

In contrast to the rather significant attention to the plight of urban youth, problems of rural youth have received little attention.[25] Rural areas have more unemployment, 38% of the country's poor, and 67% of substandard housing, although comprising only 25% of the U.S. population.[26] Furthermore, there is evidence that rural children have higher levels of injuries, drownings, and some chronic illnesses than metropolitan children.[25] In terms of mental health status, limited studies indicate that rural youth present lower rates of drug abuse than urban youth, but higher rates of alcohol abuse,[27] with urban and rural youth having roughly comparable levels of behavioral and emotional problems.[28] Impediments for rural youth to receive mental health services are significant, including geography (with fewer clinics and treatment programs spaced farther apart than in metropolitan areas), enhanced stigma for seeking mental health treatment, and significant difficulties in recruitment and retention of adequately trained mental health providers.[25]

Suburban youth (i.e., youth from suburbs and small cities and towns) are a neglected population as well. However, there is evidence that violence and carrying of weapons is increasing among suburban youth,[14] and that suburban adolescents may be more prone to abuse of hard drugs (e.g., LSD, methamphetamine) than their urban or rural counterparts.[29]

Thus, across urban, rural, and suburban settings, there is a consensus among mental health providers and analysts that youth with mental disorders are inadequately served in the current system of care. Numerous problems such as fragmentation of services, poor coordination within and between agencies, staff limitations (in numbers and quality), inadequate treatment facilities, and escalating difficulties in paying for services associated with managed care, in combination make the mental health services system for youth a "nonsystem."[6,25] Commenting on the status of children's mental health:

> The discrepancy between the conceptual model of what a system of care should be, as embraced by state policy makers and its actual implementation at a grass roots level is, in many cases, enormous. The discrepancy between the numbers of youngsters and families in need of services and the amount of services that are available is also enormous.

Community mental health clinics remain the dominant method of addressing mental health problems in youth. However, there are many barriers that prevent children and adolescents from accessing mental health services in these clinics. These include familial factors such as poor knowledge of mental health services, financial difficulties, transportation problems, and stress in families that often precludes adequate attention to children's emotional difficulties. Barriers also exist in community clinics, including long waiting lists (often 3 weeks or longer), high turnover among staff, long intake procedures, and excessive paperwork to justify even short treatment to insurance companies. These barriers often serve to prevent youth from receiving needed services. Barriers to community mental health services are particularly acute for families from other cultures, who often have little or no conception of these services or how to access them.

An additional issue of importance is that recent analyses have called into question the dominant model of treating children's emotional/behavioral disorders with weekly outpatient therapy visits. For example, Weisz, Weiss, and Donenberg conducted a meta-analysis of child and adolescent psychotherapy outcome studies and concluded that there is limited evidence for the effectiveness of such therapy as practiced with clinical samples in applied settings.[30] Another side of this issue is that youth often need to act out or show salient symptoms of emotional distress before they receive enough attention to be seen in a community clinic. As such, many youth receiving treatment in these clinics present full-blown diagnoses, meaning that prevention efforts are predominantly tertiary.[31] Moreover, the notion of once per week outpatient therapy in an artificial setting (often far removed from the child's natural environment) to address emotional/behavioral problems in youth is questionable at best.[32]

ADVANTAGES OF SCHOOL-BASED PROGRAMS

Related to recognition of inadequacies of community clinics in preventing and addressing emotional and behavioral problems in youth, there has been increasing discussion and action toward expanding mental health services for youth in schools.[33] Schools provide a single point of access to services in a familiar, nonthreatening atmosphere, and placing services in them reduces barriers that constrain the provision of community-based mental health services to youth in need. For youth from the inner city, the presence of these services in schools significantly improves their accessibility. For example, in Baltimore schools, we have found that 80% or more of youth referred for services have had no prior mental health involvement, in spite of significant presenting problems (e.g., depression with suicidal ideation).[34]

Other advantages for school-based mental health services include (1) improved capabilities to provide a full range of preventive services from primary to tertiary[35]; (2) significantly enhanced roles of therapists working in schools, for example, being able to see students in multiple settings (e.g., athletic games, assemblies, in the cafeteria) and over long periods of time (e.g., from 9th through 12th grade); (3) reduced stigma of seeking and receiving mental health services, since they are provided in an environment that is natural for the child; (4) reduced referrals to special education by providing mental health services rapidly and to all children, which serves to reduce costs to educational systems, while avoiding the labeling of children as being in "special ed"[34]; and (5) opportunities to improve the overall environment in schools through collaborative efforts between health and educational staff.[35]

In spite of these advantages, comprehensive mental health services are still not widely available to youth in schools. Although school psychologists and social workers provide the full array of mental health services to all students (including those in regular education) in some localities, in many others, these professionals work exclusively with youth in special education. In the following sections, I review issues related to these more traditional school-based mental health services for youth. This is followed by discussion of models to expand mental health services in schools to the whole student population.

MENTAL HEALTH SERVICES OFFERED THROUGH SPECIAL EDUCATION

The mandate for schools to become involved in the physical, mental, and social health of their students initially came from public laws 93-641 and 94-317, enacted in the early 1970s by the United States Congress.[36] Public Law 94-142, the Education for All Handicapped Children Act of 1975, mandated that each school system provide an appropriate educational program for all handicapped children (including those "handicapped" by emotional and behavioral disorders) in the least restrictive setting possible. It also required specific assessment approaches (e.g., based on multiple measurement strategies, nonbiased), comprehensive evaluations of handicapped children every 3 years, and adherence to due process in identifying, assessing, and developing interventions for handicapped children.[37] Public Law 94-142 was amended in 1990 and renamed the Individuals with Disabilities Education Act (IDEA).[9]

There are over 24,000 school psychologists working in school districts across the United States.[38] Since passage of Public Law 94-142, school psychologists (and in many districts, social workers) must spend a large proportion of time in special education screening, assessment, and treatment planning to ensure compliance with its provisions. For many school psychologists, these involvements have increased over the years, leaving less time for prevention and consultation activities for the whole school population.[39]

School psychologists have expressed their desire to move away from extensive involvement in psychological testing, and to be more involved in providing consultation and direct intervention services.[40,41] Although some have been successful in increasing the amount of time available for consultation,[42] most still spend only a "very small percentage" of their time in direct therapeutic activities with children or their families.[43]

Related to these constraints, some school psychologists are expressing frustration. For example, Johnston wrote:

> The literature and my experiences suggest that the present system is not working. School psychologists are overburdened with traditional caseloads. . . . Only the most severe cases receive attention, all others fall between the cracks. Classroom interventions, too, are often not

carried out, either because the teacher does not have the skill to implement the recommendations, or because the recommendations are not realistic in terms of the classroom structure or curriculum. Ultimately, many children (and teachers) reach maximum frustration levels and give up. Problems that could be dealt with in the early stages, or even prevented, become magnified, and irreversible damage is done.[44(p51)]

The picture that emerges is that traditional mental health services available for children in schools are generally limited to students in special education, and school psychologists (and other mental health staff such as social workers) are overwhelmed with demands associated with Public Law 94-142 (now IDEA) in providing these services. An additional concern is that the availability of special services to address children's emotional and behavioral difficulties decreases as children advance through grades, particularly at secondary levels. As such, services are especially limited for adolescents in regular education.

However, it is important to note that the National Association of School Psychologists (NASP) has strongly endorsed the employment of school psychologists for comprehensive mental health service delivery. Furthermore, in a growing number of school districts in the United States, school psychologists provide a wide range of services including mental health assessment, various therapeutic services, consultation with parents and school personnel, and program planning and evaluation.[38] Notwithstanding these developments, there remains a critical need for the expansion of mental health services for youth in schools.

MODELS FOR EXPANDED SCHOOL MENTAL HEALTH SERVICES

The foregoing discussion suggests a significant need for the provision of preventive (e.g., identification of incipient problems in early elementary youth) and more intensive mental health services (e.g., evaluations; individual, group, and family therapies) to youth in both special and regular education in schools. Across the nation, these "expanded" school mental health services are developing rapidly. In the following sections, I review service delivery models for mental health services for the whole school population.

Programs Developed by University Faculty

It is important to note that in the academic community, there has been long-standing recognition that schools represent a preferred site to provide mental health services to youth,[45] and there are numerous examples of innovative programs that have been developed by university faculty for schools. Prominent examples include (1) the Primary Mental Health Project (PMHP),[46,47] a program that provides supportive services by non- and paraprofessional staff (with professionals in "quarterbacking" roles) to address early behavioral and educational problems in youth identified to be at risk; (2) the Success for All program,[48] which provides intensive training in reading skills, one-to-one tutoring, and a range of mental health and social services to impoverished youth in the early elementary grades; and (3) the School Development Model (SDM),[49] which espouses a multifaceted approach (e.g., creation of school governance teams, parent outreach, curriculum change, mental health prevention, and crisis intervention services) to improve the climate in schools for disadvantaged youth.

Each of these programs is characterized by availability to all students who are determined to be in need, and fairly widespread dissemination in schools throughout the United States. There are numerous other innovative university-based school interventions that have had more limited dissemination.[50]

Efforts to Restructure School Mental Health Services

Adelman and Taylor have recommended a model for allocation of limited school mental health resources.[51] "Mental health specialists," or social workers, psychologists, psychiatrists, and other professionals trained to address emotional, behavioral, or social problems in youth serve as "catalytic agents" within schools. These specialists assist schools in developing programs that will have the broadest impact, given the school's resources. As such, mental health resource development is prioritized, followed by staff development, improving access to community resources, and providing supervision. Provision of direct service (i.e., clinical assessment and treatment) is viewed as a lower order priority "to be pursued as time allows."[51(p36)]

Recently, Adelman has promoted a conceptual model for restructuring traditional school support services (e.g., school-based psychology, social work, guidance counseling, tutoring, and other special support programs) to "enable" (i.e., facilitate, empower) children's learning.[52] A multisystemic approach is recommended, based on resource coordination and involving other elements such as classroom skill training; prevention, crisis intervention, and mental health treatment; supporting students in transition (e.g., from middle school to high school); increasing family involvement in education; and community outreach. The approach is designed to shift the view of school support services (including health and mental health services) from fragmentary and supplemental to foundational to effective learning. Beginning efforts to implement this model in the Los Angeles public schools are underway.

Collaborative Programs Between Schools and Community Agencies

The primary mission of school systems is obviously education, and many do not have the funding or resources to develop comprehensive mental health programs. Community organizations involved in health, including hospitals, community mental health centers, and some universities have the mission and resources to provide these comprehensive services.[8] The more effective school-based mental health programs involve the merging of schools and community agencies, with the latter taking primary responsibility for the development and implementation of the services.[35]

Dryfoos reviewed advantages of school-based programs developed and organized by outside community agencies versus the educational system. These include (1) increased capacity to assume responsibility for organization and delivery of services; (2) greater comprehensiveness of services; (3) knowledge of, and ability to facilitate funding for services (e.g., through Medicaid); (4) independent liability insurance, which relieves schools of a considerable financial burden and risk; and (5) better protection for students' confidentiality, leading to increased comfort by students in seeking services (since staff are viewed as being from an outside agency and not the school).

A SHIFTING LOCUS FOR PRIMARY MENTAL HEALTH SERVICES FROM COM-MUNITY CLINICS TO SCHOOLS. These school-community partnerships are leading to progressive growth in expanded school mental health services. For example, in Baltimore in 1987, there were expanded mental health programs involving such partnerships in three schools. In 1994 there were programs in over 30 schools, and in 1995, programs were operating in over 60 schools. Similarly, in the state of Maryland in 1994, there were expanded mental health services in 90 schools; in 1995, this number increased dramatically, to 140. The most significant growth was for programs placed in elementary schools, with an increase from 39 to 78 schools in the 2 years. Only small increases were shown in middle schools (plus 6) and high schools (plus 1).[53] Such local growth is congruent with regional and national trends on school-based mental health services.[34]

These programs represent a shifting locus of primary mental health care for youth from community clinics to the schools. For example, our School Mental Health Program represents a partnership between the Department of Psychiatry of the University of Maryland School of Medicine and the Baltimore City Public Schools. In this program, therapists provide focused mental health evaluation; psychological and psychiatric consultation; individual, family, and group therapy; and referral of students for more intensive services (e.g., medication, inpatient treatment) in 14 Baltimore City schools (5 elementary, 5 middle, 3 high school, and 1 school for special education students with intellectual handicaps). We also provide a range of preventive and consultative services such as support groups for students in transition (e.g., from elementary to middle school), classroom presentations on mental health issues, and consultation with teachers and health staff regarding child behavioral and emotional problems. Programs sharing this focus of providing intensive and preventive mental health services to youth in schools are operational in many other cities (e.g., Dallas, Texas; Denver, Colorado; New Brunswick, New Jersey; New Haven, Connecticut; Minneapolis, Minnesota; New York City; Memphis, Tennessee), with formal reports on these programs beginning to be circulated at national level planning meetings.

There is a continuum of services developed through these school-community agency partnerships, from augmenting services of existing school mental health staff, to "outstationing" of a mental health provider from a community clinic to a school for a small number of hours per week, to programs that essentially become school-based mental health centers. This latter concept is exemplified by programs in New Brunswick, New Jersey and Orange County, California, in which the majority of mental health services for youth have been essentially shifted away from community sites and into the schools.[8] It is important to emphasize that these school-community partnerships to develop mental health services do not seek to supplant those that already exist (e.g., services provided by school psychologists and social workers). Rather, the focus is on establishing collaborative relationships between schools and community agencies to expand the range of school-based mental health services. In fact, school psychologists and social workers can play an instrumental role in ensuring that these expanded services are appropriately developed and well coordinated.[38]

MENTAL HEALTH SERVICES PROVIDED THROUGH SCHOOL-BASED HEALTH CENTERS. A major factor in the development of expanded mental health services for youth in schools has been the growth of school-based health centers (SBHCs). This movement began in relation to general concerns about the health of adolescents, and particular concerns regarding psychological and educational risks associated with adolescent pregnancy and parenting.[54] By 1987, there were approximately 150 SBHCs operating in junior and senior high schools throughout the country.[54] In 1990, Hyche-Williams and Waszak reported that there were 178 SBHCs operating in junior and senior high schools in 32 states.[55] In 1993, the Center for Population Options reported over 500 SBHCs.[56] In the most recent survey, Schlitt, Rickett, Montgomery, and Lear reported 607 SBHCs located in 41 states and in the District of Columbia.[57] The report indicated that 46% of the SBHCs were placed in high schools, 28% in elementary schools, 16% in middle schools, and 10% in "other" schools. SBHCs are located primarily in urban, medically underserved areas, but are increasingly being developed in rural and suburban areas.[58]

Mental health services offered in SBHCs occur in the context of a range of other primary-care services including medical screening and physical examinations on site, treatment for accidents and minor illnesses, family planning services, immunizations, and a range of health education programs. Commonly, staff in SBHCs include a medical assistant, nurse practitioner or physician assistant, and a mental health professional (usually a master's level social worker) to address the psychosocial needs of the students. SBHCs are almost always run by outside community agencies, such as local health departments. The model SBHC "offers age-appropriate, comprehensive physical and mental health services through a multidisciplinary team of health professionals."[58(p101)]

Lear, Gleicher, St. Germaine, and Porter reported on a project funded by the Robert Wood Johnson Foundation, which assisted in the development of 23 SBHCs in 11 states.[59] Descriptive analyses of the programs indicated that mental health concerns were the second most frequent reason for visits to the health center (21% of visits) behind acute illness or accidents (26% of visits). In addition, the report emphasized awareness of all staff in the centers of the critically important role psychosocial issues have on adolescent health concerns. Dryfoos noted that providers in SBHCs often refer to mental health counseling as their greatest unmet need.[8] She quoted one provider: "As soon as we open our doors, kids walk past the counselor's office, past the school nurse, past the principal, and come into our clinic to tell us that they have been sexually abused or that their parents are drug users."[8(p52)] Across SBHCs, Dryfoos characterized the demand for mental health services as "overwhelming."

Baltimore currently contains 16 SBHCs. It is notable that in this city, these SBHCs were the first sites for expanded school mental health services. Since then, mental health services have been added to schools without health centers, based in large part on lessons learned from the SBHCs. As such, school-based health centers can serve as demonstration sites for expanded mental health services in cities and localities. As the health centers gain experience in the provision of mental health services, their expertise can be shared to promote the development of these services in other schools.

Although there has been growth in mental health services offered through SBHCs, gaps remain. In 1994, Advocates for Youth (AFY, formerly the Center for Population Options) reported on a survey of 231 school-based and school-linked (i.e., located off school grounds, but involving collaborative relationships between community health agencies and specific schools) health centers on their 1992–1993 activities and operations.[60] Over 85% of centers offered mental health services to address problems including substance abuse, depression, anger, sexual abuse, and dysfunctional family systems. Approximately 49% of programs offered group counseling; the most common topics were children of substance abusers (25%), self-esteem enhancement (20%), general support (16%), and coping with sexual abuse (15%). Notably, only 36% of programs providing mental health services used mental health professionals in the provision of these services; "remaining respondents used various other staff to fulfill the counseling tasks."[60(p24)]

A GROWING MOVEMENT TO INSTITUTIONALIZE SCHOOL-BASED HEALTH AND MENTAL HEALTH SERVICES. As is increasingly evident, expanded mental health services are being developed in schools as part of a broader movement to bring comprehensive health services to youth in schools. Three organizations have played an integral role in this rapidly developing movement:

1. Advocates for Youth is a national organization that aims to improve decisions by youth about sexuality. AFY has conducted annual surveys on school health programs and offers a range of technical assistance services.
2. Making the Grade, an organization sponsored by the Robert Wood Johnson Foundation, aims to develop partnerships between states and communities to expand and improve school-based health services.
3. The School Health Policy Initiative (SHPI) of Columbia University has conducted a series of national work group meetings to analyze and make policy recommendations on issues critical to the development of school health services.

These three organizations, along with professional groups such as the American School Health Association (ASHA) and federal agencies such as the Health Resources and Services Administration (HRSA) and the Centers for Disease Control (CDC) played a critical role in the development of the National Assembly on School-Based Health Care (NASBHC). The NASBHC is a new organization (inaugural meeting in June 1995) developed in response to the increasing growth of school-based health centers and the absence of a large coordinating body. It aims to improve coordination of research, technical assistance, and advocacy for school-based health care and to provide a membership organization for school health providers, planners, and supporters.

The newly formed Psychosocial Services Section of NASBHC includes providers and planners of mental health services in SBHCs. This group has begun efforts to identify a list of school mental health programs, along with descriptions of programs and presenting problems of students to begin to document the constellation of services and problems addressed by expanded school mental health services.

FULL-SERVICE SCHOOLS. Comprehensive mental health services would be one component of what Dryfoos refers to as "full-service schools." She wrote:

The vision of the full-service school puts the best of school reform together with all other services that children, youth, and their families need, most of which can be located in a school building. The educational mandate places responsibility on the school system to reorganize and innovate. The charge to community agencies is to bring into the school: health, mental health, employment services, child care, parent education, case management, recreation, cultural events, community policing, and whatever else may fit into the picture. The result is a new kind of "seamless" institution, a community-oriented school with a joint governance structure that allows maximum responsiveness to the community, as well as accessibility and continuity for those most in need of services.[8(p12)]

Dryfoos's vision for schools to become "hubs" in communities for education, health, mental health, social, and vocational services is stirring enthusiastic discussion around the country.[8] However, very few schools in the United States are approximating this vision (San Diego's New Beginnings Program and Hanshaw Middle School in Modesto, California are exceptions). Instead, there is wide variability, with some schools having no supportive services, others having singular and isolated programs, and still others having multiple service components with multiple agency involvement.[8]

As reviewed in the previous sections, expanded school mental health services based on partnerships between school and community agencies offer the best opportunity for institutionalizing these services. Although some of the earlier mentioned university-based programs have produced impressive results (e.g., Success for All),[48] these programs are unlikely to become institutionalized on a *national* level. Such university-based programs are usually characterized by adequate research methodology but a failure to extend implementation across heterogenous populations, particularly to address the array of problems of disadvantaged youth.[61] In contrast, expanded mental health services provided in the contexts of SBHCs are developing rapidly, with over 600 programs in almost every state of the United States.[57] In essence, the development of SBHCs and their associated services represents a significant national movement to bring health and mental health services to youth "where they are." This movement offers vast clinical, program development, and research opportunities for mental health professionals. In the context of this movement, critical issues attendant to these developments are reviewed next.

BROAD CRITICAL ISSUES

Limited Knowledge of Existing Programs

We conducted a recent literature review on the development of school-based mental health services.[34] This review highlighted that in spite of significant growth, little information on mental health services associated with school health services has been published or disseminated. Considerable activity has occurred to establish school mental health services nationwide, but there are few methods to capture this activity. Thus, planners and analysts of these services must rely on information provided by professional groups such as Advocates for Youth and Making the Grade. The movement to provide expanded school mental health services is so new that we do not yet know where the services are, let alone information on ideal patterns of staffing or service delivery models. Fortunately, efforts are underway through NASBHC to more systematically document the status of school-based mental health services nationwide. These assessments will serve as the preliminary step in planning to develop and improve expanded school mental health services.

Funding Issues

Funding issues are obviously critical to the development of expanded school mental health services. In Baltimore, these services are funded through at least five different mechanisms. There is considerable overlap in funding sources, and many of the local streams have state or federal support underpinning them. While enabling mental health services in more schools, this mixed funding pattern creates administrative problems related to different contractual and reporting requirements for each of the funding streams.[34]

Limited cost-efficiency data that are available suggest costs of around $8,000 per pupil per year for children receiving special education services under the classification "severely emotionally disturbed."[37] Clearly, mental health services provided through school health centers cost much less than this amount, and the diversion of children from special education to these health services is viewed as cost saving by special education administrators. Furthermore, we have seen a decrease in referrals for special education services by about one-third after clinical therapists have been placed in schools.[34] Data on cost savings to educational systems can be used by school health centers to lobby communities for funds for the development and/or expansion of mental health services.

Managed care is having a very significant impact on funding for school-based health and mental health services. For example, in Maryland, legislation has passed indicating that students in Medicaid must have a primary, coordinating medical provider. In order for services to be reimbursed, this provider (individual physician or HMO) must authorize the service, and programs are encountering significant problems in obtaining such authorization.

Perhaps more significantly, in Baltimore and other localities, "aggressive strategies" are in place to enroll students with Medicaid in managed care companies.[62] Almost uniformly, these companies have been unwilling to authorize school-based mental health services. As more and more students are enrolled in these companies, funding for school-based mental health services can be expected to decrease significantly.

To address these problems, the School Health Policy Initiative (SHPI) and other groups have recommended that school health administrators form relationships with managed care companies. This is beginning to occur, and some managed care companies are even funding SBHCs.[63] Other strategies being discussed to fund school-based health and mental health services include using surplus funds from adult-focused community mental health activities, and developing state financial support for services through excise taxes.[57]

Detailed discussion of funding issues is beyond the scope of this chapter. Needless to say, considerable activity will be needed in this area to ensure that school health and mental health services do, in fact, become institutionalized. In addition, efforts are needed at state and national levels to advocate for support of school mental health services. Unfortunately, children's mental health groups have not had the financial and political resources to significantly impact policymakers in the administration and Congress.[64]

Poor Planning of Services

Although most school-based health and mental health programs are located in lower income, urban areas, services are usually not added based on any systematic strategy (e.g., the percentage of students receiving reduced/free lunches).[8] Adelman and Taylor conducted a survey of all existing mental health programs in a Los Angeles school district.[51]

In analyzing 56 programs that targeted student adjustment problems, the most striking issue was that programs seemed to be developed in a "piecemeal" fashion, with no overall plan, and "a great deal of uncoordinated activity."[51(p33)] Services were developed at some schools but not at others with seemingly equal need. This is congruent with experiences in Baltimore, where schools appear to obtain mental health programs based on the interest of the principal versus documentation of relative need (some schools with nearly 2,000 students have no expanded mental health services, whereas schools as small as 350 contain them).

A related issue is the control principals and school administrators typically have over services offered in their building. In many school districts, the prevailing view is that education is the primary if not only function, with mental health services being viewed as beyond the reach and scope of an educational institution. One strategy to promote acceptance of mental health services by school administrators is to help them determine how these services can enhance their educational mission.[8] However, even with intensive and persuasive efforts, some school administrators continue to be resistant to expanded mental health services in their schools. This means that even with careful planning for allocation of school mental health resources, some of the more needy schools (e.g., as determined by income, unemployment, and crime statistics) will go without mental health services.

Poor Integration of School and Community Services

A serious problem is the failure of most school-based health and mental health services to be integrated with other services in the local community. Many issues are relevant here. For example, applied research programs are often developed and implemented by university faculty who fail to seek input from community representatives on the intervention. Similarly, health and mental health services are started with little, if any, input from community members. Even when services are developed with community involvement, they are often not effectively integrated into the array of other community resources and programs.[34]

Efforts to increase mental health services available to youth in schools are occurring in a broader context of reform of children's mental health services (e.g., the CASSP). These reform efforts seek to change organizational and financial structures to reduce barriers to services, improve coordination between systems, and provide a range of services tailored to the specific needs of children.[32]

Recently, considerable attention has been paid to developing comprehensive and multiple system approaches to address the needs of youth with severe emotional and behavioral difficulties. For example, multisystemic therapy (MST)[6] is a comprehensive treatment approach involving intervention at individual, family, school, and community levels that has been shown to be effective for delinquent youth.[65,66] More recent efforts have extended the model to problems of adolescent substance abuse and severe emotional disturbance, and preliminary findings are encouraging.[65]

In general, the public mental health system has identified as its top priority individuals with severe disorders,[5] and approaches such as MST appear to be the most effective for youth with severe disorders. However, it is important to not let attention to the needs of severely disturbed youth preclude the development of preventive programs for youth without, or with incipient, disturbances. Analyzing child health and mental health systems, Weissberg, Caplan, and Harwood noted that the preponderance of resources were directed at the most ill children and strongly argued for more attention to primary prevention efforts that are system or group oriented and directed toward healthy children.[67]

Analyses are needed that consider the continuum of mental health services for youth from primary to secondary to tertiary preventive activities, and where and in what fashion to provide services at various points on this continuum.[68] One plausible schema is reviewed in Table 19.1. In this scheme, primary, secondary, and some tertiary prevention activities are provided in schools. For example, services in schools would include educational activities on mental health issues; screening of students for emotional and behavioral problems; providing support groups for students under stress (e.g., during educational transitions, to address exposure to violence); assisting in the development of schoolwide programs to address pressing concerns (e.g., conflict mediation training); and individual, group, and family therapy services for youth with emotional and behavioral disturbances. These services would be developed to be complementary to services provided by school psychologists and social workers (or, in some communities, would actually be provided by school psychologists and social workers). Generally reflective of their current functions, community mental health centers would provide secondary and tertiary preventive services, such as therapy services for more severely

Table 19.1   Schema for Organizing Preventive Child Mental Health Programs.

	Prevention continuum		
	Primary	Secondary	Tertiary
School-based programs			
Mental health centers			
Multisystemic programs			

Note: Primary preventive efforts target populations at risk, before the development of the problem of concern; secondary preventive efforts target individuals showing early manifestation of the problem; and tertiary preventive efforts aim to minimize negative sequelae of established disorders.[69]

disturbed youth, psychopharmacological assessment and treatment, and referral for more intensive services such as inpatient treatment. Multisystemic programs (as in MST) would provide exclusively tertiary preventive services for youth who meet some cutoff for severity of disturbance (e.g., based on presenting diagnoses, chronicity of disorder). We are using this scheme at the University of Maryland in planning for children's mental health services and have found it useful in attempting to create a true continuum of services.

Recently, the Section on Clinical Child Psychology of the Division of Clinical Psychology of the American Psychological Association (APA) reported on a task force on Innovative Models of Mental Health Services for Children, Adolescents, and Their Families. In this report, Duchnowski reviewed innovative models of service delivery in education.[9] However, this review was restricted to services available to students in special education, because "very few schools have services for children with serious mental health needs that are part of the regular education program."[9(p13)] Thereafter, the report made almost no reference to services available to students in regular education. Reports such as this help to embed the concept that mental health services in schools are primarily for students in special education. For schools to play a significant role in addressing the continuum of children's mental health needs (as mentioned), a more expansive view of the potential for mental health services within them is needed.

Limited Evaluation of School Mental Health Services

Evaluation of school-based mental health services has been quite limited, with most of these efforts at the descriptive level. For example, the U.S. Department of Health and Human Services recently reported findings from an evaluation of seven SBHCs in rural and urban areas of the United States.[70] The report highlighted the limited access to health and mental health resources for many of the students, in spite of the high levels of health-related problems found in their communities (e.g., teenage pregnancy, infant mortality, family and community violence, child abuse and neglect). Substance abuse and mental health problems were reported to be particularly prevalent. Importantly, the report underscored the general absence of program outcome data; although there were selected reports of positive impact of the SBHCs (e.g., in reducing teenage pregnancies and school absences), these findings were based on uncontrolled evaluation designs.

Analyzing the state of affairs for assessment of outcomes of school health and mental health services, Dryfoos commented that "the limitations of published evaluations of the impact of school-based services programs on health and educational outcomes are undeniable."[8(p133)] Similarly, Barnett, Niebuhr, Baldwin, and Levine provided this cautionary note in discussing school-based mental health services: "Outcomes often have been poorly documented because of the public demand for quick remedies. As a result, these programs consume time and energy of school staff without producing convincing results."[71(p246)] Adelman and Taylor characterized evaluations of school mental health services as limited and narrowly focused, and called attention to the negligible research on cost-effectiveness of these services, as well as their possible iatrogenic effects.[51]

Prout and De Martino conducted a meta-analysis of school-based psychotherapy programs.[72] Thirty-three studies involving some type of school-based counseling services were evaluated. Results suggested that group therapies were more effective than individual approaches, behavioral approaches were more effective than others, and treatment targets most responsive to intervention were observable behaviors and problem-solving abilities. However, many of the studies cited in this review were not controlled, and a wide number of approaches were reported by relatively few studies, constraining the power of statistical analyses.

Since this review, we identified only two studies involving controlled assessment of the impact of *ongoing* school mental health services (i.e., vs. those associated with a special program). Lavoritano and Segal assessed school counseling services provided by master's level school counselors to 141 students (aged 8 to 13) in private schools in Philadelphia and the surrounding county.[73] A comparison of pre- and posttreatment responses on a measure of self-perceived competency revealed that students evidenced gains in scholastic self-perception only, and showed a small *decline* in global self-worth. In a recently completed study, we assessed the treatment outcome of mental health services for ninth graders enrolled in a school-based health clinic in Baltimore.[74] Compared to students receiving no mental health treatment ($n = 34$), treated students ($n = 39$) showed improvements in self-concept and decreased depression scores following the receipt of individual and/or group therapy services.

Numerous issues constrain the ability to track the impact of school-based mental health services in sophisticated fashion. These include pragmatic difficulties of randomly assigning children to treatment versus control conditions; high mobility of students across schools, particularly in urban areas; and difficulty in establishing causes for measured outcomes due to the coexistence of other programs and educational reform efforts.[75]

There is recognition of the need for standardization in descriptive statistics for school-based health programs. Many programs have systems in place to record presenting problems of students and the types of services rendered. Additionally, computerized systems of data collection have been implemented across school health sites in different states such as "School Health Care—On Line!!!" by David Kaplan.[8] However, such systems have generally not been established for mental health services. Programs that have systems in place to describe mental health problems and services are inadequate (e.g., use of idiosyncratic methods to record presenting problems of students). Other mental health programs have no systems in place to track students presenting problems or provided services.

There is a significant need to implement standard measures of psychosocial factors and emotional/behavioral difficulties for students who present for school mental health services. Such efforts are beginning to occur in some school-based programs. For example, clinicians in 12 schools of the University of Maryland School Mental Health Program collected standard measures of life stress, violence exposure, family support, self-concept, and emotional/behavioral functioning for youth aged 11 to 18 who presented for services. Preliminary analyses of these data indicated high levels of violence exposure for referred youth, and expected associations between life stress, violence exposure, and emotional/behavioral problems.[31]

Fortunately, developments to organize school health and mental health providers are occurring rapidly. As mentioned, the NASBHC and its Psychosocial Services Section are in the process of planning a survey of mental health service needs and programs for mental health providers from across the country. The Maternal and Child Health Bureau (MCHB) of the Health Resources and Services Administration has funded two national technical assistance and training centers to provide support to school-based health programs in developing and expanding mental health services. These centers, located at the University of Maryland at Baltimore and the University of California at Los Angeles, should be well established in mid-1996.

Need for Specialty Training in School-Based Mental Health

Juszczak, Fisher, Lear, and Friedman conducted a survey of training in school health for allied health disciplines in 9 SBHCs funded by the Robert Wood Johnson Foundation.[58] Around half of the programs included traineeships for graduate students in social work, psychology, or psychiatry. Program directors noted generally that trainees were well accepted by students, and the presence of trainees assisted the centers in providing services to more students. The study highlighted other advantages to such training programs, including experience in "front line" clinical services, hands-on exposure to the "complexities" of practicing in a SBHC, expanding the range of offered services, and decreasing feelings of isolation among school health staff.

Graduate training programs for disciplines of clinical psychology, social work, psychiatry, and psychiatric nursing generally do not include systematic preparation for trainees to work in schools as primary clinical sites. As the movement to provide expanded mental health services to youth in schools grows, there will be an increasing need for graduate-level training programs in these related disciplines to prepare clinicians for work in the school setting. The role of school psychologists in providing these expanded mental health services also needs analysis. Issues confronted by mental health professionals working in schools are next reviewed.

CRITICAL ISSUES CONFRONTING
SCHOOL-BASED CLINICIANS

Differences Between Services
in Schools and Community Clinics

In community mental health centers, a common scenario is for seven or eight children to be scheduled per day for each therapist, and for three to five 50-minute sessions to be actually held. Mental health services usually have a discrete beginning and end, and, related to pressures associated with managed care, services are often limited to six or less sessions. Children require clear diagnoses to be seen, and if they do not present clear diagnoses, they are either "creatively" fit into a diagnostic category or not seen. After termination, the therapist is unlikely to see the child again. Although this may reflect a stereotyping of children's outpatient mental health services, it begins to capture the reality of such services for most therapists.

Mental health services that are provided in schools are often dramatically different from the aforementioned picture of community mental health centers. In most school-based programs, children do not require diagnoses to be seen. Following intake sessions, which may run 50 minutes, students are seen in meaningful therapeutic encounters for briefer periods of time, such as 30 or even 15 minutes. Many of these sessions are scheduled, but others are impromptu, with students stopping in for a brief problem-solving session or to share some news with the therapist. Given that the therapist is where the children are, there is no reason for down time in his or her schedule; if one student does not show for an appointment, usually another one can be quickly found. The school therapist has contact with students not only in the therapy office, but in the hallway, at schoolwide events (e.g., assemblies), athletic games, in the cafeteria, and so on. Given these environmental factors, it is not uncommon for school-based therapists to see 10–12 children in a 7-hour day.

Unlike services provided in community mental health centers, contact with students does not have to end, with some relationships with students lasting from the 6th through 8th, or 9th through 12 grades (and sometimes longer). In such long-term relationships, at times clinicians are providing traditionally conceived therapy services, but at other times (e.g., when there are no clear presenting problems), the therapist becomes more of a mentor to the student (e.g., providing encouragement and practical support). This transitioning back and forth from the role of therapist to mentor is neither possible, nor feasible, in community mental health clinics (or in private practice).

Intensive Clinical and Administrative Demands

Related to limited funding, many school-based mental health programs are staffed by one (usually master's level) clinician. Funds for mental health services are often limited to salary support, with many funding agencies not paying for supervision or administration of the program. Generally, salary support is inadequate, creating problems in recruitment of skilled and, especially, experienced therapists. Therapists are commonly faced with intensive clinical demands associated with large caseloads and very high mental health encounters. In our program, full-time therapists usually see more than 100 children a year, maintain active caseloads of 40 or more youth, have over 40 clinical contacts (assessment and treatment sessions) per week, and over 800 clinical contacts in an academic year. In addition to clinical services, there are obvious paperwork demands, case management activities, and actions that need to be taken to arrange for contacts with students (e.g., scheduling and finding them). Furthermore, related to demands of managed care and the absence of administrative support, clinicians are forced to contact physicians to gain authorization to see youth. This can be a highly time-consuming and frustrating process.

A related issue is that mental health providers are employees of agencies outside of the educational system. As such, programs commonly need to beg and barter for office space, telephones, and so forth. Clinicians are often moved from one inadequate office space to the next and usually either do not have a phone, or have to share one with numerous other health and/or educational staff.

Low salaries, isolation, absence of support, intensive clinical, case management and administrative demands; poor office space; and limited telephone access combine to make school-based mental health services highly stressful. Clinicians are very susceptible to burnout, and turnover in these positions tends to be fairly high.

Identifying Students in Need

A challenge for school-based clinicians is developing mechanisms to receive appropriate referrals. Teachers are likely to refer children of mental health services for externalizing behaviors such as talking out of turn, being out of their seats, noncompliance, and disruptiveness.[43] In addition, there is a view among school psychologists that teachers are often not requesting assistance to develop interventions when making referrals for mental health services. Rather, the "desired intervention" is removal of the child from the classroom to be placed in special education services.[44]

Related to this, internalizing problems such as depression, anxiety, and social withdrawal do not consistently lead to referral for services by educational staff.[76] However, in programs that operate in conjunction with SBHCs, our experience has been that medical staff (e.g., nurse practitioners) regularly screen youth for depression, suicidal ideation, anxiety, and trauma symptoms, facilitating referral of youth with internalizing problems for mental health services.[34] Many SBHCs incorporate formal screening measures for these problems.

Regardless of the school setting (i.e., containing an SBHC or not), mental health staff usually need to conduct educational activities with other staff in the school to assist them in recognizing emotional/behavioral problems in youth and referring them for services.

Getting Students to Use School Mental Health Services

Lear et al. documented difficulties in some school health centers in getting students to use medical services.[59] Similarly, many youngsters in need do not utilize mental health services offered through the health center. For example, in a recent study, we found that students who used a school-based health center intensively were more likely to report significant emotional distress.[77] However, less than one-third of these distressed students were actually receiving mental health services. This finding highlights the fact that medical staff should consider intensive health center use as a marker of potential emotional/behavioral difficulties, and that staff should attempt to connect intensive users to mental health staff. We also found that students rated as socially withdrawn by their peers were much less likely to seek out the health center than more outgoing youth, pointing to the need for outreach efforts to offer mental health services to such youth.

In a survey of 471 high school juniors and seniors from Los Angeles on their use of school-based mental health services, Barker and Adelman found "low levels of utilization despite apparently widespread need."[78] The authors suggested that providing accessible mental health services in schools is "a necessary but insufficient condition for increasing the likelihood that people will seek out professional help when they need it."[78(p261)]

Integrating the Clinician into the School

School health programs implementing mental health services confront obstacles such as poor knowledge of these services and resistance or unwillingness by staff to cooperate with the new clinician. School health staff are often viewed as "outsiders" by staff hired by the Department of Education. This is particularly true for mental health staff. Generally, in the first year of mental health services, considerable efforts are needed by the clinician to meet and form alliances with school staff, and practically demonstrate the benefit of his or her services with a few salient clinical successes.

A related issue is that teachers and school personnel often form "high hopes" after referring a child for mental health services. Despite these high hopes, teachers have reported feelings of disappointment in their relationships with mental health professionals. Problems attributed to mental health staff include failing to seek teacher input, providing "already known" and simplistic formulations of children, making excessively cumbersome or vague recommendations for classroom interventions, and not reporting back to teachers on the progress of the student.[43,79,80]

Particularly in middle schools and high schools, mental health practitioners will be confronted with stigma and misconceptions about their services by students and faculty. Our experience has been that students generally do not understand the title *psychologist,* associating it with "crazy people." Similarly, the terms *therapist* and *clinician* generally do not have meaning for them. As a result, psychologists in our program refer to themselves as *counselors,* which seems to avoid the pejorative connotation of *psychologist* and is a term that most students understand and accept. However, use of this title creates some problems in distinguishing the role of the school-based clinician from guidance counselors, who also use this title.

Privacy and Confidentiality Issues

Most middle school and high school students expect their visits to the mental health provider to be kept private, and school clinicians generally do all they can to respect students' desires for such privacy. However, unique confidentiality problems arise in the school setting. There are many opportunities for students to be associated with mental health staff, which can lead to problems with other students (e.g., teasing about "being crazy"). School-based clinicians should attempt to be sensitive to these concerns by arranging for the student to receive services as privately as possible, for example, sending passes for students to attend mental health sessions without providers specified, being careful about talking to treated students in front of other students (and allowing some of them to walk 10 feet behind on the way to the therapy office!).

Most school mental health programs keep records separate from the educational record and the health records in programs having on-site health services. However, there are often requests from teachers and other school staff (including health providers) for information on students who are receiving mental health services. Standards vary across programs, with some strictly not releasing any information to anyone without a signed release of information form from the student and his or her parents, and other programs adhering to a "looser" policy. One approach that is fairly common is for mental health staff to release process information (e.g., whether a student is attending sessions), but not content information, to select staff designated by the student as important. Release of more than process information to these staff would require more formal permission from the student and his or her parents.

Issues of Race and Cultural Sensitivity

As reviewed earlier, expanded school mental health services are more likely to be found in urban, economically deprived areas, in which Caucasians are a racial minority. However, programs often have difficulty in recruiting staff of the predominant racial/cultural background of their district, or there is such heterogeneity in racial/cultural backgrounds that it would be difficult for staff to be reflective of the community. Although progress in this area has been made, a common scenario remains for a Caucasian therapist to be placed in a school that is primarily African-American. Most programs learn that issues of racial differences are relatively minor, provided that school-based clinicians are nonprejudiced, demonstrate that they truly care about their work, and are knowledgeable and sensitive about issues of cultural diversity.[81,82] However, even given these qualities, a reality is that a relatively small proportion of students and staff will avoid the clinician because of his or her race. This reality points to the need for the clinician to directly address issues of racial awareness in interactions with students and teachers, but also to accept an unfortunate limit to the boundaries of his or her work.

Coordinating Mental Health Services within Schools

As reviewed by Adelman and Taylor and Flaherty et al., mental health services within schools are often not coordinated with each other.[34,51] This leads to duplication of some services (e.g., one student seeing multiple providers) and gaps in others (e.g., the absence of substance-abuse services). Commenting on services provided in a Los Angeles school district Adelman wrote, "The ad hoc way in which programs were developed was reflected in the fragmented, piecemeal function in which they operated."[52]

As noted earlier, there are a number of disciplines that may be involved in providing mental health services to students. In most school districts (with many exceptions) assessment-oriented mental health services are provided by social workers and school psychologists to students in special education. Most districts also contain guidance counselors in middle and high schools who provide academic and career guidance, as well as some counseling for personal issues. However, most guidance counselors have responsibility for hundreds of students, which severely limits their accessibility. Also, there is variability in training background, with some guidance counselors not trained to address complex psychosocial issues.[8]

"Clinical" staff brought in to provide more intensive services (including treatment) to the whole school population must integrate their services with services provided by "traditional" mental health staff as mentioned earlier. Most commonly, these clinical staff are licensed social workers and clinical psychologists, but staff from other disciplines such as psychiatry, counseling psychology, marriage and family therapy, psychiatric nursing, and addictions counseling may be involved in the provision of expanded mental health services in a school.

There is considerable variability in mental health staffing across schools. Some may have essentially no mental health staff, some have only guidance counselors, and others have a range of traditional and clinical staff. Regardless of how limited or comprehensive mental health services in a school are, it is important for mental health staff to work closely together. In one high school in our program, the "Mental Health Team" comprises staff from the disciplines of clinical psychology, school psychology, school social work, and guidance counseling, who work closely together to avoid duplication in services, plan for difficult issues (e.g., how to handle crisis), and initiate schoolwide interventions to address pressing problems. In the past year, this team has initiated a program to promote sexual responsibility (and abstinence) for high school students, implemented a crisis-intervention plan, initiated a peer counseling program, and conducted a range of classroom presentations, assemblies, and group therapies aimed at preventing and coping with violence. Teachers have expressed appreciation for these activities and have requested the development of support groups for them to assist in stress management. These efforts have served to improve the integration of mental health staff into the school, and have also contributed to global positive impacts in the school climate.

It is important for staff from various disciplines to work together collegially, without preconceived perceptions of superiority of one discipline over another (referred to as "professional arrogance" by Conoley and Conoley).[43] For example, clinical psychologists, psychiatrists, and social workers need to be careful to not disparage the abilities of other disciplines such as school psychology and guidance counseling to provide intensive services such as individual therapy for troubled students. Rather, discussions should be held with representatives from these disciplines in which respective roles are defined. Such discussions usually lead to deference by staff such as guidance counselors to clinical staff when faced with issues such as suicidal ideation in students.

Negotiating "turf" issues is also a challenge.[8] For example, in Baltimore, a common scenario has been that outside clinical therapists are placed in schools to provide more intensive services including individual, group, and family therapy. School social workers and psychologists are tied down with administrative and assessment tasks, primarily with students in special education, and may resent the relative freedom of the clinical therapist, as well as his or her opportunity to provide treatment services. In these situations, considerable efforts are needed by the new clinical therapist to establish relationships with existing school staff, and to mutually plan for the expansion of mental health services.[43]

Involving Families in School Mental Health Services

Lack of meaningful involvement of families has been a complex issue for school-based programs. In many cases, expanded health and mental health services are placed in schools in economically disadvantaged areas. Families in the surrounding area typically must contend with a range of stressors associated with economic hardship, nonoptimal living conditions, crime, and so on. In the context of these stressors, it is often difficult for families to come to the school to work with health and mental health providers in treatment of their children. A frequent lament of health and mental health practitioners concerns the serious difficulties encountered in involving families in services, resulting in minimal or absent involvement by most families.

Difficulties in involving families are not limited to school health and mental health services. Education staff often have very limited relationships with families, with communication limited to report cards and telephone calls around specific problems. Most schools do not have established methods for schools and parents to systematically share information, and parents generally play a very limited role in educational decision making for their child. This lack of information flow can contribute to an adversarial quality between parents and school staff.[43] Efforts to involve parents as collaborators with school staff can assist with this problem. For example, some school systems have involved parents in decision making regarding school social services, outreach efforts into the community, and advocacy efforts for students.[8]

With regard to school health and mental services, there are differences in involving families of elementary versus high school aged youth.[8] Generally, involving families in mental health services is more necessary and easier with younger youth (e.g., parents are more likely to bring them to, and pick them up from, school). Mental health efforts with adolescents are often based on their choice to initiate services, and in some cases, a goal is to foster independence from a dysfunctional family. As such, services can be provided relatively independent of family involvement, which is much more difficult in traditional community settings (e.g., community mental health centers).

CONCLUDING COMMENTS

Although mental health services have been available in schools for more than four decades,[43] it is only recently that a full range of services (from primary to tertiary preventive) have become available to youth in special *and regular* education in primary and secondary schools throughout the country. For the most part, these expanded school mental health services have resulted from partnerships between schools and community agencies, with primary responsibility for the services taken by the latter. Exemplifying these partnerships are SBHCs, which are developing rapidly across the country, based on widespread support for the concept of schools as sites for primary health care for youth. Mental health services are developing lock step with SBHCs, with health staff identifying mental health problems as "overwhelming" and treatment services for them as their "greatest need." In essence, there is a significant national movement under way to "institutionalize" school health and mental health services, as provided by local community agencies working in schools. However, much activity related to this movement has not been published, and there is a prevailing view that mental health services in schools are assessment oriented and limited to students in special education. In reality, if trends continue, primary mental health care will begin to shift from community mental health centers and private offices to the schools, offering vast opportunities for those who are interested in improving mental health services for children. This review has attempted to capture this movement, its opportunities, and its limitations.

Appreciation is extended to Lois Flaherty and Beth Warner for ideas generated in an earlier paper and to Nicole Dorsey for assistance in identifying and reviewing the extant literature.

This research is supported in part by Project No. MCJ24SH02-01-0 from the Maternal and Child Health Bureau (Title V, Social Security Act), Health Resources and Services Administration, U.S. Department of Health and Human Services.

Notes

1. Knitzer J. *Unclaimed Children: The Failure of Public Responsibility to Children and Adolescents in Need of Mental Health Services.* Washington, DC: Children's Defense Fund; 1982.
2. Day C, Roberts MC. Activities of the Children and Adolescent Service System Program for improving mental health services for children and families. *J Clin Child Psychol.* 1991;20:340–350.
3. Knitzer J, Cole E. *Family Preservation Services: The Policy Challenge to State Child Welfare and Child Mental Health Systems.* New York, NY: Bank Street College of Education; 1989.
4. Henggeler SW, Borduin CM. *Family Therapy and Beyond: A Multisystematic Approach to Treating the Behavior Problems of Children and Adolescents.* Pacific Grove, Calif: Brooks/Cole; 1990.

5. Duchnowski AJ, Friedman RM. Children's mental health: challenges for the nineties. *J Ment Health Adm.* 1990;17:3–12.

6. Burns BJ, Friedman RM. Examining the research base for child mental health services and policy. *J Ment Health Adm.* 1990;17:87–97.

7. Weisz JR, Weiss B. *Effects of Psychotherapy with Children and Adolescents.* Newbury Park, Calif: Sage; 1993.

8. Dryfoos JG. *Full-Service Schools: A Revolution in Health and Social Services for Children, Youth, and Families.* San Francisco, Calif: Jossey-Bass; 1994.

9. Duchnowski AJ. Innovative service models: education. *J Clin Child Psychol.* 1994;23:13–18.

10. U.S. Congress, Office of Technology Assessment. *Adolescent Health.* Washington, DC: US GPO; 1991.

11. Zahner GE, Pawelklewicz W, Di Francesco JJ, Adnopoz J. Children's mental health service needs and utilization patterns in an urban community: an epidemiological assessment. *J Am Acad Child Adolesc Psychiatry.* 1992;31:951–960.

12. Goodwin LD, Goodwin WL, Cantrill JL. The mental health needs of elementary school children. *J Sch Health.* 1988;7:282–287.

13. Duncan G. The economic environment of childhood. In: Huston AC, ed. *Children in Poverty.* New York, NY: Cambridge University Press; 1991:23–50.

14. Prothrow-Stith D. *Deadly Consequences: How Violence Is Destroying Our Teenage Population and a Plan to Begin Solving the Problem.* New York, NY: HarperCollins; 1991.

15. Shakoor BH, Chalmers D. Co-victimization of African-American children who witness violence: effects on cognitive, emotional, and behavioral development. *J Nat Med Assoc.* 1991;83:233–238.

16. Garbarino J. A preliminary study of some ecological correlates of child abuse: the impact of socioeconomic stress on mothers. *Child Dev.* 1976;47:178–185.

17. Rutter M, Quinton D. Psychiatric disorder: ecological factors and concepts of causation. In: McGurk H, ed. *Ecological Factors in Human Development.* Amsterdam, Netherlands: Elsevier North Holland; 1977.

18. Hofferth S, Hayes C. *Risking the Future: Adolescent Sexuality, Pregnancy, and Childbearing: Statistical Appendices.* Washington, DC: National Academy Press; 1987.

19. Blum R. Contemporary threats to adolescent health in the United States. *JAMA.* 1987;257:3390–3395.

20. Elliot DS, Huizinga D, Menard S. *Multiple-Problem Youth: Delinquency, Substance Abuse, and Mental Health Problems.* New York, NY: Springer-Verlag; 1989.

21. Feigelman S, Stanton BF, Ricardo I. Perceptions of drug selling and drug use among urban youths. *J Early Adolesc.* 1993;13:267–284.

22. Pynoos RS, Nader K. Children's exposure to violence and traumatic death. *Psychiatr Ann.* 1990;20:334–344.

23. Warner BS, Weist MD. Urban youth as witnesses to violence: beginning assessment and treatment efforts. *J Youth Adolesc.* 1996;25:361–377.

24. Rhodes JE, Jason LA. *Preventing Substance Abuse Among Children and Adolescents.* New York, NY: Pergamon Press; 1988.

25. Kelleher KJ, Taylor JL, Rickert VI. Mental health services for rural children and adolescents. *Clin Psychol Rev.* 1992;12:841–852.

26. National Mental Health Association. *Invisible Children Project: Final Report.* Alexandria, Va: National Mental Health Association; 1989.

27. Alexander CS, Klassen AC. Drug use and illnesses among eighth-grade students in rural schools. *Public Health Rep.* 1988;103:394–399.

28. Offord DR, Boyle MH, Szaimarl P, et al. Ontario child health study. *Arch Gen Psychiatry.* 1987;44:832–855.

29. Way N, Stauber HY, Nakkula MJ, London P. Depression and substance abuse in two divergent high school cultures: a quantitative and qualitative analysis. *J Youth Adolesc.* 1994;23:331–357.

30. Weisz JR, Weiss B, Donenberg GR. The lab versus the clinic. *Am Psychol.* 1992;47:1578–1595.

31. Weist MD, Myers MP, Baker ME. Violence exposure and behavioral functioning in inner-city youth. Presented at the Maryland Psychiatric Research Center; June 1995; University of Maryland School of Medicine; Baltimore, Md.

32. Henggeler SW. A consensus: conclusions of the APA Task Force report on innovative models of mental health services for children, adolescents, and their families. *J Clin Child Psychol.* 1994;23:3–6.

33. Adelman HS, Taylor L. Early school adjustment problems: some perspectives and a project report. *Am J Orthopsychiatry.* 1991;61:468–474.

34. Flaherty LT, Weist MD, Warner BS. School-based mental health services in the United States: History, current models, and needs. *Community Ment Health J.* 1996;32:341–352.

35. Knitzer J, Steinberg Z, Fleisch B. *At the Schoolhouse Door: An Examination of Programs and Policies for Children with Behavioral and Emotional Problems.* New York, NY: Bank Street College of Education; 1990.

36. Thomas PA, Texidor MS. The school counselor and holistic health. *J Sch Health.* 1987;57:461–463.

37. Butler JA. National special education programs as a vehicle for financing mental health services for children and youth. Presented at the Financing

of Mental Health Services for Children and Adolescents workshop; August 1988; National Institute of Mental Health, Washington, DC.

38. National Association of School Psychologists. *School Psychologists: Helping Educate All Children.* Bethesda, Md: National Association of School Psychologists; 1995.

39. Thomas A. School psychologists: an integral member of the school health team. *J Sch Health.* 1987;57:465–468.

40. Abel RR, Burke JP. Perceptions of school psychology services from a staff perspective. *J Sch Psychol.* 1985;23:121–131.

41. Stewart KJ. Innovative practice of indirect service delivery: realities and idealities. *Sch Psychol Rev.* 1986;15:466–478.

42. Fisher GL, Jenkins SJ, Crumbley JD. A replication of a survey of school psychologists: congruence between training, practice, preferred role, and competence. *Psychol Sch.* 1986;23:271–279.

43. Conoley JC, Conoley CW. Collaboration for child adjustment: issues for school- and clinic-based child psychologists. *J Consult Clin Psychol.* 1991;59:821–829.

44. Johnston NS. School consultation: the training needs of teachers and school psychologists. *Psychol Sch.* 1990;27:51–56.

45. Cowen EL. Emergent approaches to mental health problems: an overview and directions for future work. In: Cowen EL, Gardner EA, Zax M, eds. *Emergency Approaches to Mental Health Problems.* New York, NY: Appleton-Century-Crofts; 1967.

46. Cowen EL, Trost MA, Lorion RP, Dorr D, Izzo LD, Isaacson RV. *New Ways in School Mental Health: Early Detection and Prevention of School Maladaptation.* New York, NY: Human Sciences Press; 1975.

47. Farie AM, Cowen EL, Smith M. The development and implementation of a rural consortium program to provide early preventive school mental health services. *Community Men Health J.* 1986;22:94–103.

48. Slavin RE, Madden NA, Karwelt NL, Dolan LJ, Wasik BA. *Success for All: A Relentless Approach to Prevention and Early Intervention in Elementary Schools.* Arlington, Va: Educational Research Service; 1992.

49. Comer JP. Educating poor minority children. *Sci Am.* 1988;259:42–48.

50. Kellam SG, Rebok GW. Building developmental and etiological theory through epidemiologically based preventive intervention trials. In: McCord J, Tremblay RE, eds. *Preventing Antisocial Behavior: Intervention from Birth Through Adolescence.* New York, NY: Guilford Press; 1992.

51. Adelman HS, Taylor L. School-based mental health: Toward a comprehensive approach. *J Ment Health Adm.* 1993;20:32–45.

52. Adelman HS. *Restructuring Support Services: Toward a Comprehensive Approach.* Kent, Ohio: American School Health Association; 1996.

53. Maryland Department of Health and Mental Hygiene. *School-Based Mental Health: Charting Program Development and Exploring Issues in Service Delivery.* Baltimore, Md: Department of Health and Mental Hygiene; 1995.

54. Dryfoos JG. School-based health clinics: three years of experience. *Fam Plann Perspect.* 1988;20:193–200.

55. Hyche-Williams J, Waszak CS. *School-Based Clinics: 1990.* Washington, DC: Center for Population Options; 1990.

56. Center for Population Options. Survey of school-based and school-linked clinics [unpublished]. Washington, DC: Center for Population Options; 1993.

57. Schlitt JJ, Rickett KD, Montgomery LL, Lear JG. *State Initiatives to Support School-Based Health Centers.* Washington, DC: Robert Wood Johnson Foundation; 1994.

58. Juszczak L, Fisher M, Lear JG, Friedman SB. Back to school: training opportunities in school-based health centers. *J Dev Behav Pediatr.* 1995;16:101–104.

59. Lear JG, Gleicher HB, St Germaine A, Porter PJ. Reorganizing health care for adolescents: the experience of the school-based adolescent health care program. *J Adolesc Health.* 1991;12:450–458.

60. Advocates for Youth. Survey of school-based and school-linked health services [unpublished]. Washington, DC: Advocates for Youth; 1994.

61. Schoenwald SK, Henggeler SW, Pickrel SG, Cunningham PB. Treating seriously troubled youths and families in their contexts: multisystemic therapy. In: Roberts MC, ed. *Model Programs in Child and Family Mental Health.* Hillsdale, NJ: Erlbaum; 1996.

62. School Health Policy Initiative. *Ingredients for Success: Comprehensive School-Based Health Centers.* Bronx, NY: School Health Policy Initiative; 1993.

63. Rosenthal B, Hinman E. Negotiating relationships between managed care and SBHCs. Presented at the first annual meeting of the National Assembly on School-Based Health Care; June 1995; Washington, DC.

64. Theut SK, Bailey HG. What is the outcome for children's mental health needs in national health care reform? *J Am Acad Child Adolesc Psychiatry.* 1994;33:1219–1222.

65. Henggeler SW, Schoenwald SK, Pickrel SG, Rowland MC, Santos AB. The contribution of treatment outcome research to the reform of children's mental health services: multisystemic therapy as an example. *J Ment Health Adm.* 1994;21:221–239.

66. Henggeler SW, Melton GB, Smith LA. Family preservation using multisystemic therapy: an effective alternative to incarcerating serious juvenile offenders. *J Consult Clin Psychol.* 1992;60:953–961.

67. Weissberg RP, Caplan M, Harwood RL. Promoting competent young people in competency-enhancing environments: a systems-based perspective on primary prevention. *J Consult Clin Psychol.* 1991;59:830–841.

68. Winett RA, Anderson ES. HIV prevention in youth: a framework for research and action. In: Ollendick TH, Prinz RJ, eds. *Advances in Clinical Child Psychology,* vol 16. New York, NY: Plenum Press; 1994:1–44).

69. Caplan G. *The Principles of Preventive Psychiatry.* New York, NY: Basic Books; 1964.

70. Public Health Service. *School-Based Clinics That Work.* Rockville, Md: US Department of Health and Human Services; 1994.

71. Barnett S, Niebuhr V, Baldwin C, Levine H. Community-oriented primary care: a process for school health intervention. *J Sch Health.* 1992; 62:246–248.

72. Prout HT, De Martino RA. A meta-analysis of school-based studies of psychotherapy. *J Sch Psychol.* 1986;34:285–292.

73. Lavoritano J, Segal PB. Evaluating the efficacy of a school counseling program. *Psychol Sch.* 1992;29:61–70.

74. Weist MD, Paskewitz DA, Warner BS, Flaherty LT. Treatment outcome of school-based mental health services for urban teenagers. *Community Ment Health J.* 1996;32:149–157.

75. Dolan LJ. *Models for Integrating Human Services into the School.* Tech. Rep. No. 30. Baltimore, Md: Johns Hopkins University Center for Research on Effective Schooling for Disadvantaged Students; 1992.

76. Ritter DR. Teachers' perceptions of problem behavior in general and special education. *Except Child.* 1989;55:559–564.

77. Weist MD, Proescher EL, Freedman AH, Paskewitz DA, Flaherty LT. School-based health services for urban adolescents: psychosocial characteristics of clinic users versus nonusers. *J Youth Adolesc.* 1995;24:251–265.

78. Barker LA, Adelman HS. Mental health and help-seeking among ethnic minority adolescents. *J Adolesc.* 1994;17:251–263.

79. Lusterman DD. An ecosystem approach to family school problems. *Am J Fam Ther.* 1985;12:22–30.

80. Pryzwansky WB. Private practice as an alternative setting for school psychologists. In: D'Amato RC, Dean RS, eds. *The School Psychologist in Nontraditional Settings.* Hillsdale, NJ: Erlbaum; 1989:76–87.

81. Lee CC. *Counseling for Diversity: A Guide for School Counselors and Related Professionals.* Needham Heights, Mass: Allyn & Bacon; 1995.

82. Sue S, Zane N. The role of culture and cultural techniques in psychotherapy: a critique and reformulation. *Am Psychol.* 1987;42:37–45.

CHAPTER 20

School-Based Teen Pregnancy Prevention Programs

A Review of the Literature

Helina H. Hoyt and Betty L. Broom, 2002

⌇⌇ Teenage pregnancy is a well-documented problem in the United States. Although teen birth rates remain high, they have fallen gradually since 1991.[1,2] Despite this decline, recent statistics indicate that teen birth rates remain higher than they were during the early to mid-1970s and continue to exceed the rates in most developed countries.[1,3] The teen birth rate in the United States is fourfold that of European countries.[4] Approximately 890,000 pregnancies occur each year among U.S. adolescents.[2] These pregnancy rates include live births, induced abortions, and fetal losses. The high rates of teenage pregnancy and childbearing occur among almost all races and ethnic groups in the United States. Socioeconomic conditions and the family appear to influence early teenage sexual activity more than race.[5]

Substantial morbidity and social problems result from adolescent pregnancies.[3,6] Adolescents who give birth are more likely to have

This chapter originally appeared as Hoyt HH, Broom BL. School-based teen pregnancy prevention programs: a review of the literature. *J Sch Nurs*. 2002; 18(1):11–17. Copyright © 2002. Reprinted with permission from the National Association of School Nurses.

lower educational and occupational attainment, remain single parents, and suffer poverty.[7] The children of teenage mothers experience more cognitive and behavioral problems by the time they reach school age, and they have less stimulating home environments, poorer educational outcomes, and higher teen pregnancy rates when they become adolescents than children of adult mothers. Society as a whole experiences high costs associated with public assistance and health care for adolescent parents and their children.[7]

Teen pregnancy prevention is currently a public health priority. Many efforts to decrease teen pregnancies have failed over the past 40 years. Current interventions include pregnancy prevention education, access to contraceptive services, and community-based life option programs. Each effort uses a variety of approaches, including clinical and school-based services.[6] Although there have been multiple approaches designed to prevent adolescent pregnancy, few programs have demonstrated significant pregnancy reductions, in part because outcomes have not adequately been evaluated.[6] As prevention efforts multiply, there is need for research that examines not just program outcomes but also the processes by which programs create change in participants. The recent decline in teen pregnancy, birth, and abortion rates has been attributed to many factors. Abstinence and voluntary contraception are both on the rise. Use of condoms among sexually active teens has risen fourfold in the last 15 years, from 11% to 44%, mostly due to HIV and AIDS. In addition, a strong economy allowed teens to perceive more life options and delay childbearing to prepare for a career.[4]

REVIEW OF THE LITERATURE

For almost a century, schools have been developing programs to reduce sexual behavior in youth at risk for pregnancy or sexually transmitted diseases (STDs). The following section reviews the common approaches to and characteristics found in pregnancy prevention programs.

Pregnancy prevention education is a common strategy. These programs are often labeled *family life education.* Most of them provide information about sexuality, reproduction, decision making, and sexual relationship issues. They focus on teaching about the reproductive process and how to avoid an STD or pregnancy, using either abstinence or contraceptives.[6] Curricula have been diverse and implemented primarily in junior and senior high schools. Historically, most of the programs contain activities or elements reflecting a variety of approaches. These approaches can be divided into five groups[8,9]:

1. Programs that increase knowledge and emphasize the risks and consequences of pregnancy

2. Programs that clarify values and provide skills, especially decision-making and communication skills

3. Abstinence-only curricula

4. HIV/AIDS education

5. Theoretically based programs building on the successes and failures of previous programs, with more rigorous evaluation

In the early 1990s, several new approaches and modifications of earlier methods appeared. These included (1) a renewed emphasis on abstinence, (2) a more positive view of responsible sex, and (3) a greater emphasis on character development. Many collaborative programs among schools, community groups, and family planning clinics have been implemented to coordinate educational efforts and youth development programs for the prevention of initial and repeat teen pregnancies.[4] In addition, initiatives in the form of sex education, statutory rape laws, and media campaigns with a variety of messages promoting teen pregnancy prevention have come from both local and state governments. At the national level, the National Campaign to Prevent Teen Pregnancy was founded in 1996 to prevent teen pregnancy by supporting values and stimulating actions that are consistent with a pregnancy-free adolescence. The campaign goal is to decrease teen pregnancy rates by one third by the year 2005.[2]

The acceptance of scientifically evaluating teen pregnancy prevention programs has been slow. By 1990, several hundred teen pregnancy prevention programs had been developed and implemented; however, even today only a few have been adequately evaluated. A consensus is growing that program development should include rigorous outcome evaluation.[4]

Based on the evaluation that has been done, current programs that demonstrate the most improvements in teen pregnancy rates share the following nine characteristics[4,10]:

1. They focus on reducing sexual behaviors that lead to unintended pregnancy or STD.

2. They include behavioral goals, teaching methods, and materials that are age and culturally appropriate, so that the problem is always seen through the eyes of the students whom the programs seek to serve.

3. They are based on theoretical approaches, such as social learning theories, which have been demonstrated to be effective in influencing health-related risky behaviors.

4. They are of appropriate length to allow participants to complete important activities. For example, a program does not merely consist of an assembly, but includes multiple components with sufficient time for follow-up.

5. They provide accurate and basic information about the risks of unprotected sex and methods of avoiding unprotected sex.

6. They use teaching methods that are designed to actively involve the participants so as to personalize the information.

7. They include activities that address social pressures related to sex.

8. They provide models of and practice in communication, negotiation, and refusal skills.

9. They provide training and practice sessions to teacher or peer program leaders who are selected because they believe in the program.

In programs judged exemplary by the Program Archive on Sexuality, Health and Adolescence, a panel of noted scientists in the field of pregnancy/STD/HIV/AIDS prevention found eight prevalent elements (see Table 20.1).[4] Techniques that were involved with successful program delivery are identified in Table 20.2.[4] The elements and techniques of the exemplary programs provide insight into what works and offer a guide to future program development and implementation, especially within the school system.

Table 20.1 Elements of Exemplary Programs.

Abstinence education
Behavioral skill development
Community outreach
Contraceptive access
Contraceptive education
Life option enhancement
Self-efficacy/self-esteem education
Sexuality/STD/HIV/AIDS education

Table 20.2 Delivery Techniques of Exemplary Programs.

Adult involvement
Case management
Group discussion
Lectures
Peer counseling/instruction
Public service announcements
Role playing
Video

PROMISING PRIMARY PREGNANCY PREVENTION PROGRAMS

The following section reviews specific school-based programs reported in professional journals. The programs described appear to have the potential to reduce exposure to unintended pregnancy. Each program varies in components, length, and intensity.

Abstinence-Based Programs

Postponing Sexual Involvement (PSI) is a program designed for students aged 16 years and younger and is aimed at deterring teens from having sexual intercourse. Participants learn about human relationships, sources of sexual pressure, and assertive responses to use in high-risk situations in order to remain abstinent. Trained peer leaders direct repeated role-playing and student interaction over a 10-session period. Video presentations demonstrating refusal and negotiation skills are also used. A field study of PSI was conducted with 1,005 8th-grade students from low-income communities in Atlanta, Georgia. Compared with a control group of peers, male PSI participants who had not had sexual intercourse before the program were found to be 3 times more likely than the comparison group to remain abstinent through the end of the 9th grade. PSI females were 15 times less likely to have engaged in sexual intercourse at the end of the 8th grade than the comparison group. The effects had declined by the end of the 9th grade, but comparison-group girls were still more likely to engage in sexual intercourse than were girls who had participated in the program. Although PSI participants were more likely to delay sexual activity, pregnancy rates were disappointing. No significant differences were found between the comparison group (18%) and the program participants (16%) at either time period.[4,11,12]

Project Taking Charge was developed for junior high school home economics classrooms. It integrates family life education with vocational exploration, interpersonal and family relationships, and decision-making and goal-setting lessons. The program promotes abstinence as the correct choice for teens. No material on contraception is included. A field study was conducted with 136 youths from three low-income communities with high rates of teen pregnancy. Six months following the intervention, program participants showed significant gains in knowledge of sexual development, STDs, and the risks of adolescent pregnancy, relative to a comparison group of peers. There was also some evidence that participation was associated with a delay in the initiation of sexual intercourse. However, the evidence fell short of statistical significance at the .05 level. No long-term follow-up of pregnancy rates was presented.[4,13,14]

Abstinence- and Contraceptive-Based Programs

Reducing the Risk is a 16-week program for high school students. The sexuality education curriculum is designed to reduce the frequency of unprotected intercourse through delaying or reducing the frequency of intercourse and increasing contraceptive and STD protection. A field study of the risk reduction program was conducted in 13 California high schools, with 1,033 health education students as participants. Participation in the program significantly increased teens' knowledge and communication with parents about abstinence and contraception. The program also significantly ($p < .05$) reduced the likelihood that students who had not had intercourse at the beginning of the program would become sexually active by the 18-month follow-up assessment. Unfortunately, program participation did not affect the frequency of sexual intercourse or the use of contraceptives among teens who were already sexually active at the start of the program. No long-term follow-up of pregnancy rates was reported.[4,8,12]

Safer Choices is a multicomponent, HIV, STD, and pregnancy prevention program for high school youth. This 2-year, school-based intervention is based on social cognitive theory, social influence theory, and models of school change. The intervention is unique because of its focus on schoolwide change and the influence of the total school environment on student behavior. The program consists of five primary components: (1) school organization, (2) curriculum and staff development, (3) peer resources and school environment, (4) parent education, and (5) school-community linkages. Safer Choices was first implemented during the 1993–1995 school years. The evaluation used a randomized trial involving 10 schools in northern California and 10 schools in southeast Texas with an average of 1,767 students. Five schools from each state were randomly assigned to the Safer Choices program, whereas the other schools were assigned to a comparison program of standard, knowledge-based HIV prevention curriculum. No significant differences, as detected by *t* tests, existed between intervention and comparison schools on any demographic variables used in randomization. Cohort data were collected through trained data collectors using student self-report surveys. Baseline data were collected in the fall of 1993, and the initial follow-up data collection was performed in spring 1994. The evaluation questionnaire consisted of items assessing demographic characteristics, sexuality-related psychosocial factors, sexual behaviors, and program exposure. The three primary behavioral outcomes included (1) whether students delayed sexual intercourse, (2) the number of times students had intercourse without a condom in the previous three months, and (3) the number of sexual partners with whom students had intercourse without a condom in the previous 3 months.

The survey gathered data on numerous secondary behavioral outcomes, such as use of a condom at first intercourse, use of protection at last intercourse, number of sexual intercourse in the past 3 months, number of sexual partners in the past 3 months, use of alcohol or drugs before intercourse in the past 3 months, being tested for HIV, and being tested for other STDs. The analyses examined the impact of the intervention from baseline to the first follow-up measurement, approximately 7 months later. Significant differences ($p < .05$) were found for 9 of the 13 psychosocial scales including knowledge, self-efficacy for condom use, normative beliefs and attitudes regarding condom use, perceived barriers to condom use, risk perceptions, and parent–child communication. Safer Choices also reduced selected risk behaviors, specifically, reducing the frequency of intercourse without a condom and increasing the use of selected contraceptives at last intercourse. Although results from this study are encouraging, several methodological limitations were evident: (1) self-report questionnaires were used to measure outcomes, (2) students retained in the cohort differed in some aspects from students dropped from the cohort and lost to follow-up, and (3) the data were collected at 7 months, evaluating only the short-term impact of the program. The authors indicate, however, that planned 19-month and 31-month follow-ups will provide an opportunity to examine the long-term impact of Safer Choices.[15]

Life Option Enhancement Program

Teen Outreach was designed for teens between the ages of 12 and 17. The program was formulated to prevent early pregnancy and encourage academic progress. The two main program components are small-group discussion sessions with a facilitator and participation in volunteer service learning in the community. An experimental study was conducted with 695 high school students in 25 states who were randomly assigned to either the Teen Outreach program or a control group. Each was assessed at program entry and at program exit 9 months later. Rates of pregnancy, school failure, and academic suspension at exit were substantially lower in the Teen Outreach group ($p < .01$).[16]

Another study evaluating this program was conducted with mostly female students between 11 and 21 years of age. The program was implemented around the country, with 985 students participating. Overall, participants had fewer pregnancies and used contraception more regularly than a control group of peers. They also had higher rates of school attendance and greater academic success.[4,17–19]

Role-Playing Program

Baby Think It Over is a computerized infant simulator program introduced in 1994. This modular program was designed to be incorporated within and complement other subject curriculum. Ideally, the program reaches teens before they become sexually active and pregnant. Through the use of the Baby Think It Over, a 6 $1/_2$-pound infant simulator, adolescents can experience parenting a newborn. The simulator is designed to replicate the sleeping, waking, and feeding patterns and the random crying episodes of a young infant. The student inserts a "care key" into the baby's electronic box and holds it in place for a specific length of time to simulate feeding, bathing, diaper changing, and comforting. The baby can be programmed for easy, normal, or cranky episodes. An electronic device monitors all handling episodes and records any neglect or rough handling. The recommended minimum for a parenting simulation is 2 days for middle school students and 4 to 7 days for high school students. The experience is intended to include student assignment of the baby with its care key, baby care activities, and related worksheet assignments, including pre- and postcare experience questionnaires. The hypothesis is that introducing young people to the realities of caring for an infant will delay sexual activity and reduce teenage pregnancies.

A quasi-experimental study of 48 high school students demonstrated the impact of Baby Think It Over on adolescents' attitudes and beliefs regarding future parenting experiences. The Parenting Attitude Scale, a 10-item measure, was used to determine realistic parenting expectations. It was assessed to be adequately reliable among the study's sample with a Chronbach's alpha of .73. Results indicated that after the 3-day intervention, the teenagers who participated had much more realistic notions about the responsibilities and demands involved in childrearing.[21]

Another study conducted with 68 6th-grade and 41 8th-grade girls in an urban middle school in a predominantly lower socioeconomic, Hispanic neighborhood had conflicting results. The students cared for the Baby Think It Over doll for 3 days and 2 nights. Responses to a three-part, self-administered questionnaire developed for this investigation and written at a 4th-grade reading level were used to assess the girls' understanding of the responsibilities and difficulties related to parenting. The questionnaire also evaluated the similarity of the Baby Think It Over care and students' view of real infant care and the student's childbearing intentions before and after caring for the baby. Only 29% of the 109 girls participating thought that real infant care would be like Baby Think It Over care. Sixth-grade students were more likely than the 8th-grade students to endorse statements suggesting that real infant care would be easier than Baby Think It Over care. Caring for Baby Think It Over had no significant effect on the intent of students to become teen parents. Of the 109 students, 12% wanted to be teen parents before they cared for the doll, and 15% wanted to be teen parents after they cared for the doll. In discussing these somewhat surprising results, the authors reported that the doll was implemented without the recommended educational program intended by the manufacturer of the Baby Think It Over simulator.[22]

DISCUSSION

According to the findings of these recent studies, some pregnancy prevention programs appear to delay the onset of sexual activity and increase contraception use by sexually active teens. Although some program evaluations have found changes in attitudes regarding sexual behavior or increased knowledge about reproduction and contraception, few programs have demonstrated a long-term impact on pregnancy prevention.

Common characteristics and components of effective programs have been identified. It appears that programs with a more comprehensive approach have the greatest potential for success.[4,6] That should not be surprising because many variables are thought to affect the success of educating teens and decreasing the teen pregnancy rate. Gender, age, previous sexual experience, socioeconomic status, and ethnicity are just a few examples of variables that should be included in studies evaluating program effectiveness.

Several significant limitations are noted in this review of multiple programs. First, most of the programs aimed at reducing teenage pregnancy have not been guided by a theoretical framework. In general, programs are more likely to be successful if they are based on theoretical approaches that have been demonstrated to be effective in influencing other health-risk behaviors.[4,6] For example, social influence and learning theories allow a program to go far beyond the cognitive level. They focus on recognizing social influences, changing individual values, changing group norms, and building social skills.

A second limitation is that many of the evaluations have had methodological flaws and constraints. For example, experimental design use has been infrequent, sample sizes are small, and few have used random assignment. As a result, it is difficult to determine whether programs effective for one group will be effective for another. Programs, particularly Baby Think It Over, have reported inconsistent results, indicating the need for more research. Another limitation is that in comprehensive programs with multiple components, it is difficult to differentiate effective from ineffective components or to determine the level of intensity required of the participating students. More complex comparison studies need to be undertaken to answer these questions.

The third limitation among pregnancy prevention programs is that most programs are developed without regard for prior knowledge of sex education or for parental involvement. Several of the program reports identified the need for further evaluation of previous sex education history, grade-level in which students have received this education, and what parental roles have been.

A final limitation among the programs is that not all studies include pregnancy as an outcome measure. This is probably because evaluations only measure the short-term impact of the programs. For example, Project Taking Charge and Reducing the Risk both identify that participation in their programs was associated with a delay in initiation of sexual intercourse but did not provide long-term follow-up measuring pregnancy rates. Programs need to share the results of their evaluations, whether successful or not, to enhance the development of new and innovative interventions.

There are many unanswered questions, beyond the limitations identified, in adolescent pregnancy prevention. Pregnancy prevention efforts need to address issues that go beyond individual decisions about contraceptives and fertility. The influence of family, neighborhood, and community must be recognized as having a major impact on reproductive behavior. Few programs have included male participants or family members in their interventions. In addition, future programs should be developmentally and culturally sensitive. They must address the specific needs of adolescent subgroups, younger and older adolescents, as well as those from different ethnic backgrounds. Program evaluation and replication are crucial in the area of teen pregnancy prevention. As program effectiveness is demonstrated, replication studies are needed to examine these promising results with more diverse samples.

IMPLICATIONS FOR
SCHOOL NURSING PRACTICE

During the teen years, young people are at constant risk for behaviors that will negatively shape their lives. The school nurse is in a prime position to lead the way in protecting American youth and decreasing the national teen pregnancy problem. Teenage sexuality and pregnancy prevention are indeed complex issues facing school nurses. Although teenage pregnancy rates have declined, the battle is not won. School nurses have the unique ability to make a difference in students' lives and in the choices that they make.[23] As health educators, nurses must educate and counsel based on research findings. Furthermore, it is imperative that nurses play an active role in following pregnancy rates to identify trends, reviewing district curriculum and helping to select appropriate programs, and scientifically evaluating outcomes of prevention programs.

Although the effects of the programs identified in this article have been modest, future prevention programs should incorporate the identified components of effective programs. Existing programs can continue to be strengthened by building on what is known to work. The school nurse should base programs on the age, culture, and level of risk of the target population. A logical connection should exist in the program between the components and the length and intensity of each prevention program. Measurable short-term and long-term outcomes that the intervention hopes to achieve should be identified from the beginning. School nurses have much to offer in the link among theory, program design, implementation, and evaluation. Rigorous evaluation of programs is desperately needed.

CONCLUSION

The national focus on lowering teenage pregnancy rates has been somewhat successful, but much remains to be done. The most promising prevention programs appear to be comprehensive in content and varied in delivery techniques. However, uniform scientific evaluation of the effectiveness of these programs is lacking. School nurses have a vital role to play in the fight to reduce teen pregnancy. They have a responsibility to help select or develop appropriate programs, scientifically evaluate program outcomes, and support the implementation of effective programs in their schools and community.

Notes

1. March of Dimes. Teenage pregnancy [Web page]. 2000. Available at: http://www.noah.cuny.edu/pregnancy/marchofdimes/prepreg.plan/teen-fact.html. Accessed February 29, 2000.

2. National Campaign to Prevent Teen Pregnancy. Facts and stats [Web page]. 2000. Available at: http://www.teenpregnancy.org/fedprate.htm. Accessed December 16, 2000.

3. Kann L, Kinchen SA, Williams BI, et al. Youth risk behavior surveillance—United States, 1997. *J Sch Health.* 1998;68:355–369.

4. Card JJ. Teen pregnancy prevention: do any programs work? *Annu Rev Public Health.* 1999;20:257–285.

5. Clifford J, Brykczynski K. Giving voice to childbearing teens: views of sexuality and the reality of being a young parent. *J Sch Nurs.* 1999;15(1):4–15.

6. Nitz K. Adolescent pregnancy prevention: a review of interventions and programs. *Clin Psychol Rev.* 1999;19:457–471.

7. Maynard RA. *Kids Having Kids: A Robin Hood Foundation Special Report on the Costs of Adolescent Childbearing.* New York, NY: Robin Hood Foundation; 1996.

8. Kirby D. School-based programs to reduce sexual risk-taking behaviors. *J Sch Health.* 1992;62:280–286.

9. Kirby D. Reducing adolescent pregnancy: approaches that work. *Contemp Pediatr.* 1999;16:83–94.

10. Kirby D. Reflections on two decades of research on teen sexual behavior and pregnancy. *J Sch Health.* 1999;69:89–94.

11. Howard M, McCabe J. Helping teenagers postpone sexual involvement. *Fam Plann Perspect.* 1990;22:21–26.

12. Kirby D, Short L, Collins J, et al. School-based programs to reduce sexual risk behaviors: a review of effectiveness. *Public Health Rep.* 1994; 109:339–360.

13. Jorgensen SR. Project Taking Charge: an evaluation of an adolescent pregnancy prevention program. *Fam Rel.* 1991;40:373–380.

14. Kelly JA. Sexually transmitted disease prevention approaches that work: interventions to reduce risk behavior among individuals, groups, and communities. *Sex Transm Dis.* 1994;21:73–75.

15. Coyle K, Basen-Engquist K, Kirby D, et al. Short-term impact of safer choices: a multicomponent school-based HIV, other STD, and pregnancy prevention program. *J Sch Health.* 1999;69:181–188.

16. Allen JP, Philliber S, Herrling S, Kuperminc GP. Preventing teen pregnancy and academic failure: experimental evaluation of a developmentally based approach. *Child Dev.* 1997;68:729–742.

17. Allen JP. Programmatic prevention of adolescent problem behaviors: the role of autonomy, relatedness, and volunteer service in the teen outreach program. *Am J Community Psychol.* 1994;22:617–638.

18. Allen JP, Philliber S, Hoggson N. School-based prevention of teenage pregnancy and school dropout: process evaluation of the national replication of the teen outreach program. *Am J Community Psychol.* 1990;18:505–524.

19. Philliber S, Allen JP. Life options and community service: teen outreach program. In: Miller BC, Card JJ, Paikoff RL, Peterson JC, eds. *Preventing Adolescent Pregnancy: Model Programs and Evaluations.* Newbury Park, Calif: Sage; 1992:139–155.

20. *Baby Think It Over* [brochure]. Eau Claire, Wis: Baby Think It Over Inc; 2000.

21. Strachan W, Gorey KM. Infant simulator lifespace intervention: pilot investigation of an adolescent pregnancy prevention program. *Child Adolesc Soc Work J.* 1997;143:1–5.

22. Krawelski J, Stevens-Simon C. Does mothering a doll change teens' thoughts about pregnancy? *Pediatrics.* 2000;105(3):1–5.

23. Dychkowski L. A national decline in the teen pregnancy rate: what do the latest numbers mean for school nurses? *Sch Nurs News.* 1999;163:3–4, 6, 18, 33.

Pregnancy Prevention Among Urban Adolescents Younger Than Fifteen

Results of the "In Your Face" Program

Lorraine Tiezzi, Judy Lipshutz, Neysa Wrobleski,
Roger D. Vaughan, James F. McCarthy, 1997

D ata from a pregnancy prevention program operating through school-based clinics in four New York City junior high schools suggest that an intensive risk-identification and case-management approach may be effective among very young adolescents. Among students given a referral to a family planning clinic for contraception, the proportion who visited the clinic and obtained a method rose from 11% in the year before the program began to 76% in the program's third year. Pregnancy rates among teenagers younger than 15 decreased by 34% over four years in the program schools. In the fourth year of the program, the pregnancy rate in one school that

This chapter originally appeared as Tiezzi L, Lipshutz J, Wrobleski N, Vaughan RD, McCarthy JF. Pregnancy prevention among urban adolescents younger than 15: results of the "In Your Face" program, *Fam Plann Perspect*, 1997;29(4):173–176. Copyright © 1997 the Alan Guttmacher Institute. Reprinted with permission.

was unable to continue the program was almost three times the average rate for the other three schools (16.5 pregnancies per 1,000 female students vs. 5.8 per 1,000).

The problem of teenage pregnancy in the United States is far from resolved, especially among very young adolescents and minorities. In 1990, an estimated one million pregnancies occurred among U.S. teenagers; 28,000 of these were among adolescents younger than 15.[1] Although the overall pregnancy rate for adolescents has declined, the rate for those younger than 15 continues to climb. Among the 39 states that reported pregnancy rates for teenagers younger than 15 in 1991–1992, 20 reported increases, nine reported no change and 10 reported a decrease. In contrast, only five of the 42 states that reported pregnancy rates among 15–19-year-olds reported an increase for that age-group.[2]

The pregnancy rate among minority youth is twice as high as that among white teenagers, and appears to be rising: Between 1980 and 1988, it increased from 181 to 184 per 1,000 among nonwhites, while it decreased from 96 to 93 per 1,000 among whites.[3] Minority adolescents are disproportionately represented among teenagers who give birth; of the 38 states that reported rates for 1991–1992, 27 reported an increase in birthrates among Hispanic adolescents, whereas only six of 50 states reported an increase in birthrates among non-Hispanic white teenagers.[3]

Although no research has been conducted on factors contributing to the risk of pregnancy specifically among the youngest teenagers, some studies have examined the issue among all adolescents. Nonuse or inconsistent use of contraceptives is a major factor: Approximately 35% of unmarried, sexually active teenagers use no form of birth control at first intercourse,[4] and a sexually active teenager who does not use birth control has a 90% chance of becoming pregnant within a year's time.[5]

One reason for nonuse of contraceptives may be an imbalance of negotiating power resulting from the age discrepancy between many teenage women and their partners; approximately 60% of mothers aged 15–17 report that their partner is at least three years older than they are.[6] Young minority adolescents are especially at risk of pregnancy, as nonwhites are likely to engage in sexual intercourse at a younger age than whites.[4]

Programs aimed at reducing or preventing teenage pregnancies, especially among younger adolescents, must overcome several formidable financial and logistical barriers.[7] School-based clinics have long been regarded as an effective means of overcoming some of these barriers by providing convenient, affordable, comprehensive health care to adolescents, and have been the site of several successful prevention programs.[8-10] Many of these clinics, however, are prohibited from dispensing contraceptives. Rather, students must obtain contraceptives by prescription from an off-site source, a requirement that presents them with yet another barrier. Even if school-based clinics are able to provide contraceptives on-site, they need a rigorous follow-up mechanism to ensure that each adolescent receives counseling regarding the decision to become sexually active, chooses and receives an appropriate contraceptive, and is using the chosen method.

In 1986, the Center for Population and Family Health (CPFH) at the Columbia University School of Public Health, in collaboration with the Presbyterian Hospital in the City of New York and with New York City School District 4 established its first comprehensive school-based clinic. It now operates school-based clinics in four junior high schools and one high school in economically disadvantaged and medically underserved areas of New York City. These clinics, their services and their client population have been described elsewhere.[11-15]

In 1992, CPFH introduced a health education pilot program focusing on pregnancy prevention as part of clinic services. The pilot was then expanded in all four of the junior high schools served by CPFH. These schools have approximately 3,500 students, the majority of whom are immigrants from the Dominican Republic. This article describes the pregnancy prevention program and reports on the outcomes in its first four years of operation.

PROGRAM DESCRIPTION

The "In Your Face" pregnancy prevention program was designed to reduce the risk of unintended pregnancy by providing information, counseling, support and referral for reproductive health care. Students were targeted for this health education intervention in a variety of ways.

A confidential schoolwide health and risk factor screening survey[15] was administered annually by CPFH staff; typically, the screening captured about 85% of the student population. The survey, which was available in English and Spanish and took 25–30 minutes to complete, identified students who were sexually experienced and those who had characteristics correlated with sexual activity. These characteristics included alcohol and substance use by students or by their parent or guardian, having run away from home or having manifested some indicator of an underlying psychiatric or mental health problem, such as a suicide attempt or chronic depression.

Students who reported sexual activity or characteristics correlated with sexual activity were referred to the health educator. If the health educator determined that a student's survey responses were accurate, the student was invited to participate in the In Your Face health education program.

Other students entered the program after visiting the health educator because of referrals from the clinic-based medical providers and social workers, teachers and guidance counselors, or through self-referral. Many of the students who came on their own had heard a classroom presentation given by the health educator, informing students of the clinic location, hours and services.

From the pool of students identified as being at risk of pregnancy, the health educator in each school formed a number of groups, each consisting of 5–10 students. The groups met at least once a week during the school year. The program relied on group meetings as well as individual counseling; groups made efficient use of the health educator's time, created peer groups in which new norms could be established and provided a support group to reinforce positive attitudes and behavior.

The In Your Face intervention consisted of several components—group education, individual education and counseling, interdisciplinary support (i.e., a team approach, with input from social workers, medical providers and psychiatrists), referrals and classroom interventions, plus other special events and projects. In the group setting, the health educator delivered a series of 15 lessons based on the "Reducing the Risk" curriculum,[16] which had been reviewed and modified to be sensitive to the culture and language of the students. The lessons focused on such topics as knowledge, behavior and decision-making skills. However, since purely didactic lessons usually "turn off" adolescents, the intervention incorporated role-playing exercises, group games, brainstorming exercises and audiovisual presentations. Throughout the sessions, students explored ways to assess their own risks and identify behavioral cues of risk.

Saying no to sex was explored as an important and valid option. Students already involved in sexual activity were encouraged to abstain. For those continuing sexual activity, individual sessions were scheduled to discuss the available array of contraceptive methods, offer counseling about each option and provide referrals to obtain contraceptives. Each of these options was discussed in an open, honest, nonjudgmental way.

Dispensing contraceptives and prescriptions in junior high school clinics is prohibited in New York City; therefore, a referral mechanism enabled sexually active students to receive contraceptives at one of two satellite hospital clinics—the Young Adult Clinic and the Young Men's Clinic—which are jointly operated by CPFH and the Ambulatory Care Network Corporation of Presbyterian Hospital. The clinics, which offer a full range of medical and mental health services, are staffed and administered by CPFH health care workers.

The benefits of this arrangement are enormous: The students see the same staff they see in their own school-based clinics; record-keeping, transfer of information, compliance and follow-up are greatly enhanced, and students receive greater continuity of care. The health educator in the school-based clinic who refers a student to either of the satellite clinics acts as a case manager for that student; the educator organizes all documentation and paperwork required, meets the student at the clinic, oversees the visit at the clinic and tracks any lab test or follow-up needed. In this way, the health educator serves as a mediator and a guide for the student, essentially removing structural barriers to appropriate contraceptive services.

Sexual activity is related to and may indeed result from other events or conditions in an adolescent's life. Therefore, the health educator's ongoing case management is supplemented by regular follow-up meetings of an interdisciplinary team of nurse practitioners, social workers and physicians who work in the school-based clinic. A student who has been identified as having a serious medical or psychosocial problem is referred to the appropriate clinic provider, and the case is co-managed by all the providers involved. This "whole-person" approach to pregnancy prevention is a key component of the In Your Face program: trustworthy, competent and caring health providers are "in the student's face" to ensure that he or she obtains appropriate care.

RESEARCH DESIGN

Adolescent health programs in general, and pregnancy prevention programs in particular, are often designed and implemented without the benefit of a thorough and rigorous evaluation of the effectiveness of specific program approaches. However, the research designs that are typically seen as the best present serious challenges to community health programs such as the one described in this article. The best research design would have entailed random assignment of students to treatment and control groups, with the treatment group receiving the intensive In Your Face program and the control group receiving only services routinely available through the school-based clinics. We did not use this approach because we could not justify withholding this potentially useful intervention from a portion of the students for the sole purpose of implementing a strong research design.

Another option was to select a control group consisting of junior high schools that were as similar as possible to the experimental schools in every aspect and dimension, both demographic and programmatic, except for the In Your Face program. However, it would have been difficult, if not impossible, to find a second group of junior high schools that had a student population predominantly made up of immigrants from the Dominican Republic, that had school-based clinics and that had environmental and economic conditions that were comparable to those of the program schools.

In addition, we could have compared the outcomes of students who participated in the In Your Face program to the outcomes of those who did not participate. However, because we attempted to reach all students at risk through multiple outreach mechanisms, a control group composed of those who were not involved in the program would tend to be at lower risk and would therefore bias the estimate of program effectiveness.

Another possibility was to assign students to different levels of the intervention. We chose not to use this approach because we believed that all students should have access to the full program. Inferences about "dose" effects could not be based on student attendance because such an approach would seriously confound program effects with student characteristics related to attendance.

Given these constraints, we decided to rely on what Cook and Campbell refer to as a one-group pre- and post-test design.[17] Although Cook and Campbell caution that one should not try to draw "hard-headed causal inferences" from studies using this design, they consider that "inferences may be possible."

DATA AND ANALYSIS

CPFH maintains its own tracking and data analysis system. Each time a student makes an individual visit to a school-based clinic, the provider records the reason for the visit, diagnoses, sexual behavior, problems identified, services rendered and referrals (among other information) on a comprehensive clinic visit form. Logs are kept of group attendance and visits to the hospital satellite clinics.

Pregnancy data for this analysis were compiled from clinic records. Young women who suspected that they were pregnant were referred to the clinic for testing, or came on their own. In addition, sexually active students who had symptoms consistent with pregnancy when they visited the clinic for other reasons were offered pregnancy tests and were referred to the health educator and social worker for counseling and follow-up. Although this data collection method may have missed some pregnancies, conversations with students and staff indicated that students were likely to come to the clinic if they were pregnant, because they felt that they would be treated with respect and that the clinic "was the place to go to get help."

The data from student clinic visits and the results from the schoolwide risk survey were linked by a unique nine-digit identification number assigned to each student by the school system. Using data sets that were linked across visit type, locations and years, we were able to compile a variety of descriptive statistics and cross-tabulations.

RESULTS

Table 21.1 describes the population of students in the schools served by the In Your Face program during its first year (1992–1993); the social and demographic characteristics; of the population remained relatively stable over the study period. A substantial majority (81%) of the students described themselves as Hispanic (generally Dominican), 10% as black and 9% as members of other racial groups. Despite their young age (mean, 12.9 years), 20% had already had sexual intercourse, 18% had assaulted someone and 14% had thought about suicide.[18]

Because so-called "problem behaviors" tend to cluster, we expected that students enrolled in the program—whom we had actively recruited because they had been identified as being at risk of pregnancy—would report more risk factors in the schoolwide screening survey than would those who either did not use the school-based clinic services or who used the clinic but were not enrolled in the program. Indeed, the data presented in Table 21.2 show much higher risk profiles among students who were in the program (approximately 250 each year). Differences across categories for each risk variable in the table are significant (by the chi-square test) at the $P < .001$ level.

Table 21.1 Percentage Distribution of Students in Program Schools, and Percentage with Selected Risk Factors, All by Demographic Characteristics, 1992–1993 (N = 3,738).

Characteristic	Total	Ever Had Sex	Ever Considered Suicide	Assaulted Someone in Past Year
All	100	20	14	18
Gender				
Female	46	7	19	8
Male	54	31	10	27
Race/ethnicity				
Hispanic	81	18	14	17
Black	10	33	12	32
Other	9	16	13	17
Grade level				
6	35	16	14	19
7	33	18	14	19
8	32	25	14	17

One of the goals of the In Your Face program was to reach as many as possible of the adolescents identified as sexually active. Because there was only one health educator in each school, and because the daily absentee rates in the four schools ranged from 10% to 20%, we

Table 21.2 Percentage of Students in Program Schools, by Use of Clinic Services and Program Participation, according to Year and Risk Factor.

Year and Risk Factor	All	Never Used Clinic	Used Medical Social Work Services Only	Participated in Program
1992–1993				
Ever had sex	20	7	9	33
Ever considered suicide	14	11	16	26
Involved assault in past year	18	6	9	27
1993–1994				
Ever had sex	16	8	11	42
Ever considered suicide	3	2	2	6
Involved assault in past year	7	6	7	20
1994–1995				
Ever had sex	18	8	12	48
Ever considered suicide	2	1	2	3
Involved assault in past year	7	4	7	12

were unable to achieve this goal. Information gathered by the health educators about sexually active students who were not reached by the program indicated that the vast majority could not be contacted because of what the schools classified as "consistent absenteeism" or "ongoing truancy." However, the success rate of the program in enrolling students classified as "currently sexually active" (defined as having had sex in the past three months) increased by nearly half over the first three years, from 50% of sexually active students in 1992–1993 to 74% in 1994–1995.

Changes in several outcome measures suggest that the program was effective. As we noted earlier, one of the program's objectives was to encourage sexually active students to consider abstinence. In 1994–1995 25% of the students in the program who had ever had sex indicated that they had chosen to become abstinent (this question was not asked in previous years).

In addition, among students who chose to remain sexually active but were not using contraceptives consistently, the proportion who were successfully referred to the off-site family planning clinic increased from 25% (14 of 56) during the year before the program began to 85% (80 of 94) in the program's third year (see Table 21.3). The majority of these students were female: In 1993–1994, for example, only 7% of those who completed referrals were male (not shown). Overall, among students who were referred to the clinic, the proportion who adopted a method increased from 11% (6 of 56) in the year before the program began to 76% (71 of 94) in the program's third year.

We calculated the overall pregnancy rate for the four junior high schools served by the In Your Face program by dividing the number of pregnancies occurring in the school as a whole by the number of

Table 21.3   Among Sexually Active Students Who Were Not Consistently Practicing Contraception, Number Who Were Referred to Family Planning Clinic, Who Visited the Clinic and Who Adopted a Method, by Year.

Year	Referred to Clinic	Visited Clinic	Adopted a Method
1991–1992	56	14	6
1992–1993	79	35	26
1993–1994	94	85	80
1994–1995	94	80	71

female students enrolled midway through the year, regardless of whether they participated in the program. The rate decreased from 8.8 per 1,000 female students in 1992–1993 to 5.3 per 1,000 in 1993–1994 and then increased to 6.8 per 1,000 in 1994–1995. (Unfortunately, the number of pregnancies in prior years had not been recorded.) The decrease in the pregnancy rate mirrors the corresponding increases in the rates of referral for and acceptance of contraceptives.

In 1995–1996, one of the four schools was unable to operate the program because of a one-year lapse in funding. For that year, the three participating schools had a pregnancy rate of 5.8 per 1,000 female students, compared with a rate of 16.5 per 1,000 in the non-participating school. Thus, the removal of the In Your Face program components from the fourth school may have been associated with an increase in the pregnancy rate.

Comparisons between the pregnancy rate in the program schools and the regional rate for adolescents younger than 15 are not possible because regional data for the period of our study are not available. Between 1990 and 1993, however, the pregnancy rate for adolescents younger than 15 in Manhattan rose from 6.2 per 1,000 to 7.4 per 1,000, a 19% increase (R. Lewis, personal communication, May 3, 1996). The rate in the schools operating the program declined by 34% between 1992 and 1996.

DISCUSSION

The results presented in this article demonstrate that well-designed, well-implemented programs may be able to lower pregnancy rates among very young, high-risk adolescents. The In Your Face program used approaches based on commonly accepted standards of quality public health and clinical practice. The program draws on the public health principle of taking a population-based approach to the diagnosis and treatment of a given condition.

The In Your Face program collected risk factor information from the great majority of students in four junior high schools through the use of a schoolwide screening survey. This information was used to identify students who were in need of the program services; program staff then sought out and invited students identified as at risk to participate in the program. Once in the program, these students were provided, in effect, with both intensive case management and continuity of care, two hallmarks of quality medical care.

The pregnancy prevention program described in this article was not expensive. Its cost consisted of the salary of one health educator placed in each school, serving approximately 1,500 students. The health educators worked in existing school-based clinics, and clearly benefited from the infrastructure available through those clinics. Fortunately, school-based clinics are now available in many schools, and this model of intensive pregnancy prevention efforts, with its emphasis on aggressive case identification and management, can be applied in such schools.

Our study has some major limitations that must be acknowledged. It was not designed as a controlled trial; therefore, alternative explanations for the decrease in pregnancy rates must be explored. The program may simply have documented a natural or ecological decline in pregnancy rates.

Several factors, however, argue against this explanation. First, the most recent New York State Department of Health statistics indicate that state and city pregnancy rates were on the rise among all adolescent age categories in the four years prior to the inception of the In Your Face program (1990–1993). It seems unlikely that a natural decrease in pregnancy rates started the same year the program began.

Second, the decrease in pregnancy rates corresponded with the increase in factors that seem necessary for pregnancy reduction—identification of "at-risk" students and increases in referral rates and family planning acceptance rates. Third, the unintentional "crossover" design, in which one of the four program schools dropped out of the treatment group and was transformed into a control group, provides a comparison that demonstrates that the pregnancy rate dramatically increased in the school from which the program components were removed, while it continued to decrease in the schools that retained the program. Although none of these factors alone is powerful enough to prove that it was the program that caused the decrease in pregnancy rates, rather than some combination of unmeasured factors, the available evidence argues against alternative explanations and for program effectiveness.

The design on which our evaluation is based is limited; however, CPFH's strategy for monitoring and evaluation helped compensate for many of these constraints. First, it monitored changes in behavior and other outcomes over time. Second, we collected and analyzed not only data on program inputs (process data) and results (impact data), but also information on intermediary data that lie in the hypothesized causal pathway of the outcome of interest. Therefore, an important part of our overall approach to program evaluation is the collection of extensive data on the various phases of the program, to ensure that the entire process of the program worked as hypothesized.[19]

Early childbearing is a symptom and a consequence of the extreme poverty that pervades urban, minority communities in the United States. The long-term solution must address the basic economic conditions that give rise to early childbearing and to limited opportunities. However, results from this study demonstrate that public health programs, in the absence of fundamental economic change, can help some adolescents to avoid early pregnancies and to delay the start of childbearing.

Notes

1. Maternal and Child Health Bureau, Public Health Service. *Child Health USA '94*. DHHS Publication No. HRSA-MCH-95–1. Washington, DC: US Department of Health and Human Services; 1995.

2. Centers for Disease Control and Prevention. State-specific pregnancy and birth rates among teenagers, United States, 1991–1992. *MMWR*. 1995;44: 677–684.

3. National Center for Health Statistics. Trends in pregnancies and pregnancy rates, United States, 1980–88. *Monthly Vital Stat Rep*. 1992;41(6):1–7.

4. Forrest JD, Singh S. The sexual and reproductive behavior of American women, 1982–1988. *Fam Plann Perspect*. 1990;22:206–214.

5. Harlap S, Kost K, Forrest JD. *Preventing Pregnancy, Protecting Health: A New Look at Birth Control Choices in the United States*. New York, NY: Alan Guttmacher Institute; 1991.

6. Landry DJ, Forrest JD. How old are US fathers? *Fam Plann Perspect*. 1995; 27:159–165.

7. Beachler MP. Improving health care for underserved infants, children, and adolescents. *Am J Dis Child*. 1991;145:565–568.

8. Kirby D, Waszak CS, Ziegler J. Six school-based clinics: their reproductive health services and impact on sexual behavior. *Fam Plann Perspect*. 1991;23: 6–14.

9. Howard M, McCabe JB. Helping teenagers postpone sexual involvement. *Fam Plann Perspect*. 1993;14:553–561.

10. Zabin LS, Hirsch MB, Smith EA, Streett R, Hardy JB. Evaluation of a pregnancy prevention program for urban teenagers. *Fam Plann Perspect*. 1986;18:119–126.

11. Walter HJ, Vaughan RD, Armstrong B, et al. Sexual, assaultive, and suicidal behaviors among urban minority junior high school students. *J Am Acad Child Adolesc Psychiatry.* 1995;34:73–80.

12. Vaughan RD, McCarthy JF, Armstrong B, Walter HJ, Waterman PD, Tiezzi L. Carrying and using weapons: A survey of minority junior high school students in New York City. *Am J Public Health.* 1996;86:568–572.

13. Walter HJ, Vaughan RD, Armstrong B, Krakoff RY, Tiezzi L, McCarthy JF. School-based health care for urban minority junior high school students. *Arch Pediatr Adolesc Med.* 1995;149:1221–1225.

14. Walter HJ, Vaughan RD, Armstrong B, Krakoff RY, Tiezzi L, McCarthy JF. Characteristics of users and nonusers of health clinics in inner-city junior high schools. *J Adolesc Health.* 1996;18:344–348.

15. Vaughan RD, McCarthy JF, Walter HJ, et al. The development, reliability, and validity of a risk factor screening survey for urban minority junior high school students. *J Adolesc Health.* 1996;19:171–178.

16. Barth RP, Leland N, Kirby D, Fetro JD. Enhancing social and cognitive skills. In: Miller BC, Card JJ, Paikoff RL, Peterson JC, eds. *Preventing Adolescent Pregnancy: Model Program and Evaluations.* Newbury Park, Calif: Sage; 1992:53–82.

17. Cook TD, Campbell DT. *Quasi-Experimentation: Design and Analysis Issues for Field Settings.* Boston, Mass: Houghton Mifflin; 1979.

18. The wording of the question asking about thoughts of suicide was changed after the first year to more accurately identify students who had actually tried to commit suicide or had considered doing so. Consequently, the proportions reporting thoughts of suicide are considerably lower in subsequent years.

19. Ward VM et al. A strategy for the evaluation of activities to reduce maternal mortality in developing countries. *Evaluation Rev.* 1994;18:438–457.

Grant Report Summaries from the Robert Wood Johnson Foundation

TRAINING, EVALUATION, AND DOCUMENTATION OF HIV/AIDS PREVENTION AND CONDOM AVAILABILITY PROGRAMS AT NEW YORK CITY SCHOOLS

(last updated October 2001)

Grants from the Robert Wood Johnson Foundation (RWJF) provided partial funding for evaluation, documentation, and training activities associated with the implementation of HIV/AIDS prevention and condom availability programs at public high schools in New York City. In February 1991, the New York City Board of Education approved a plan for expanded HIV/AIDS education that included making condoms available on request to the 261,000 students in the city's 120 public high schools. One grant provided partial support for a project director to lead a team of HIV/AIDS trainers to assist New York City high schools in implementing the education and condom availability program. Project staff prepared a manual—*HIV/AIDS Education Training Design for High School HIV/AIDS Education Teams*—used in training school-based HIV/AIDS teams and health resource staff, and a handbook, *Protecting Youth, Preventing AIDS: A Guide for Effective High School HIV Prevention Programs.* A second grant funded an evaluation of the program in 12 schools, using 10 Chicago schools as a comparison group. Findings, published in a report and journal articles, included that students enrolled in New York City schools for 1 year or more were more likely to have used a condom during their last intercourse than similar students in Chicago, students in New York City who had had three or more sexual partners within the past 6 months were more likely than students with fewer partners to have used a condom at last intercourse, and making condoms available at schools does not lead to increased sexual activity. A third grant funded a project directed by Jill Blair, the former chief adviser to the New York City schools' chancellor on HIV/AIDS education, to document the design, development, and implementation of the HIV/AIDS education and condom availability program. The researchers published four journal articles.

ENGAGING HIGHER EDUCATION IN REGIONAL HEALTH PROBLEMS

(last updated January 2003)

The National Commission on Partnerships for Children's Health held a conference of southeastern state officials and higher education representatives on ways to form regional child health collaborations in October 2000. The National Commission on Partnerships for Children's Health aims to engage higher education in working with state and local agencies on the health and welfare of children and families. The Robert Wood Johnson Foundation (RWJF) provided a $49,050 grant to the Harvard School of Public Health in support of the conference.

EVALUATING THE EFFECTIVENESS OF HEALTH BEHAVIOR CHANGE INTERVENTIONS IN CHILDREN AND ADOLESCENTS

(last updated March 2003)

Investigators at the Behavioral Medicine Laboratory at the State University of New York at Buffalo evaluated the effectiveness of school-based interventions to increase physical activity or aerobic fitness among children and adolescents. The study was conducted in 2001 and 2002 under a $20,525 grant from the Robert Wood Johnson Foundation.

MERGING SCHOOL-BASED SUPPORT GROUPS AND OTHER SERVICES FOR TEEN PARENTS

(last updated June 1998)

This grant supported a replication in New Jersey of the MELD (originally, the Minnesota Early Learning Design) self-help support program for teen parents. To address the needs of new teen parents, MELD was created in Minneapolis in the 1970s with support from the Lilly Endowment and the Carnegie Foundation. MELD programs were operational in 80 sites around the country as of 1992. This Robert Wood Johnson Foundation grant was aimed at expanding the MELD program from an earlier pilot phase in the state and implementing it within the context of existing school-based youth services in 12 high schools in New Jersey. It became the first program in the nation to combine peer support for adolescent parents with school-based services. The focus on service delivery specifically in school-based settings had originated in 1986 through the School-Based Youth Services Project (SBYSP) of the New Jersey Department of Human Services, which established school-based youth services programs in 29 districts. Services varied across sites but included health care, mental health services, family planning, employment services, child care, transportation, and recreation. Prevent Child Abuse—New Jersey (PCANJ), an organization with prior experience in replicating MELD, collaborated on this project as well. MELD's goal was to develop confidence and competence in teen parents' child-rearing and life skills. The replication of MELD at existing SBYSP sites allowed MELD participants to benefit from the spectrum of services already offered at those sites. Although the original intent of the grant was to provide programs for young mothers, the grantee also established some programs for young fathers after they starting coming to the sites. Between May 1992 and April 1997, MELD served 2,600 young parents at nine sites through 13 new programs. Nine programs served young mothers, and four served young fathers.

ELEMENTARY SCHOOL PROGRAMS TO PREVENT SUBSTANCE ABUSE AND OTHER PROBLEMS

(last updated August 1998)

This project was based on the premise that public schools are crucial institutions in American life for imparting the social values and skills young people need to prevent the onset of problem behaviors, including substance abuse. One promising model, developed by the Social Problem Solving (SPS) Unit of the University of Medicine and Dentistry of New Jersey (UMDNJ), is based on an eight-step clear-thinking strategy designed to help children identify problems and generate alternative solutions for solving them. Previous research suggests that children who learn such interpersonal cognitive problem-solving skills in the elementary grades are less likely than peers to be involved in substance abuse and other problem behaviors when they reach middle school and high school. This project sought to expand SPS's social-skills-development and problem-solving program, which was being used only in the fourth and fifth grades, to a schoolwide model to be institutionalized in 14 elementary schools in New Jersey. Shortly after the grant began, investigators amended the SPS curriculum to improve its effectiveness with the largely African American school population it was serving, adding two components to increase the students' knowledge of their history and strengthen their belief that they can achieve and succeed. Over the 5-year grant, more than 2,000 children in 15 New Jersey schools received training, and 142 educators participated either in graduate-level courses developed by the SPS Unit or in school-based, in-service minicourses. In a published paper, investigators reported on the program's impact on 60 Jersey City fourth graders. A posttest comparison with a control group who did not take the course found that participants showed better knowledge of course content, greater self-esteem, and improved problem-solving ability. The grant did not result in instituting the program schoolwide at any of the 15 schools. Upon the termination of Robert Wood Johnson Foundation funding, SPS received contracts with school districts in Newark, Orange, and Piscataway, New Jersey, which pay for teachers to receive graduate-level training in the curriculum in a summer institute and for SPS to work directly with students.

ORGANIZED MEDICINE SUMMIT ON SCHOOL AND YOUTH VIOLENCE

(last updated March 2003)

From 1997 to 1999, school shootings in the United States resulted in the deaths of 26 students and three teachers, and many more were wounded. The Commission for the Prevention of Youth Violence, established by the American Medical Association (AMA), conducted research and dissemination activities during 2000 and 2001. These activities included five meetings of commission members, a literature review on youth and school violence, and publication of the commission's recommendations in a report and in a training and outreach guide. The Robert Wood Johnson Foundation (RWJF) provided a $197,745 grant to the AMA for the project; the AMA and its commission provided in-kind support.

ANALYZING DATA ON UNIVERSAL SCHOOL-BASED DRUG EDUCATION PROGRAM EVALUATIONS

(last updated January 2004)

From 2000 to 2002, researchers at Social Capital Development Corporation, a community development and social science research firm, analyzed outcome data from more than 200 school-based drug education and prevention programs. The analysis was designed to help the field understand which programs work with which students and how best to deliver the programs. In contrast to earlier findings, the researchers found that comprehensive life skills programs were no more effective than social influences programs at all grade levels and with all types and levels of substance use and that the difference between the effectiveness of interactive and noninteractive programs across all grade levels was not statistically significant. The Robert Wood Johnson Foundation supported the research with two grants, from April 2000 through January 2003, totaling $299,712.

BUILDING A COLLABORATIVE TO IMPROVE CARE FOR CHILDREN WITH ATTENTION DEFICIT HYPERACTIVITY DISORDER

(last updated January 2004)

The National Initiative for Children's Healthcare Quality, a nonprofit organization that works to transform the quality of care for children in the United States, developed a learning collaborative designed to improve care for children with attention deficit hyperactivity disorder (ADHD) and held an international summit on the subject to disseminate the results further. The initiative began as a program of the nonprofit Institute for Healthcare Improvement and is now independent. The two organizations maintain a close working relationship. From September 2001 through February 2002, the Robert Wood Johnson Foundation (RWJF) provided $367,890 for this project. The U.S. Agency for Healthcare Research and Quality, the David and Lucile Packard Foundation, the Alza Corporation, and the North Carolina Department of Medical Assistance provided additional support.

Financing

Reprints of Key Reports and Articles

CHAPTER 22

Collision or Collaboration?

School-Based Health Services Meet Managed Care

Paula Armbruster, Ellen Andrews, Jesse Couenhoven, and Gary Blau, 1999

The World Health Organization report *Mental Health Programmes in Schools* stated, "Schools have a central position in many children's lives and potentially in their development, especially when families are unable to assume a leading role. Therefore, schools, for many children, may be the most sensible point of intervention" for mental health services.[1(p1)] In *At the Schoolhouse Door*, Knitzer, Steinberg, and Fleisch, in their examination of national policies for children with behavioral and emotional problems, concluded that close collaboration between schools and children's mental health services is the optimal effective intervention to reach behaviorally and emotionally disordered children, who otherwise might not have access to treatment. Furthermore, according to the findings of the Great Smokey Mountain Study of Youth, schools were clearly "the major player in the *de facto* system" for the delivery of children's mental health services.[3(p155)] Hence, the national movement of the past decade toward school-based mental health services is gaining momentum as an effective and accessible means of meeting the needs of the almost 8 million children who are underserved.[4,5]

Just at the time that school-based health centers (SBHCs) were moving toward becoming a partner in the children's mental health delivery system, health-care reform was instituted and managed care became a reality.[6] More importantly, managed care in some states, including Connecticut, affected the disadvantaged, underserved communities before reaching those who could afford commercial insurance. Hence, those not-for-profit institutions and agencies—child guidance clinics, community mental health centers, and school-based mental health programs, in particular—who historically provided services to disadvantaged populations and who had the least experience with the for-profit corporate culture were immediately affected. Are these differences irreconcilable? Will this confluence of events lead to collision or collaboration in implementing programs that affect America's neediest children, adolescents, and families? In this article we describe some of the interactions of for-profit managed care with SBHCs and provide an illustration of this interaction in Connecticut.

Before proceeding further, some clarification is in order. There are two prominent models for school mental health programs: one has off-site services delivered in a school by a child guidance clinic, children's outpatient psychiatric clinic, or a community mental health center; the other is the mental health component of an SBHC. An SBHC is a free-standing health clinic based in a school that provides a range of primary health-care services, including treatment of acute illnesses and accidents, health screening and physicals, and, in some cases, management of chronic illnesses, and family planning.[4,7,8] Most, *but not all,* SBHCs have a mental health component, in addition to these physical health services. In the following discussion, when SBHC is mentioned, implicit in the discussion is the assumption that a mental health component is an integral part of the SBHC. Since child guidance clinics and community mental health centers have had fewer struggles with negotiating contracts with managed-care organizations (MCO), the greater challenge has been negotiations between SBHCs and MCOs. Hence, the issues between SBHCs and MCOs are the primary focus in this overview.

SCHOOL-BASED HEALTH CENTERS AND MANAGED CARE

In his review of the school mental health movement, Weist noted that a major problem for the relationships between SBHCs and other organizations, such as MCOs, is that little is known about the school-based movement.[4] This lack of information may be responsible, in part, for the lack of coordination between school mental health programs and managed-care entities.[9] Weist suggested a solution may be for SBHCs to form relationships with MCOs and other organizations.[4] He emphasized that the school-based movement must not be allowed to develop in a haphazard fashion; rather, school-based centers must learn to integrate their services with the schools and the larger community, which includes managed-care companies. Furthermore, he challenged school mental health programs to improve their political presence. His concern, and his solution, has been echoed by others (e.g., Schlitt et al.[10]).

Zimmerman and Reif, based on their experience with managed care in Minnesota, have also concluded that a major reason for the difficulty in developing contractual relations with MCOs is that it is hard to obtain and share information about school-based clinics.[8] These authors proposed that it is crucial for school-based clinics to educate managed-care companies about access issues for adolescents and about the scope of the services offered by these clinics. They suggested meetings, extensive exchange of written information, and even clinic tours. Additionally, they called on school-based clinics to be involved with the legislative process at the state and national levels in order to influence policy decisions and develop links with managed-care systems.

While managed-care companies have often been unwilling to authorize school-based services, evidence suggests that this is changing and that managed-care companies may be increasingly open to working with and funding SBHCs.[4] One of the best ways to develop a positive relationship with a managed-care company is to demonstrate the merits of SBHCs. A number of authors have emphasized the continuing gap between need and utilization of children's mental health services and the role of SBHCs in closing the gap.[4,11–13] Based on an overview of the relationships that seven SBHCs in different states formed with managed-care companies, Schlitt et al. suggested that SBHCs offer benefits including accessibility to children, ability to intervene early, and assistance to MCOs in fulfilling state requirements for comprehensive care.[10] Similarly, Brindis et al. emphasized benefits of partnership with school-based clinics to MCOs to increase access to parents and children.[13] Even where there is high or near universal insurance coverage, access remains vitally important.

Although there is some optimism about an improvement in relations between SBHCs and managed care, Schlitt et al. predicted that some plans will resist forming relationships with SBHCs and that states will have to intervene in order for such relationships to be formed.[10] Brindis and Wunsch also noted that, thus far, very few contractual agreements have been made between SBHCs and MCOs.[9] They too affirmed the importance of the state in creating incentives for interaction between managed care and school-based centers. However, several models of partnership and agreements with managed-care companies exist, and authors agree that there is no one way that works best.[8–10]

Another major issue is the financial relationship between SBHCs and managed care. Lear, Montgomery, Schlitt, and Rickett noted that many SBHCs have been established without a clear understanding of how they will continue to be funded.[14] It is relevant that since their inception in the early 1970s, SBHCs have remained outside the mainstream organizational and financial arrangements that characterize the prevailing health-care system.[10] Traditionally, SBHCs have relied on private foundations, local health departments and Maternal and Child Health block grants. Further deviant from the mainstream model is that many school centers chose not to bill clients or to seek third-party reimbursement, as they sought a continuing relationship with Medicaid as the foundation for future funding.[10,15]

As SBHCs begin to develop relationships with MCOs for funding, Brindis and Wunsch cautioned that SBHCs should expect only partial funding from managed care, with recognition of this reality enhancing relationships with MCOs.[9] There is consensus that in order to strengthen their position, it is critical that school-based clinics must have data on the utilization of their services, on cost and on outcome measures.[8–10,14] According to the Massachusetts Department of Public Health, quality assurance standards must be comparable to those of clinics and mental health agencies. Since SBHCs are competing with other providers for dollars,[14] they must define their services clearly and provide information on how they fill service gaps to children, while at the same time remaining flexible and open to addressing needs of the communities they serve.

Schlitt et al. expressed the view that SBHCs may never be self-supporting.[10] Many students are uninsured, and many services provided by SBHCs are not reimbursable, or are the kind of services that MCOs are highly reluctant to reimburse. For example, in SBHCs, mental health providers, because they are located in the schools, spend time collaborating with educational staff, both formally and informally, regarding the needs and behaviors of particular students. Additionally, more time is spent in family outreach. This may require making home visits to engage other family members or to have a permission form signed. Since the provider also functions as a referral source to more acute or supplementary care (e.g., hospitalization, day hospital, residential care), additional time is spent making such referrals. Also, school mental health practitioners often conduct prevention programs, both with students and staff. These programs might include workshops on substance abuse, violence, conflict resolution, peer pressure and other issues relevant to students. Schlitt et al. suggested that SBHCs would have to relinquish too much of what makes them effective (i.e., flexible, productive, proactive approach) if they were to completely conform to managed-care specifications.[10]

Another barrier to developing relationships between MCOs and SBHCs is philosophical differences between the two. Relevant here is the "managed-care mindset." Managed-care companies tend to see partnership with SBHCs as a *business venture*. If SBHCs do not understand this managed-care perspective, collaboration will be impossible.[10] Brindis and Wunsch noted that while the primary interests of SBHCs are to increase access and address the needs of the students, the primary concern of MCOs are to contain costs and serve only those individuals who are part of their service plan.[9]

However, in spite of the aforementioned challenges, linkages are currently being established between MCOs and SBHCs. In 1993, the U.S. Department of Health and Human Services reported on the status of efforts to coordinate SBHCs and managed care. This report indicated that the level of coordination *varies widely* across the country. In some instances, SBHCs acted as a limited provider, needing prior authorization from the managed-care plan before providing a restricted number of services. In other instances, SBHCs provided primary care and were reimbursed for all services they delivered to children and adolescents in the plan. A promising development is that some states are passing laws requiring linkage between SBHCs and MCOs. For example, state law requires Medicaid managed-care providers to coordinate with SBHCs in Multnomah County, Oregon. In other states, such as Maryland, protocols for referral and treatment between SBHCs and managed-care providers have been encouraged by legislation.

In order to build the trust necessary for collaboration, it is important to focus on the common goals shared by MCOs and SBHCs, including improving access, having a primary medical home and a focus on wellness.[8,9] In the following we elaborate on these goals.

Access. Specific to improved access, many health-care reformers believe that school-based and school-linked health-care services have proven themselves to be an effective means for reaching high-risk populations that would otherwise go unserved.[16,17] Thus, for vulnerable populations, such as children eligible for Medicaid, school-based services may be the preferable treatment modality.[18,19]

Although any Congressional national health-care reform movement appears to be stalled, the Clinton administration's original proposal would have expanded school health programs (including mental health) across the country. The President's Fiscal Year (FY) 1996 budget provided for $100 million in SBHC expansion grants, increasing to $400 million dollars in FY 1999. These grants would have been used to establish nearly 3,500 new school-based or school-linked health centers nationally, increasing access to health-care services for thousands of children and adolescents, and enhancing opportunities for SBHCs to participate actively in emerging national health and managed-care movements.[20] Despite the reality that broad health-care reform has not occurred, child advocates are encouraged by the increasing national interest in comprehensive school health and mental health services. Further, there are now funding mechanisms in place through the recently established State Children's Health Insurance Program (SCHIP), which will significantly expand health insurance coverage for youth over the next 10 years. Experts predict that in many states, school-based programs will be centerpieces in expanded services for children.

Medical home. It is not unreasonable to believe that if the prevailing health-care delivery system continues its current movement toward increased managed care, SBHCs could emerge as a gatekeeping system for children and adolescents. In an evolving health-care delivery system, increasingly reliant on principles of managed care, the SBHC offers the distinct advantage of providing initial care and entry point services, with referrals to providers of specialty care. Dowden, Calvert, Davis, and Gullotta (1997) emphasized that SBHCs can provide a medical home for children and adolescents by functioning as a primary care facility for both physical and behavioral health-care needs.

Wellness and prevention. Preventing future illness, and thereby reducing health-care costs associated with illness, should be a basic element of managed-care activities. Prevention is more clearly a goal of SBHCs, which offer a natural site for such activities to take place. Schools offer the unique opportunity for health-care professionals to develop positive relationships with youth while they are still healthy, and SBHCs can promote healthy lifestyles via education and modeling.[21,22] School-based health centers can also be a focal point for preventive activities aimed at reducing drug, alcohol, or tobacco use; depression; suicide; teen pregnancy and sexually transmitted diseases; accidents; and interpersonal violence.

However, while many, if not most, MCOs will espouse the benefits of prevention, a reality is that few fund preventive activities. In fact, there is a concern that managed-care will curtail prevention and focus care on those with clearly demonstrated need.[4] Time will tell whether MCOs will continue to pay lip service to prevention, or begin to engage in prevention activities at more meaningful levels. Should MCOs show interest in the latter, SBHCs present a natural vehicle for the implementation of prevention programs.

These goals pertaining to access, having a medical home, and wellness and prevention represent some congruity between MCOs and SBHCs. Ideally, closer linkages could emerge between managed-care entities and school health clinics, ultimately improving the physical and behavioral health-care services delivered to children and adolescents. With this overview of the current interactions between SBHCs and managed care, we turn now to the experience of Connecticut, a state that is in the forefront of managed care and health services for children.

SCHOOL-BASED HEALTH CENTERS AND MANAGED CARE IN CONNECTICUT: A CASE EXAMPLE OF COLLABORATION IN PROCESS

There is a high level of utilization of school health services in Connecticut; in 1996, over 12,000 students had over 60,000 documented visits to SBHCs in the state.[21] For medical services, the most common visits were for a medical history, health education, physical exam or health screening, and medication administration. For mental health, the majority of visits were for counseling, support, referral, or advocacy.

Fortunately, Connecticut has a long history of experience with SBHCs providing behavioral and physical health care to high-risk children living in medically underserved communities. Most policy makers, both in the legislative and executive branches, are aware of the successes and unique opportunities that these sites offer, and have been supportive over the years. That history of support has been an advantage in the switch to managed care, but it has also presented certain challenges.

Connecticut has required, since their inception in 1995, that Medicaid Managed Care plans include SBHCs in their provider networks as a condition of their contracts with the state. Connecticut is not alone in this support for SBHCs—Maryland, Minnesota, New York, Oregon, and Rhode Island all include contract language that requires plans to contract with SBHCs as their primary care provider. Many states require or strongly encourage plans to include historic community-based Medicaid providers (in behavioral health this means SBHCs, Child Guidance Clinics, and community mental health centers) in managed-care networks. It is up to *advocates* to ensure that these protections are reflected in contract language and that contract provisions are enforced by the state. Particular attention must be paid to the inclusion of mental health services in these contracts.

Despite provisions requiring SBHC–managed care contracting in Connecticut, SBHCs reported *severe* drops in Medicaid revenue under managed care, jeopardizing their ability to serve both Medicaid and uninsured students.[23] One year after the implementation of Medicaid Managed Care, all 19 SBHCs that responded to a survey had signed contracts with at least one plan, but only 12 were billing. Even fewer were billing for mental health services. While virtually all of Connecticut's 59 SBHCs provided care to Medicaid recipients prior to the implementation of managed care, few billed Medicaid for those services. The vast majority of SBHCs and their mental health service providers were funded by grants from public and private sources. When Medicaid moved to managed care, SBHCs were expected to enter managed-care provider networks and to bill for reimbursement. Some of the stress on Connecticut's SBHCs is due to this shift in funding and not to Medicaid managed care per se.

As has been described, SBHCs and their mental health staff are often not familiar with formal negotiations in a corporate environment; this lack of sophistication has reportedly led some Connecticut centers to sign contracts with terms that are at odds with the long-term financial health of the clinic. For example, in some clinics, fees since the switch to managed care have been reduced by as much as 75%.[23]

In Connecticut and elsewhere, limits on the scope of services that plans are willing to certify and reimburse is a barrier to developing working relationships. Contracts typically include primary, acute, and episodic care services. Behavioral health services, group counseling, outreach, and health education are sometimes omitted from contracts, but these services are at the heart of the mission of SBHCs and are the keys to their success.[23,24] As yet, some of the MCOs perceive these services to be outside of their purview, but the state had taken a firm stand to ensure that these services are properly funded. The issue of parity between health and mental health at the forefront of federal discussion has been taken up by child advocates, providers, and consumers locally, as is the case in Connecticut. This will likely have a positive impact, ensuring that all SBHCs provide mental health services.

Zimmerman and Reif stated that "perhaps the most complex issue for school-based health center providers around the country is the need to form relationships with all plans that serve the school population."[8(p39)] Connecticut is no exception. As noted, poor communication is the biggest barrier to collaboration between SBHCs and managed-care plans. Without effective communication, suspicions can grow and productive relationships are impossible both in contracting and in day-to-day functions. *Advocacy is optimized by individual personal relationships between mental health clinicians and utilization reviewers and care managers of plans.* Recognizing this, some plans in Connecticut route claims from specific mental health providers to the same care manager over time. Other plans have implemented tours and meetings between health-plan personnel in order to discuss concerns and resolve issues.

In Connecticut, there have been significant efforts to educate health plans about the mental health needs of Medicaid clients and the unique opportunities for access to preventive care and health education that SBHCs provide. This education of MCOs is critical, as they are unfamiliar with this population because they have traditionally served healthy, low-risk, commercial populations. Managed-care organizations must appreciate the variety of providers and techniques employed by SBHCs in the collaborative environment of a school, working with teachers, administrators, parents, communities, and students to optimize health. It has been equally challenging to educate SBHCs and mental health providers about the potential benefits of managed care and overcoming suspicions and horror stories concerning managed-care companies.

While the increased administrative burden of managed care is a universal complaint among providers, these difficulties represent a special problem for SBHCs. In contrast with mental health programs that operate out of community mental health centers (CMHCs), programs connected to SBHCs often have little administrative support. Hence, increased efforts associated with managed care, such as obtaining authorizations for services, maintaining necessary paperwork, conducting utilization reporting, and billing can be very difficult for SBHCs to handle. Thus, it is critical that procedures in each of these areas be thoughtfully designed and coordinated, and supported by the state. For example, in Connecticut, under the leadership of the legislative Medicaid Managed Care Council, plans and providers (including SBHCs) collaborated to develop a standard reporting form for mental health services applicable to all plans and providers.

Credentialing processes are a particular burden for mental health providers in SBHCs. In Connecticut, the Department of Social Services has notified plans that facility credentialing is sufficient for their purposes. Facility credentialing allows a state-licensed facility to maintain credentials for all its providers rather than requiring each clinic provider to submit extensive documentation to each plan, as in individual credentialing. However, state licensure implies compliance with all state regulations, involving substantial administrative work. With limited support staff, compliance with these regulations can bootstrap a program, limiting the number of children that can be served by it. On the other hand, if an SBHC opts for individual versus facility credentialing, relatively few providers may be credentialed by the MCO.

Confidentiality is also a problem for SBHCs, and is a particularly sensitive issue in the delivery of mental health services. While managed-care plans need information about services provided to clients, and will not provide reimbursement unless this information is obtained, SBHCs must respect the privacy of adolescents accessing services at school, at times without parental knowledge. This must be addressed by state policy-makers with thoughtful attention to the needs of all interested parties.[23] Connecticut is in the process of discussions between managed-care plans and providers to try to resolve issues of confidentiality and privacy. The reality of diagnoses for children entering MCO databases is a very complicated issue, not only in Connecticut but nationwide. In the case of the Medicaid population, psychiatric diagnoses are assigned for problems that are often reactive to environmental issues rather than intrinsically psychiatric. Such diagnoses will follow the child for life and risk being misinterpreted to the detriment of the child as he or she becomes an adult.

Connecticut is also grappling with another problem for SBHCs and other public health providers—identifying funding for preventive programs, such as outreach and health education. While these services are an important part of the mission of public health institutions, they are not typically reimbursed by MCOs. In Connecticut, advocates, consumers, and providers are lobbying the legislature to require MCOs to reimburse for preventive programs so essential for this population. Our argument is that by supporting preventive programs, more expensive, acute care may be avoided. By this argument we are hoping to address the fiscal concerns of the MCOs. It is critical, however, that groups band together to emphasize to MCOs the importance of reimbursing preventive programs, which are viewed as essential to school-based health care.[4,25]

In Connecticut, there are protections against health plans "creaming" or enrolling only healthy, low-risk, low-cost clients, but no plan is required to seek out high-cost clients, such as adolescent substance abusers or teens with mental illnesses. It is vital that SBHCs, with their links to schools and other community organizations, ensure that these clients are not ignored by the system. This is made more difficult by the above-described administrative and financial pressures of managed care on SBHC staff. Cooperation with other community organizations on behalf of the children and adolescents and their families is even more important in a time of scarce resources.

Uninsured students represent a large financial drain on SBHCs, which, like most other public health institutions, do not turn anyone away. Significant health-care needs of uninsured children often determine where SBHCs are established. Typically a provider in a SBHC will see any child who is referred and determine who to bill for those services after they are provided. In a random class of 24 American children, approximately eight were uninsured for a month or more and four of those were uninsured for at least a year.[26] Two or three of those children were actually eligible for Medicaid, but not enrolled.[27] In Connecticut, this figure represents 80,000 children. When an uninsured child presents in a SBHC, the clinic should determine whether that child can enroll in Medicaid. This is important not only for the financial health of the Center, but for the future health-care needs of the child. This question of lack of insurance is a particular problem for adolescents who are estranged from their families and "on their own" or for reasons of privacy do not wish to use their parents' insurance, particularly for mental health. However, clinics must be sensitive to families' reluctance to apply for public assistance. In whatever way these issues are resolved, children should not be denied care because of insurance.

COMMONALITIES AMONG STATES

While we have been discussing Connecticut's singular experience, common issues emerge across states. Schlitt et al. noted that among SBHCs, there is consensus on three primary lessons learned in building partnerships with managed care[10]:

1. Understanding the managed-care perspective and taking the initiative in educating the plans on the role and services of the school-based model;

2. Marketing the strengths of the centers, particularly underscoring their role in providing access to traditionally underserved populations; hence, having a preventive role in decreasing the need for more acute services;

3. Collecting, analyzing, and using data. The importance of the collection and use of data cannot be overly emphasized in order to demonstrate the strength of the centers and in helping the MCOs understand the SBHCs' perspectives.

Schlitt et al. emphasized that most critical to the future success of the partnership between managed-care plans and SBHCs, is the role of the states in taking a facilitation or promotional role by either encouragement or regulatory mechanisms.[10] We favor the latter, as we believe encouragement is not enough. In Connecticut, the Department of Social Services required managed-care plans to contract with SBHCs in their service area. Leaders and advocates in child health and mental health in the state view this requirement as being essential to the delivery of effective health and mental health services and, as such, were necessary ingredients in the state's contracts with MCOs.

In addition to commitments to SBHCs by the states, grant dollars must be made available to cover the cost of serving students in the centers.[10,28] At a recent meeting of federal and state health policy-makers, and representatives from SBHCs and MCOs, it was agreed that "to survive, school-based health centers and their sponsors, must secure reliable sources of funding."[29(p1)] Hence, the recently established SCHIP, which expanded health insurance for uninsured, low-income children may have important implications for SBHCs because they serve the children identified by the federal legislation.

A major implication of the above is that SBHCs need to work hard to reach proportionally more children with insurance. In addition, SBHCs need to attend to three other major issues as SCHIP unfolds[28]:

1. The degree to which the 10% set-aside will be used to strengthen the existing delivery system including SBHCs. Under SCHIP, states are allowed to spend 10% of the total budget on activities other than insurance coverage, including direct payments to providers (e.g., SBHCs) for activities such as outreach.

2. The development of effective enrollment strategies necessary to engage the estimated 25% of children eligible but not enrolled in Medicaid. School health clinics are in a key position to enroll students in programs developed under SCHIP, given their high percentage of uninsured students.

3. Benefit packages under SCHIP may not match the services delivered by SBHCs. Hence, while SBHCs may reduce the number of uninsured children, reimbursement for services may not increase.

Florida conducted an expensive outreach campaign to enroll families in either Medicaid or in the SCHIP program—notably, program administrators found that 90 to 95% of the families whose children enrolled learned of the program from materials distributed at schools. Hence, it is critical that SBHCs seize this opportunity to underscore their role as important conduits for outreach.

The SCHIP legislation may be an extraordinary opportunity for SBHCs to assure continuity of funding. However, much will depend on how effective supporters, advocates, and SBHCs are in convincing state legislatures, state officials, and MCOs that school-based health care should become a prioritized solution to addressing the needs of uninsured children. It is vital that SBHCs and all client advocates work to ensure that consumers have a voice in the design, implementation, and ongoing development of Medicaid managed-care programs. There are many mechanisms for consumer input, including consumer advisory boards, public hearings, hotlines, ombuds programs (independent advocacy organizations that can intervene in individual cases on behalf of clients), input into outside quality assurance processes (e.g., consumer surveys, focus groups, or direct communication), grievance procedures (internal managed-care plan grievance programs and state agency fair hearings), and by hiring Medicaid recipients as employees of plans, subcontractors, and enrollment brokers.[30] It is important that historic providers advocate for mechanisms allowing consumer input into systems of care and that they inform and support clients in accessing those mechanisms. The most important advocates are consumers themselves; providers are often able to help consumers take on this role. Additionally, providers need to become advocates, as well as be aware of advocacy groups in the state, such as those associated with the National Alliance for the Mentally Ill, the Federation of Families for Children's Mental Health, and the Human Service Association.

A SCHOOL-BASED MENTAL HEALTH PROGRAM WITHIN THE CONTEXT OF MANAGED CARE

We would like to turn to a case example of a child guidance clinic providing school-based services while navigating the managed-care environment. The program was created as a direct outgrowth of our work in the New Haven community, which emphasized to us the number of children who need mental health services but do not receive them. Nationally, we know that two thirds of the children needing mental health services do not receive such services.[5,31] In New Haven, a recent children's mental health needs assessment found that almost 40% of its children were at risk for psychiatric disorder, but that only 11% of these at-risk children had utilized mental health services.[32] These findings became very real for us when, in addition to the increasing number of referrals to the Outpatient Clinic, the Yale Child Study Center's outreach programs were uncovering children and families with acute mental health needs who had never contacted a clinic. In addition, our study of attrition in the Outpatient Clinic found that the inner-city family is at risk of dropping out during the first few weeks of contact with the clinic.[33,34] In response to these challenges and with the support of the New Haven Public Schools, the clinic developed a school-based mental health program to bring its services to the inner-city schools. The goal of the program was to provide more effective access and outreach to underserved, disadvantaged children and to collaborate more closely with the schools in this endeavor.

In January of 1992, the Outpatient Clinic, in collaboration with New Haven Public Schools and the Connecticut Department of Children and Families, established mental health services in 4 inner-city schools; this number increased to 37, or almost 80% of the schools by September of 1997. The Clinic, the largest child guidance clinic in the state, serves approximately 1,500 children annually, and 50% (750) of these children were seen in the schools between 1996 and 1997. The project responded to clinical need and was built on the legacy of school collaboration instituted by the School Development Program in our university developed by James Comer.[35,36] The Comer Project addressed school climate; the clinic provided direct services. The World Health Organization Division of Mental Health noted that effective school intervention can implement an "environment centered" model (such as the Comer Project), a "child centered" model (such as the Clinic's service) or, optimally, both.[1] In our case, both programs worked in concert to provide supplementary services to the school.

Children and families seen in the schools are considered clinic cases. They are assured the same evaluation and treatment they would receive if they had entered the central clinic. All children seen in the schools are assigned to the clinic's weekly interdisciplinary clinical treatment team, and hence are subject to the identical review and quality assurance program, as the cases seen in the clinic. In addition to the clinic's weekly interdisciplinary treatment team, a school clinic team meets bimonthly. This team ensures integration of all school-based services both within and outside our institution, as it is comprised of clinicians in the schools and consultants from the Yale Child Study Center (such as those from School Development Project), as well as representatives from schools and community agencies. A child psychiatrist provides medication consultation on site.

The program was envisioned as an outreach program of the clinic and started with one basic service; clinicians from the Outpatient Clinic went to the school to bring the clinic services to the schools in order to improve access for disadvantaged children and adolescents. Since then, three other approaches have evolved, creating the four we have presently. In the three newer programs, the Outpatient Clinic (1) provides the mental health component to three SBHCs and receives a grant; (2) supplements the mental health component of the SBHCs and receives no grant; (3) and provides school-linked services in a suburban school system. In the school-linked approach, there is close collaboration with the school, with a formal referral mechanism, but services are provided at the clinic, not off site in the school.

Funding and referral mechanisms depend on the service approach. For the off-site services from the central clinic and services supplementing the mental health component of SBHCs (neither of which have grant support), billing is done through the central clinic, as these services are considered clinic services provided off site (e.g. school, home, hospital, or other). Since the advent of managed care in October 1995, the central clinic has contracted with all 11 managed-care companies in the state. Hence, reimbursement for these school-based services has not been a problem, as the services rendered are regarded by the MCOs as services of the central clinic.

When the clinic receives a grant to provide the mental health component for a funded SBHC, the clinician is there full time, and until recently no billing was instituted. All children needing services were seen for no fee. However, two issues have arisen. First, the SBHCs have had difficulty acquiring contracts with the MCOs for reasons discussed earlier (e.g., credentialing, documentation). Second, grant funding for the majority of the SBHCs will end, since the private foundations that provided the initial funding for them expected the state to assure and institutionalize permanent funding. In anticipation of the loss of grant support, starting in September 1997, we have been asked to bill through the central clinic for the mental health services in these SBHCs. Fortunately, due to our experience with providing off-site services in our other programs, we were able to initiate billing procedures with little difficulty. Our history of providing services without grants has stood us in good stead in the environment of fewer grants and the expansion of MCOs.

Students seen in high schools have presented us with billing challenges. One of the largest issues for this underserved population is lack of insurance. A significant number of the adolescents who are seen are disconnected from their families either physically, emotionally, or both. Many of the teens we see do not live at home; they live with friends either at their homes or make other arrangements. Even if they live at home, emotional estrangement from their families is often notable. We have used the term *adolescents at large* or, to quote others, *adolescents on their own* to describe this population.

This disconnection from family has a direct impact on payment for service. Generally, whether or not the teen is at home, if family conflict is present, either the family refuses to have the teen use their insurance, or the teen does not want their family to know they are seeking mental health services. Often teens "on their own" are not knowledgeable about their health or mental health benefits. We have found that educating certain teens about their benefits can be helpful. There are also teens whose families simply have no insurance, public or private. If an adolescent is in a group home or shelter, the situation is much better, as the State Department of Children and Youth Services is responsible for linking the adolescent with a MCO.

The number of uninsured students we serve collectively in the school and central clinic has increased from 0% in 1993–94 to 20% in 1995–96. We suspect that this increase is a result of our school-based services, because by providing access to service to a heretofore underserved population, we have "uncovered" many children who have no insurance or who are Medicaid eligible but whose families have not utilized it. Also, this was a year of transition from Medicaid to Medicaid managed care and there was much confusion both on the part of the clients, as well as in the databases of the billing systems in both the clinic and the various MCOs. We anticipate this situation to improve. Another contributing factor is that in the schools, we have encountered parents who will not let us bill for a mental health problem, as they do not want their child to have a diagnoses in the MCO database.

Another function we provide to the school is that of a referral source for medical care, specialized or acute care, and also for recreational activities and tutoring. Hence, in many schools we become the informal gatekeepers to a range of services, approximating a "medical home" for students.[21] The central clinic also has an Immediate Access Service for visits at the clinic within 24 hours if the family chooses not to receive services in school during a crisis. This Immediate Access Clinic has replaced what was in the past a visit to the hospital Emergency Room. It is also noteworthy that in some schools the clinicians spend almost 50% of their time in crisis intervention. This service has significant cost savings implications for which MCOs need to be made aware.

Perhaps most importantly, our services are reaching the targeted disadvantaged population and are effective. Since the data collected in the schools and in the clinic is the same, recent investigations compared children seen in the central clinic with those seen in the schools. When compared with the central clinic sample ($N = 304$), the school sample ($N = 44$) was found to be comparable in terms of socioeconomic status and psychiatric impairment.[12] At the time of the study (1994) only four schools were served. By September 1996, 80% (36) of the city's public schools received mental health services. Since impressions of school and mental health personnel affirmed the effectiveness of such services, an evaluation of this program was conducted. A clinic sample ($N = 220$) was compared with a school sample ($N = 168$).[37] Findings revealed that clinician ratings for psychiatric disturbance and functional adjustment were comparable for children seen at the clinic and those seen at the school.

IMPLICATIONS BASED ON OUR EXPERIENCES

The fact that the school-based service was spawned by the clinic service has had major implications for the school-based service. Perhaps most importantly, clinicians who provide services in the central clinic are the same ones who serve the children and adolescents in the schools. Hence, the issue of credentialing is automatically assured, since the clinic has contracts with all the MCOs, which mandate that all the clinicians are credentialed. Thus, one issue programs may struggle with MCOs over is automatically eliminated. In addition, since clinicians working in the central clinic must seek the MCO's authorization for service and are accustomed to its documentation requirements, another potential obstacle is also overcome. Further, since the billing and the data collection done for school cases is the same as that done in the clinic, again the school service met the requirements of the MCO. Finally, having clinicians provide services both in the schools and in the clinic has prevented "burn-out." Providing mental health services in schools is often challenging. However, by working both in the schools and the clinic, therapists are afforded a different perspective, which can be energizing, stimulating, and supportive. They experience a sense of back-up from the central clinic so they do not feel isolated in the school environment.

All clinicians receive training to reflect the work in the schools; also included is a focus on working in the managed-care environment. Hence, the training essentially reviews three cultures, that of the school, the clinic, and the managed-care environment, each of which is a critical system with which they must interact.

A great deal of diversity exists among the clinicians. At least half of our clinicians come from similar ethnic and racial backgrounds as the students, their families, and school personnel. As a result, trust has developed both on the part of the clients and the schools, as well as fostering communication on cultural, ethnic, and racial issues among the clinicians. MCOs also prefer to refer to our clinic because our clinicians are diverse racially, ethnically, and linguistically. We believe we have a critical role in educating the MCOs on the importance of cultural competence and diversity.

Before closing, it is important to describe another offshoot of the clinic's program. To reiterate, the program was created to provide access to mental health services to underserved, disadvantaged children and families. Because of the school-based programs, the clinic has become identified with outreach. This has led to requests for mental health services from other community-based agencies. For example, the clinic now provides services to a homeless adolescent drop-in center, to adolescent group homes, and to adolescent shelters. Most recently, a neighborhood community center that serves five elementary schools and one intermediate school has requested the clinic's services. The mission of the clinic is to close the gap between children in need of services and those who receive them. The school is a critical point of departure in implementing this mission. Thus, the clinic is becoming a model of proactive delivery of services to youth where they are, an approach that is consistent with natural innovations.[7]

Experience has shown us that, once in the schools, a snowball effect takes place and mental health services heretofore never available to those in need are provided to the neighborhoods and community agencies who request them. A corollary to this has been reimbursement

for children seen in these community settings because they are perceived as clinic interventions rendered off site.[15] Since community
agencies have requested our services, they have also taken the initiative
in obtaining information from parents, so that our clinicians have had
the necessary documentation to request and obtain authorization from
MCOs for their services.

We have identified at least eight benefits of our school-based services
to the child and adolescent mental health delivery system. These contributions include (1) access to services for disadvantaged and underserved youth, (2) system wide collaboration, (3) prevention of acute
psychiatric intervention, (4) assuming a gatekeeper role for more acute
or specialized care, (5) systematic program evaluation, (6) training in
working with a range of systems and cultures, (7) cultural competence
and diversity, and (8) outreach and community-based care. We have
become advocates for our school-based program and its benefits to the
MCOs and the children and families in their charge. We have presented
that providing access and early intervention is cost-effective in the long
run.[6] We have demonstrated that our school-based service is as effective as that of the clinic.[37] We believe we have the responsibility to take
on the role of educating for-profit MCOs on the importance to them,
in terms they understand, of not-for-profit community-based mental
health services, such as those provided by SBHCs. We would like to educate them further of the value of *pro bono* work.

SUMMARY AND FUTURE CHALLENGES

School-based mental health services perform a vital function in the
children's mental health delivery system in assuring that high-risk, disadvantaged, and underserved children have access to care. Often students seen in the schools would otherwise not receive needed services.
Further, in our school population, we have found that approximately
12% of the students present serious psychiatric disorders or are significantly cognitively impaired.[37] Without the school-based services, it is
likely these disorders would have remained undetected until a more
acute phase emerged. Furthermore, providing services in schools has
led to a snowball effect. Once access is provided and the benefits perceived, other neighborhood-based agencies are requesting that services
come to their sites as well. As the African proverb states, "it takes a village to raise a child," our commitment is to go into the village to facilitate the process. Managed care must join us in the "village."

It is the responsibility of child and family mental health programs, advocates, and children and families utilizing these services to convince and educate the MCOs of the importance of providing accessible services in the community, with school-based programs exemplifying this quality. As mentioned earlier, access is purportedly a major tenant of managed care. The dialogue must continue between SBHCs and MCOs so that the latter become more responsive to the needs of the children with behavioral health problems, particularly disadvantaged children. The MCOs must recognize that SBHCs, as well as other community-based services, are a critical link in accessing services for those children and families who may need them most.

The Connecticut experience is still a work in progress. Our goals have not been achieved. However, untiring advocacy groups, a committed legislature, and knowledgeable state department leadership offer optimism. Above all, it is essential that consumer groups be informed and enlisted in the advocacy process. They are the groups that MCOs target for enrollment. The more educated a consumer base, the better the services. State and agency administrators, clinicians, school personnel, legislators, and other groups need to join with consumers in advocacy for school-based mental health care.

Finally, this is a reciprocal process and an ongoing dialectic. We believe that both providers and planners of school-based mental health programs and managed-care leaders can learn from one another, and both have major contributions to make to the overall delivery system. Service providers contribute knowledge and skills in working with this population; MCOs bring administrative and fiscal expertise and a focus on and mandate for quality and cost-effective care. For-profits and not-for-profits must enter into a dialogue to educate and understand each other so that they may become collaborators in the service of children and youth. If we fail, so will our children. If we succeed, so will our children.

Notes

1. World Health Organization, Division of Mental Health. *Mental Health Programmes in Schools.* Geneva, Switzerland: World Health Organization; 1994.
2. Knitzer J, Steinberg Z, Fleisch B. *At the Schoolhouse Door: An Examination of Programs and Policies for Children with Behavioral and Emotional Problems.* New York, NY: Bank Street College of Education; 1990.

3. Burns BJ, Costello EJ, Angold A., et al. Children's mental health service use across service sectors. *Health Aff.* 1995;14:147–159.

4. Weist MD. Expanded school mental health services: a national movement in progress. In: Ollendick TH, Prinz RJ, eds. *Advances in Clinical Child Psychology.* New York, NY: Plenum Press; 1997:318–352.

5. US Congress, Office of Technology Assessment. *Children's Mental Health: Problems and Services.* Washington, DC: US GPO; 1986.

6. Kaplan DW, Calonge BN, Guernsey BP, Hanrahan MB. Managed care and school-based health centers. *Arch Pediatr Adolesc Med.* 1998;152, 25–33.

7. Flaherty LT, Weist MD, Warner BS. School-based mental health services in the United States: history, current models, and needs. *Community Ment Health J.* 1996;32:314–352.

8. Zimmerman DJ, Reif CJ. School-based health centers and managed care health plans: partners in primary care. *J Public Health Manag Pract.* 1995;1:33–39.

9. Brindis CD, Wunsch B. *Finding Common Ground: Developing Linkages Between School-Linked/School-Based Health Programs and Managed Care Health Plans.* Sacramento, Calif: Foundation Consortium for School-Linked Services; 1996.

10. Schlitt JJ, Lear JG, Ceballos C, et al. *School-Based Health Centers and Managed Care: Seven School-Based Health Center Programs Forge New Relationships.* Washington, DC: Making the Grade National Program Office; 1996.

11. Adelman HS, Taylor L. School-based mental health: toward a comprehensive approach. *J Ment Health Adm.* 1993;20:32–45.

12. Armbruster P, Gerstein SH, Fallon T. Bridging the gap between service need and service utilization: a school-based mental health program. *Community Ment Health J.* 1997;33:199–211.

13. Brindis CD, Kapphahn C, McCarter V, Wolfe AL. The impact of health insurance status on adolescents' utilization of school-based clinic services: implications for health care reform. *J Adolesc Health.* 1995;16:18–25.

14. Lear JG, Montgomery LL, Schlitt JJ, Rickett KD. Key issues affecting school-based health centers and Medicaid. *J Sch Health.* 1996;66(3):83–88.

15. Koyanagi C, Brodie JR. *Making Medicaid Work to Fund Intensive Community Services for Children with Serious Emotional Disturbance: An Advocacy Guide to Financing Key Components of a Comprehensive System of Care.* Washington, DC: Bazelon Center for Mental Health Law; 1994.

16. Davis WE. School-linked mental health services for children: overcoming common obstacles. Presented at the annual convention of the American Psychological Association;Chicago, Ill.; 1997

17. Davis WE, Becene S. *School-Linked and School-Based Mental Health Services: A Selected Bibliography.* Orono, Maine: University of Maine, College of Education, Institute for the Study of Students at Risk; 1996.

18. Gullotta TP, Noyes L, Blau GM. School-based health and social service centers. In: Blau GM, Gullotta TP, eds. *Adolescent Dysfunctional Behavior: Causes, Interventions, and Prevention.* Thousand Oaks, Calif: Sage; 1996:267–283.

19. Reissman J. *School-Based and School-Linked Clinics: The Facts.* Washington, DC: Center for Population Options; 1991.

20. Koppleman J. *Delivering Health and Social Services at School: A Look at the Full-Service School Movement.* Washington, DC: George Washington University; 1994.

21. Dowden SL, Calvert RD, Davis L, Gullotta TP. Improving access to health care: school-based health centers. In: Weissberg RP, Gullotta TP, Hampton RL, Ryan BA, Adams GR, eds. *Establishing Preventive Services.* Thousand Oaks, Calif: Sage; 1997:154–182.

22. Levy J. Shepardson W. A look at current school-linked service efforts. *Future Child.* 1992;2:44–55.

23. Langhill D, Dubois S, Martin K, Perkins J, Rivera L. *Medicaid Managed Care: An Advocate's Guide for Protecting Children.* Washington, DC: National Association of Child Advocates; 1996.

24. Children's Health Council. *Evaluation of the Connecticut Access Medicaid Managed Care Program: Impact on Recipient Access to Quality Care.* Hartford, Conn: Children's Health Council; 1997.

25. Durlak JA. *School-Based Prevention Programs for Children and Adolescents.* Thousand Oaks, Calif: Sage; 1995.

26. Families USA Foundation. *One out of Three Kids: Kids Without Health Insurance.* Washington, DC: Families USA Foundation; 1997.

27. Congressional Budget Office. *Health Insurance for Children: Private Insurance Coverage Continues to Deteriorate.* Washington, DC: US GPO; 1996.

28. Making the Grade. *Insurance Expansions and School-Based Health Centers.* Washington, DC: Making the Grade National Program Office; 1997.

29. Making the Grade. *Medicaid, Managed Care, and School-Based Health Centers: Proceedings of a Meeting with Policy Makers and Providers.* Washington, DC: Making the Grade National Program Office; 1995.

30. Perkins J, Olson K, Rivera L, Skatrud J. *Making the Consumer's Voice Heard in Medicaid Managed Care: Increasing Participation, Protection, and Satisfaction.* Washington, DC: National Health Law Program; 1996.

31. US Congress, Office of Technology Assessment. *Adolescent Health.* Washington, DC: US GPO; 1991.

32. Zahner GEP, Pawelkiewicz W, De Francesco JJ, Adnopoz J. Children's mental health service needs and utilization patterns in an urban community: an epidemiological assessment. *J Am Acad Child Adolesc Psychiatry.* 1991;31:951–960.

33. Armbruster P., Schwab-Stone M. Who are the child guidance clinic dropouts? *Hosp Community Psychiatry.* 1994;45:804–808.

34. Armbruster P, Fallon T. Clinical, sociodemographic, and systems risk factors for attrition in a children's mental health clinic. *Am J Orthopsychiatry.* 1994;64:577–585.

35. Comer JP. The Yale-New Haven primary prevention project: a follow-up study. *Am Acad Child Psychiatry.* 1985;24:154–160.

36. Comer JP. Educating poor minority children. *Sci Am.* 1988;259(5):42–48.

37. Armbruster P, Lichtman J. Are school-based mental health services effective? Evidence from 36 inner-city schools. *Community Ment Health J.* 1999;35:493–504.

CHAPTER 23

An Elementary School-Based Health Clinic

Can It Reduce Medicaid Costs?

E. Kathleen Adams and Veda Johnson, 2000

S chool health services, most often provided by nurses, have existed in this country for more than 100 years. Although these activities initially consisted primarily of communicable disease control, a broader comprehensive view of school health programs began to emerge in the 1970s. The concept of comprehensive school health programming in which direct services, education, and improvement of school environment are considered complementary efforts is now accepted in the public health and educational communities. A recent national survey found that community-based health care providers often play a key role in school health services, while school nurses continue to operate in a traditional fashion.[1]

The Whitefoord Elementary School-Based Health Clinic (WESBHC) has been in operation in metro Atlanta since November of 1994. Its purpose, like other school-based health clinics (SBHCs), is to overcome

The chapter originally appeared as Adams EK, Johnson V. An elementary school–based health clinic: can it reduce Medicaid costs? *Pediatrics*. 2000; 105(4): 780–788. Copyright © 2000. Reproduced by permission of *Pediatrics*.

barriers to care for the wide range of medical and social problems that confront children residing and attending school in a relatively poor community. The purpose of this analysis is to assess the effect of the WESBHC on the children's use of expensive health care services, such as emergency department and inpatient hospital, while potentially increasing the use of preventive and other primary care services funded by the Medicaid program.

As noted, the concept of school-based services has grown in popularity during the past 2 decades. In a recent survey, the services provided by school nurses included primarily direct service/intervention, screening, special education, and prevention.[1] One national survey documented that school nurse practitioners diagnosed 87% of the presenting health problems, achieved 96% resolution of those problems, and avoided unnecessary duplication of services.[2] There are also school-based clinics, which encompass the regular supervision and visitation by physician providers of service, such as the ESBHC.

School-based and school-linked health centers now serve as comprehensive centers for medical and mental health screening and treatment for children on or near the school grounds. They are designed to address barriers to care, such as transportation, inconvenient appointment times, burdensome out-of-pocket costs, and other personal barriers to seeking care. School-based clinics are being widely used to reach children for preventive and other routine care; there are currently over 1,100 operating across the country. Forty-six percent serve high school students, 16% serve middle school students, 28% serve elementary school children, and 10% serve some combination.[3] In addition to their broad design, these clinics are often serving a large number of uninsured children. One report showed that nearly 40% of all school-based and school-linked health center users are completely uninsured; at a California SBHC, 93% of clinic enrollees reported no other source of medical care.[4] Children without insurance are less likely to receive any ambulatory care, even when medically indicated, than their privately insured counterparts.[5]

WESBHC in Atlanta, Georgia is an expanded model of an SBHC serving preschool and elementary school-aged children. It is a joint effort of the public schools, Emory University School of Medicine, and several other community, state, and private organizations. Its overall goal is to integrate relevant programs to serve the children of Whitefoord Elementary School and their preschool siblings in such a manner that their overall health and well being are sustained and/or improved. Ultimately, the program is aimed at improving school attendance and classroom performance and the longer-term prospects for these children as they mature.

This SBHC was organized by the Department of Pediatrics, Emory University School of Medicine and is located within the Whitefoord Elementary school. The clinic was initially opened in November of 1994; the clinic services were expanded to include preschool children (0–4-year-olds) in July of 1996. By its immediate proximity to the child during the day, the WESBHC removes major access barriers to primary care (eg, transportation time and costs, lost work time, etc.) that other providers cannot. The child can immediately enter the health care system because the WESBHC is located within the school walls. It is open all year and does have after hour (24 hours) phone triage by a nurse with physician backup. Further, the WESBHC strives to promote wellness through an interdisciplinary approach and to provide education to help parents take responsibility for their child's health and health care. The key services provided by the clinic include (1) diagnosis and treatment for acute illnesses and injuries, (2) management of chronic illnesses, (3) preventive care and screening, (4) mental health screenings and management, (5) dental care, (6) health promotion/education, (7) social services, and (8) referrals to medical subspecialties and community agencies.

While there have been earlier evaluations of the effects of SBHCS, these are relatively few in number, lack comprehensiveness, and have sometimes been based on simulated data rather than the actual experience of those served by a SBHC. For example, earlier studies have concluded that school nurse practitioner services and school-based high school health services can result in savings for the schools and families.[6] This study found lower costs for parent and child of a visit to a SBHC compared with a physician's office. Further, service costs are believed to be lower for some services at a SBHC because of the greater substitution of nursing for physician time. There is also some evidence that their outcomes are as good or better than those achieved by physician's primary care.[7] One study on the cost-effectiveness of school nurse practitioner services reported that multiple case histories involving medical problems could be cited in which school nurse practitioners had averted unnecessary adaptive education placements while freeing placement slots for students in real need of those programs.[8]

Another earlier study focused on outcomes and found that comprehensive elementary school health education programs increased the health knowledge of younger groups but not older ones.[9] Still other studies have asked more comprehensive questions about the costs and benefits of such programs, while not carrying out a specific evaluation.[10] Most studies have not included all costs affected by school clinics or chosen appropriate comparison groups for evaluating effects. None, to our knowledge, have focused on Medicaid program savings.

METHODS

The overall goal of this analysis is to evaluate and compare the Medicaid health care costs per child for those children whose primary caregiver is the WESBHC to children in an area without a SBHC. In completing this analysis, we are taking the perspective of Medicaid, a publicly financed program designed to care for the poor and recently expanded to cover more children at or near poverty. To achieve this overall goal, we ask:

- Have the types of services used (e.g., preventive care, ER) for those whose primary care provider is the WESBHC changed over time? How does this change compare to the change in utilization over time for a similar group of children whose primary care provider is not a SBHC?

- Are Medicaid health care expenses lower for those whose primary source of care is the WESBHC before and after the start of the clinic and/or compared with those whose primary care is not a school-based clinic?

Our major underlying hypothesis is that the increased access to primary care provided by the WESBHC will reduce children's emergency department use as well as maintain the child's health so that hospitalizations are avoided and Medicaid expenses are lowered.

Our overall design involves using Medicaid claims data to measure the health care use and expenses of children served by the WESBHC in 1995, compared with those used by them in 1994 and to those used by children who do not have access to a SBHC. The Medicaid program is designed to fund, rather than directly deliver care and hence patterns of delivery will vary across children served in different areas. We use data for periods before and after (1994–1996) the implementation of the clinic's service. These data include information on all outcomes of interest (e.g., use of emergency room, hospitalizations) for our analysis.

The 1994 period is largely before the implementation of the WESBHC and provides a baseline or control period for the Whitefoord and comparison children. We assembled data from the Georgia Department of Medical Assistance (DMA) or Georgia Medicaid program for children served by the Whitefoord clinic and for a comparison group of children over the 1994–1996 period. We are only able to study the use/expense of either group while they are enrolled in Medicaid. Because these children are in high poverty areas, they are likely to qualify for Medicaid coverage. Indeed, over 90% of the Whitefoord children were enrolled in Medicaid sometime during this period.

The Medicaid identifications of the children enrolled (having parental approval for care) and/or using the Whitefoord SBHC were obtained from the clinic, while Medicaid identifications for the comparison group were drawn from the DMA files. Using these identifications, we matched the WESBHC children to the Medicaid enrollment files; of the 696 listed, between 598 and 646 were enrolled in Medicaid at some time during the 1994–1996 period. Enrollment and claims histories were pulled for the Whitefoord and comparison children for the 1994, 1995, and 1996 periods. The claims history provides all outpatient and inpatient utilization by date of service and includes details on diagnoses (*International Classification of Diseases, 9th Revision* [ICD-9] coding), procedures (*Current Procedural Terminology-4* and state-specific), amounts billed/paid, provider type, place of service, category of service, etc. The Medicaid enrollment files provide data on age, sex, race, residential zip, and Medicaid eligibility group. We constructed monthly enrollment and utilization records for each child.

We then drew a sample of children believed to be similar in their sociodemographic background to those with access to the WESBHC, enrolled in Medicaid, and without access to a SBHC. To do this, we drew from a geographic area with similar household characteristics (e.g., income and family education) that generally affect a child's health status and utilization by using a set of 5-digit zip codes. These zip codes comprise the school district for a nearby school, East Lake Elementary, which has no SBHC program. The 1990 census data indicated that 63% of the children in the East Lake Elementary census tracts were in poverty, whereas 68% of those served by Whitefoord Elementary were in poverty; from 92% to 93% of each group were in the school lunch program.

Children found on the Medicaid enrollment files anytime during 1994, 1995, or 1996 and residing in the zip codes served by East Lake Elementary comprised our comparison group. The total number of children enrolled in Medicaid residing in the East Lake Elementary zip codes during both 1994 and 1995 or 1994–1996 and in the same age group (4–12 years old in 1994) totaled a little less than 500 in some years. This sample size more than satisfied our criteria for detecting 30% to 40% differences in emergency department use based on an α of .05 and power of 80.

As noted, we used all those children whose participation in the clinic was approved by their parents as the initial cases for our analysis. Most of these children are actual users of the clinic during the year but some are not. We were, therefore, interested in identifying the subset of Whitefoord children for whom the Whitefoord clinic is their usual provider of primary care. To define usual providers, we first arrayed the claims data associated with primary care. We used physician visit codes, all Early and Periodic Screening, Diagnostic and Treatment (EPSDT) claims, all immunization claims, and all those claims with category of service equal to nurse practitioner as primary care. In addition, all claims with a V diagnostic code were included to capture all well-child visits in this definition.

For each child, we identified the (unique) provider identification on most claims of the above types. A tie between 2 providers was broken by using the provider with the most dollars paid. We expected to find stronger evidence of our hypothesized effects, such as reduced emergency department use, for WESBHC children who use the clinic as their medical home. Although the comparison group children generally had physicians as their usual provider, followed by public health departments, these entities cannot reduce access barriers in the same manner as the WESBHC.

In the above process, we found that a large number of the Whitefoord clinic claims for EPSDT and other primary care services had not been billed properly during late 1996 and the volume of the Whitefoord clinic was understated. The 1996 data for these categories of service overstate our case, because the Whitefoord children look less expensive because of the underbilling. Therefore, we focus on the identification of the usual provider during the 1995 period and although we present 1996 data for all categories of service, we focus on those not affected by the billing problem, such as emergency room and inpatient services. Finally, we were also interested in the effects of the Whitefoord clinic for children with a chronic and costly condition, such as asthma. Additional analyses are shown for children with this diagnosis. We identified asthmatic children as those with an ICD-9 diagnosis code of 493 anytime during the year.

Our primary statistical methods include testing for differences in means for the Whitefoord and comparison sample before and after the clinic opening. We also use multivariate analysis. In the multivariate analysis, we derive a measure of the differences in differences for the 2 groups and test its significance. That is, we derive a measure of the difference between 1994 and 1995 for Whitefoord and comparison children's groups and then compare this difference across the 2 groups. The coefficients on the interaction of a dummy variable denoting membership in the Whitefoord group and the time variable (1994–1995) are used to derive this measure.

Specifically, the regression coefficients are as follows:

$$\frac{(\$_{t=\text{post},D=W} - \$_{t=\text{pre},D=W}) - (\$_{t=\text{post},D=C} - \$_{t=\text{pre},D=C})}{X},$$

where

$\$_{t=\text{post},D=W}$ is the 1995 or post period expense per Whitefoord child;

$\$_{t=\text{pre},D=W}$ is the 1994 or pre period expense per Whitefoord child;

$\$_{t=\text{post},D=C}$ is the 1995 or post period expense per comparison child;

$\$_{t=\text{pre},D=C}$ is the 1995 or pre period expense per comparison child; and

X = a vector of control variables in the form of characteristics of the child and a time dummy variable.

Throughout the descriptive and multivariate analyses, the Medicaid expense data are adjusted for the relative length of Medicaid enrollment of each child in the WESBHC and comparison groups.

RESULTS

Overall, the results indicate that the introduction of the WESBHC did alter the utilization and expense patterns of children enrolled in Medicaid and residing in the area served by the WESBHC and program.

Descriptive Data

In Table 23.1 the average Medicaid amounts paid in 1994 and 1995 for children who were enrolled in Medicaid in 1994 and 1995 and in the comparison zip code or the WESBHC during 1995 are shown. In the third column, we provide the ratio of the Medicaid expenses for the comparison group to those for the WESBHC children and in the last column

Table 23.1   Average 1994 Costs for Whitefoord Children
(Ever Used in 1995) Versus Comparison Children.

	Average 1994 Costs			
	Whitefoord (*n* = 269)	Other (*n* = 594)	Ratio	*t* Test
Total yearly expense per individual (including drugs)	$1,741.97	$1,772.38	1.02	−.155
Category of service breakdowns				
Inpatient	$126.15	$212.48	1.68	−.821
Outpatient	$188.84	$228.79	1.21	−.576
Nonemergency transport	$504.22	$480.44	.95	.358
Mental health	$1.69	$0.97	.58	.655
Physician	$384.07	$349.16	.91	.678
EPSDT	$93.67	$91.44	.98	.264
Drug	$244.69	$302.77	1.24	−.746
Other	$198.63	$106.33	.54	1.104
Emergency department	$103.40	$101.34	.98	.139
	Average 1995 Costs			
	Whitefoord (*n* = 262)	Other (*n* = 632)	Ratio	*t* Test
Total yearly expense per individual (including drugs)	$1,206.46	$1,493.74	1.24	−1.090
Category of service breakdowns				
Inpatient	$132.82	$272.25	2.05	−1.389
Outpatient	$155.05	$358.45	2.31	−1.153
Nonemergency transport	$150.12	$178.08	1.19	−.941
Mental health	$2.46	$5.43	2.21	−.746
Physician	$260.75	$250.56	.96	.234
EPSDT	$101.67	$80.97	.80	2.718*
Drug	$242.73	$200.96	.83	1.119
Other	$160.87	$147.05	.91	.160
Emergency department	$84.67	$112.24	1.33	−1.732

*t value significant at .01 level.

we provide the value of the *t* test on the difference in these mean Medicaid amounts. We note that these data are for children who were 4 to 12 years old in 1994, enrolled in Medicaid, and users of some services in the year. The children identified as Whitefoord in Table 23.1 are those who used the clinic at least once during 1995. Although the comparison group does not include children enrolled in Medicaid and never using services during the year, this is the appropriate comparison group because the Whitefoord children are users by definition. The Medicaid

Table 23.1   Average 1994 Costs for Whitefoord Children (Ever Used
             in 1995) Versus Comparison Children (*Continued*).

	Average 1996 Costs			
	Whitefoord ($n = 262$)	Other ($n = 632$)	Ratio	*t* Test
Total yearly expense per individual (including drugs)	$898.98	$2,360.46	2.63	4.133*
Category of service breakdowns				
Inpatient	$197.24	$748.97	3.80	2.129
Outpatient	$129.57	$175.74	1.36	1.118
Nonemergency transport	$56.82	$122.28	2.15	2.077
Mental health	$.96	$14.25	14.78	1.985
Physician	$137.75	$287.49	2.09	3.177*
EPSDT	$59.81	$119.77	2.00	5.609*
Drug	$217.79	$393.31	1.81	3.440*
Other	$99.03	$491.06	4.96	4.627*
Emergency department	$52.97	$143.64	2.71	3.608*

*t value significant at .01 level.

expenses of both groups are adjusted for the length of time they were enrolled during the year.

As these data show, the average amount paid by Georgia Medicaid for health care for the WESBHC children in 1994, before the implementation of the clinic, was lower than for the comparison children. Medicaid expenses for the WESBHC children equaled $1,742, whereas for the comparison children, the average was $1,772. However, this difference was not statistically significant, and there were no statistical differences in the mean expenses of the 2 groups in any single service category in this pre-period.

The second bank of data in Table 23.1 shows that although Medicaid expenses declined for both groups of children, they declined more for the WESBHC children. The decline from 1994 to 1995 was $536 for the Whitefoord children versus $277 for the comparison children. Much of the decrease in Medicaid expenses per child in both groups was in nonemergency transportation, a category of service in which the Georgia DMA sought cost savings during these years. The substantially greater decline in non-emergency expenses for the Whitefoord versus comparison children is likely attributable to better access to primary care services provided by the clinic after 1994.

These results also show 2 findings important to our basic hypothesis. First, the WESBHC children have higher expenses for EPSDT preventive care services in 1995 than they did in 1994 and higher than the comparison children in 1995; this difference is statistically significant ($p = .01$). Second, their emergency department expenses are lower than those of the comparison group by 1995, and this difference is also statistically significant ($p = .10$).

We also show in Table 23.1 the 1996 inpatient, non-emergency transport, drug, and emergency department expenses per child for the Whitefoord (user of Whitefoord in 1995) and comparison groups. We note that the comparison group of children is markedly lower in number in 1996 attributable to (1) disenrollment of the child from the Medicaid program, (2) movement out of the zip code, or (3) nonuse of any Medicaid service in 1996. The Medicaid amounts presented in Table 23.1 are generally lower in 1996 and the differences are statistically significant at either the .01 or .05 level. These data indicate that the WESBHC users cost the Georgia Medicaid program only $197 per child-year enrolled in 1996 inpatient care expenses, whereas the comparison group cost the program $749. The difference in emergency department expenses is also significant. Recall that the 1996 EPSDT and physician primary care data are understated because of missing claims for the Whitefoord clinic.

Similar types of data are shown in Table 23.2. The children listed as Whitefoord children in this table, however, are those for whom the clinic is the usual provider of primary care during 1995. We expect stronger effects for this subset of the Whitefoord children examined in Table 23.1. Although this classification is perhaps a better measure of the impact of the clinic on the child's health care utilization, we note that the children so identified are smaller in number and that there may be some overstatement of the effect of the clinic on emergency department use. Our identification of the WESBHC as the usual provider means it provides the most primary care services to the child during 1995. By definition, then, their use of a non-WESBHC physician in the emergency room for primary care has to be smaller than their use of the WESBHC. Still, the child's use of the emergency room for any services in 1995 could be higher or lower than that use in 1994 and it is this change that is the focus of the analysis.

These data also show a statistically significant difference in the total expenses of the 2 groups over the 1994–1995 period and significant changes in their utilization patterns. Medicaid expenses per child drops from $1,797 in 1994 for the WESBHC usual provider group to only $901 in 1995; total Medicaid expenses are significantly lower ($p = .01$)

for the WESBHC than for the comparison children whose expenses are almost $1494 in 1995. Underlying this overall change for the Whitefoord children is a drop in Medicaid expenses for all categories of service except mental health and EPSDT. Moreover, although the only statistically significant difference between the 2 groups in 1994 was for other services, by 1995, the WESBHC usual provider group has significantly lower nonemergency transportation, physician, and emergency room expenses paid by Medicaid. The lower emergency room and inpatient expense also hold in 1996.

The equality of expenses between the 2 groups of children in 1994 reflects, in part, a comparability of their underlying characteristics as we had desired. The mean age in 1994 was just over 6 years old for both groups and both groups were predominantly black (97%–98%). Children in both groups were enrolled in Medicaid ~11.5 months of the year. The children were also comparable in terms of their distribution across eligibility groups within the Medicaid program in 1994. We do note, however, that the comparison group of children was comprised of relatively more disabled children by 1995; 3.5% of the comparison group fell into this eligibility category as opposed to 1.2% of the Whitefoord (usual provider) children in 1995. Given that disabled children have more chronic and high-cost medical conditions, this would make the comparison group of users more expensive. Yet, we would not expect them to have greater use of the emergency room unless their care is not well managed. This points to the need to examine the impact of the WESBHC in a multivariate context, holding constant the percentage of disabled children.

REGRESSION ANALYSIS

In Table 23.3, we show the results of multivariate regression analysis of the total, emergency department, and inpatient expenses per child-year enrolled for the pooled 1994 and 1995 observations for the WESBHC (usual provider) and comparison children. By using multivariate analysis, we are able to hold constant certain characteristics of the child that may affect their use of Medicaid services and expenses. We include the child's age, sex, race, and Medicaid eligibility category as covariates; the means and standard deviations of these variables for the pooled 1994 and 1995 samples are shown in Table 23.4.

The results in Table 23.3 are largely consistent with the descriptive analyses, although there is not generally statistical significance on the

Table 23.2   Average 1994 Costs for Whitefoord Children (Ever Used in 1995) Versus Comparison Children.

	Average 1994 Costs			
	Whitefoord ($n = 166$)	**Other** ($n = 594$)	**Ratio**	t **Test**
Total yearly expense per individual (including drugs)	$1,796.62	$1,772.38	.99	.101
Category of service breakdowns				
Inpatient	$173.79	$212.48	1.22	−.291
Outpatient	$121.17	$228.79	1.89	−1.269
Nonemergency transport	$491.17	$480.44	.98	.141
Mental health	$1.65	$0.97	.59	.536
Physician	$374.50	$349.16	.93	.415
EPSDT	$95.91	$91.44	.95	.444
Drug	$253.57	$302.77	1.19	−.501
Other	$284.86	$106.33	.37	1.767†
Emergency department	$103.40	$101.34	.98	.139

	Average 1995 Costs			
	Whitefoord ($n = 166$)	**Other** ($n = 632$)	**Ratio**	t **Test**
Total yearly expense per individual (including drugs)	$901.26	$1,493.74	1.66	−3.003*
Category of service breakdowns				
Inpatient	$112.39	$272.25	2.42	−1.398
Outpatient	$114.71	$358.45	3.12	−1.103
Nonemergency transport	$92.63	$178.08	1.92	−3.547*
Mental health	$2.51	$5.43	2.16	−.586
Physician	$194.04	$250.56	1.29	1.830‡
EPSDT	$103.31	$80.56	.78	2.385*
Drug	$172.04	$200.96	1.17	−.678
Other	$109.63	$147.05	1.34	−.348
Emergency department	$70.05	$112.24	1.60	−2.557*

*Significant at .01 level.
†Significant at .05 level.
‡Significant at .10 level.

Whitefoord effect. Although the coefficient on the time variable (TIME) indicates an overall downward trend in total Medicaid expenses in the first equation, it is not significant. Being in the WESBHC usual provider group (WHITEPROV) shows no significant effect for total Medicaid nor emergency department expenses. The coefficient of most interest is that

Table 23.2 **Average 1994 Costs for Whitefoord Children (Ever Used in 1995) Versus Comparison Children (*Continued*).**

	Average 1996 Costs			
	Whitefoord (*n* = 169)	Other (*n* = 349)	Ratio	*t* Test
Total yearly expense per individual (including drugs)	$727.30	$2,360.46	3.25	−4.619*
Category of service breakdowns				
Inpatient	$110.39	$748.97	6.78	−2.454†
Outpatient	$104.13	$175.74	1.69	−1.449
Nonemergency transport	$45.18	$122.28	2.71	−2.295†
Mental health	$.00	$14.25	NA	−2.140†
Physician	$118.59	$287.49	2.42	−3.589*
EPSDT	$61.54	$119.77	1.95	−5.004*
Drug	$203.44	$393.31	1.93	−3.594*
Other	$84.02	$491.06	5.84	−4.680*
Emergency department	$36.19	$143.64	3.97	−4.414*

*Significant at .01 level.
†Significant at .05 level.

Table 23.3 **Determinants of Expenses per Child-Year Enrolled, Pooled 1994–1995 Data for Whitefoord and Comparison Children.**

	Total Expense per Child-Year Enrolled	Emergency Expense per Child-Year Enrolled	Impatient Expense per Child-Year Enrolled
TIME	−276.67	11.73	63.43
AGE	212.02	9.37	61.56
NONWHITE	−1,343.06‡	−98.12	198.61
Male	17.60†	6.31	−40.29
AFDC	−1,728.21	−117.65*	−508.27†
Foster	−1,162.51	−60.40*	−759.12‡
POVREL	−2,143.97*	−133.05*	−660.67*
WHITEPROV	21.56	13.07	−48.88
TIME* WHITEPROV	−505.13	−52.39‡	−96.18
(Constant)	4,682.13*	305.97*	517.96
r^2	0.21	.014	.010
	n = 1556	*n* = 1556	*n* = 1556

*Significant at .01 level.
†Significant at .05 level.
‡Significant at .10 level.

Table 23.4   **Means and Standard Deviations, Pooled Data.**

Definition	Mean	Standard Deviation
Dependent variables		
Total expense per child-year enrolled	$1,569.12	$3,289.54
Emergency expense per child-year enrolled	$276.58	$333.87
Emergency and inpatient expense per child-year enrolled	$860.30	$2,722.10
Independent variables		
AGE 1	.56	.50
NONWHITE	.99	.11
Male	.49	.50
AFDC	.81	.40
POVREL	.14	.35
Foster	.02	.13
WHITEPROV	.21	.41
TIME*WHITEPROV	.11	.31

on the time and Whitefoord group interaction (TIME * WHITEPROV); this coefficient, as noted in our "Methods" section, measures the differences in differences, or the difference between the Whitefoord and comparison children in the change in Medicaid expenses over the pre and post period. This coefficient is negative and significant ($p = .10$) in the emergency department expense equation.

Other results shown in Table 23.3 are consistent with expectations but not generally significant. Expenses are generally higher for younger (4–7 years old in 1994 [AGE 1]) children relative to older (8–12 years old in 1994) children. Younger children have greater periodicity of preventive care and also tend to have more acute care illnesses than older children. Although there is a negative coefficient on the race variable (NONWHITE), there is so little variation in this variable this result is hard to interpret. The findings with regard to Medicaid eligibility group are also not surprising. They indicate that the nondisabled children's groups, those related to the Aid to Families With Dependent Children (AFDC) or in the newer poverty-related expansion groups (POVREL) are generally less expensive than children in the (omitted) disabled child category, as expected.

ASTHMATIC CHILDREN

Asthma is a chronic condition that affects a large and growing number of minority children across the country. It is a particular problem for inner-city youth and numerous efforts are being made to better manage the clinical manifestations and costs of this condition. We chose to look further at this condition by subsetting the children based on evidence that they suffered from asthma. To do so, we flagged children with an ICD-9 code of 493 on any inpatient or outpatient claim during the study. As the data in Table 23.5 show, there were relatively few of these children in the WESBHC and comparison groups in the 1994–1996 period and the percentage of children affected was similar.

The descriptive data on asthmatic children (see Table 23.5) again indicate there are not significant differences for the Whitefoord and comparison children in the period before 1994. Total Medicaid expenses per asthmatic child-year enrolled are higher, as expected, than the average (Table 23.1), ranging from $2,373 to $2,414 for the WESBHC and comparison groups in 1994. By 1995, the expenses of those asthmatic children served by the WESBHC were lower, equal to $1,758, whereas expenses per asthmatic child for those in the comparison group had increased to $2,541. Although neither the 1994 nor 1995 total Medicaid expense were significantly different across the 2 groups, there was a statistically significant difference in inpatient hospital expenses by 1995. In 1995, the WESBHC asthmatic cost the Medicaid program an average of $352 in inpatient expenses, the comparison group cost over 3 times that or $1,259. Although we cannot control for possible differences in asthma severity, the results do indicate the pattern of care changed from the 1994 to the 1995 period to lower costs for the Whitefoord asthmatics relative to the comparison group asthmatics. The 1996 data also indicate inpatient and drug expenses for the Whitefoord asthmatic children were significantly lower.

DISCUSSION

The foregoing data and analysis indicate that the placement and operation of the WESBHC in the Whitefoord Elementary community had an impact on Medicaid expenses for the state of Georgia. A major effect of the clinic was the reduction in the probability that children use the emergency department, and hence, emergency room expenses. The data also indicate the clinic enhanced the downward trend in total Medicaid expenses taking place for children in these inner-city Atlanta communities over the 1994–1995 period. The overall downward trend likely reflects the continued implementation of primary care case management within Georgia's Medicaid program and the implementation of controls on nonemergency transportation expenses over this

Table 23.5   **Average 1994 Costs for Whitefoord Asthmatic Children (Ever Used in 1995) Versus Comparison Children.**

	Average 1994 Asthma Costs			
	Whitefoord ($n = 26$)	Other ($n = 68$)	Ratio	t Test
Total yearly expense per individual (including drugs)	$2,372.77	$2,414.42	1.02	−.052
Category of service breakdowns				
Inpatient	$422.36	$727.35	1.72	−.469
Outpatient	$260.83	$112.26	.43	1.563
Nonemergency transport	$394.43	$272.84	.69	1.093
Physician	$304.64	$379.56	1.25	−.624
Drug	$501.57	$591.94	1.18	−.531
Other	$488.94	$330.48	.68	1.231
Emergency department	$221.60	$226.71	1.02	−.059

	Average 1995 Asthma Costs			
	Whitefoord ($n = 34$)	Other ($n = 81$)	Ratio	t Test
Total yearly expense per individual (including drugs)	$1,757.80	$2,540.93	1.45	−1.030
Category of service breakdowns				
Inpatient	$351.94	$1259.35	3.58	−1.966[†]
Outpatient	$212.85	$125.13	.59	.968
Nonemergency transport	$87.50	$113.48	1.30	−.350
Physician	$294.00	$218.34	.74	1.269
Drug	$447.32	$363.02	.81	.652
Other	$364.19	$461.60	1.27	−.732
Emergency department	$197.16	$279.72	1.42	−.726

[†]t value significant at .05 level.

period. The WESBHC enhanced this overall trend by lowering emergency department expenses.

Another important effect of the clinic was an increase in the EPSDT expenses per child. It seems that the WESBHC, by increasing access, had the expected effect on increased primary care. This is consistent with the belief of the WESBHC that they were able to shape the parent's perceptions of the importance of primary care and having a medical home for their child. Staff members at the WESBHC report spending significant time educating and reenforcing these concepts for the parents in what are often dysfunctional homes in these poor

Table 23.5 Average 1994 Costs for Whitefoord Asthmatic Children (Ever Used in 1995) Versus Comparison Children (*Continued*).

	Average 1996 Asthma Costs for 1995 Patients Who Used Services at Whitefoord or Other			
	Whitefoord ($n = 34$)	Other ($n = 81$)	Ratio	*t* Test
Total yearly expense per individual (including drugs)	$1,966.77	$4,078.38	2.07	−2.176
Category of service breakdowns				
Inpatient	$706.88	$2,311.52	3.27	−1.899[‡]
Outpatient	$256.53	$201.84	.79	.462
Nonemergency transport	$56.36	$106.57	1.89	−.534
Physician	$348.93	$375.34	1.08	−.246
Drug	$260.44	$441.12	1.69	−2.139[†]
Other	$337.63	$591.61	1.75	−1.746
Emergency department	$212.32	$388.44	1.83	−1.106

[†]*t* value significant at .05 level.
[‡]*t* value significant at .10 level.

neighborhoods. If the parent does come to see the clinic as the child's medical home, this allows the WESBHC to shape the parents' response to an illness and better control the child's overall care.

These are important and encouraging findings for the potential of SBHCs to save money while improving the use of preventive care. We note, however, that we have only focused here on the costs of services and clinic revenues for those who are Medicaid enrolled. Hence, we have not looked at the total costs of running a SBHC such as the WESBHC. This clinic, as well as others, must cover their total costs through Medicaid revenues plus subsidies from the taxpayers of the federal and/or state governments.

Although our findings indicate that public or private investment in a SBHC has the potential to produce savings for public programs such as Medicaid, we are not able to analyze total costs for either group or compare total costs when a clinic is the usual provider to that of an office-based physician. We do note, however, that there is significant evidence of a lack of physician practices in inner-urban areas,[12,13] and hence, the alternative source of care for these children is likely to be another subsidized clinic rather than a physician's office. From a societal perspective, the private subsidization of the Whitefoord clinic might reflect a cost-shift from the public to private sector if these children would have otherwise been served in a public clinic.

Just as we have not examined all costs, we also have not examined full benefits of the WESBHC. For example, if students and their families are assured better access to health care services, this can reduce travel time, parent's lost time at work, and increase the child's school attendance. If conditions such as asthma are better managed/controlled, the student may actually be able to achieve more in the time they are attending school. Beyond this, there are other less readily measured benefits to the child, family, and community that likely accrue with the presence of a program such as the Whitefoord Community program and WESBHC.

The findings here also have relevance to broader health policy issues. In 1989, Congress sought to achieve the improvement of children's participation in the Medicaid EPSDT program through the Omnibus Budget Reconciliation Act of 1989 in a number of ways,[14] including increased provider participation. An analysis of EPSDT before and after the implementation of the Omnibus Budget Reconciliation Act of 1989 found increases in the Medicaid child case-loads of clinic providers inclusive of school-based clinics.[14] Because school attendance is mandatory and SBHCs do not typically turn anyone away, they serve as a ready source of access for children's primary and preventive care.

Although states may, therefore, see SBHCs as an avenue through which to increase access and participation in the EPSDT program, they will need to carefully maintain them as a source of care if they are expanding enrollment in capitated managed care. As noted, the WESBHC and others like it are at least partially dependent on Medicaid as a source of revenue. However, these clinics will not be reimbursed for services provided to Medicaid children unless they become part of the provider network of health maintenance organizations (HMOs). They are often not set up as billing entities, and hence, may need to become affiliated with others to enroll in networks. Unless states carve out the types of services provided by SBHCs or require HMOs to include these providers in their network, SBHCs may see diminished Medicaid revenues without diminished children's needs, causing increased financial stress. A more constructive policy might integrate the SBHC into the HMO network of providers to pay for its services and to allow for the exchange of clinical information for the better management of the child's health and well being. We recognize, however, that HMOs will not likely be able to pay the full costs of these clinics and that subsidizations from taxpayers or other sources will likely be necessary to cover their full costs.

Notes

1. Hacker K, Fried LE, Bablouzian L, Roeber J. A nationwide survey of school health services delivery in urban schools. *J Sch Health.* 1994;64:279–283.

2. Meeker RJ, De Angelis C, Berman B, Freeman HE, Oda D. A comprehensive school health initiative. *Image J Nurs Sch.* 1986;18:86–91.

3. School Health Resources Services. *School-Based Health Centers: The Facts: 1995 Resource Packet Series.* Denver, Colo: University of Colorado Health Sciences Center; 1995.

4. Health Resources and Services Administration, Bureau of Primary Health Care. *School-Based Clinics That Work.* Washington DC: Health Resources and Services Administration, Division of Programs for Special Populations; 1993.

5. Weinick RM, Weigers ME, Cohen JW. Children's health insurance, access to care and health status: new findings. *Health Aff.* 1998;17:127–136.

6. Siegel LP, Krieble TA. Evaluation of school-based high school health services. *J Sch Health.* 1987;57:323–325.

7. Igoe JB, Giordano BP. *Expanding School Health Services to Serve Families in the 21st Century.* Denver, Colo: School Health Resources Services, University of Colorado Health Sciences Center; 1995.

8. Sobolewski SD. Cost-effective school nurse practitioner services. *J Sch Health.* 1981;51:585–588.

9. Du Shaw ML. A comparative study of three model comprehensive elementary school health education programs. *J Sch Health.* 1984;54:397–400.

10. Newman IM, Newman E, Martin GL. School health services: what costs? What benefits? *J Sch Health.* 1981;51:423–426.

11. Hurley RE, Freund DA, Taylor DE. Emergency room use and primary care case management: evidence from four Medicaid demonstration programs. *Am J Public Health.* 1989;79:843–847.

12. Fossett, JW, Perloff JD, Peterson JA, Kletke PR. Medicaid in the inner city: the case of maternity care in Chicago. *Milbank Q.* 1990;68:111–139.

13. Goldstein A. Many doctors in few places: where doctors work, health care in Washington. *Washington Post.* July 31, 1994.

14. Gavin NI, Adams EK, Herz EJ. The use of EPSDT and other health care services by children enrolled in Medicaid: the impact of OBRA89. *Milbank Q.* 1998;76:207–250.

ᲐᲕᲕ Name Index

⟶ Subject Index